CARDIAC
Functioning, Disorders, Challenges and Therapies

CARDIAC
Functioning, Disorders, Challenges and Therapies

Editor

Mahira Parveen MPhil PhD

Professor
Department of Zoology
Government PG College
Bina, Madhya Pradesh, India

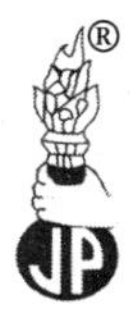

JAYPEE BROTHERS MEDICAL PUBLISHERS (P) LTD

New Delhi • Panama City • London • Philadelphia (USA)

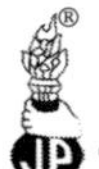

Jaypee Brothers Medical Publishers (P) Ltd

Headquarters
Jaypee Brothers Medical Publishers (P) Ltd
4838/24, Ansari Road, Daryaganj
New Delhi 110 002, India
Phone: +91-11-43574357
Fax: +91-11-43574314
Email: jaypee@jaypeebrothers.com

Overseas Offices

J.P. Medical Ltd
83 Victoria Street, London
SW1H 0HW (UK)
Phone: +44-2031708910
Fax: +02-03-0086180
Email: info@jpmedpub.com

Jaypee-Highlights Medical Publishers Inc.
City of Knowledge, Bld. 237, Clayton
Panama City, Panama
Phone: +507-301-0496
Fax: +507-301-0499
Email: cservice@jphmedical.com

Jaypee Brothers Medical Publishers (P) Ltd
17/1-B Babar Road, Block-B, Shaymali
Mohammadpur, Dhaka-1207
Bangladesh
Mobile: +08801912003485
Email: jaypeedhaka@gmail.com

Jaypee Brothers Medical Publishers (P) Ltd
Shorakhute, Kathmandu
Nepal
Phone: +00977-9841528578
Email: jaypee.nepal@gmail.com

Website: www.jaypeebrothers.com
Website: www.jaypeedigital.com

Inquiries for bulk sales may be solicited at: jaypee@jaypeebrothers.com

Cardiac Functioning, Disorders, Challenges and Therapies

First Edition: **2013**

ISBN 978-93-5090-306-3

Printed at Rajkamal Electric Press, Plot No. 2, Phase-IV, Kundli, Haryana.

Contributors

A Ricart MD
Hospital Universitari de Bellvitge
Barcelona, Spain

Ahmet Baydin MD
Department of Emergency Medicine
Faculty of Medicine, Ondokuz Mayis
University, Samsun, Turkey

Ali Kemal Erenler MD
Department of Emergency Medicine
Faculty of Medicine, Ondokuz Mayis
University, Samsun, Turkey

Andrea Viggiano MD PhD
Faculty of Motor Sciences, University
of Naples "Parthenope", Naples, Italy

Andrés Ricardo Perez Riera MD
Incharge of Electrovectocardiographics
Sector - Cardiology Discipline - ABC
Medical Faculty - ABC Foundation -
Santo André - São Paulo. Brazil

Béatrice Peperstraete MD
Cardiology Department, Brugmann
Hospital, Place Van Gehuchten 4, 1020
Brussels, Belgium

Bilel MD
Cardiology Department, Brugmann
Hospital, Place Van Gehuchten 4, 1020
Brussels, Belgium

C Javierre MD PhD
Department de Ciències Fisiològiques
II. Facultat de Medicina, Universitat de
Barcelona, Spain

Catalin Boiangiu MD
Department of Medicine, Newark Beth
Israel Medical Center, Newark, NJ, USA

Christophe Janssen MD
Cardiology Department, Brugmann
Hospital, Place Van Gehuchten 4, 1020
Brussels, Belgium

D Rodríguez-Castro MD
Hospital Universitari de Bellvitge,
Barcelona, Spain

Denis Abramochkin PhD
Department of Human and Animal
Physiology, Moscow State University
of MV Lomonosov, Moscow,
119311, Russia

Domenico Tafuri MD
Faculty of Motor Sciences, University
of Naples "Parthenope", Naples, Italy

E Farrero MD
Hospital Universitari de Bellvitge,
Barcelona, Spain

Emmanuel Catez MD
CHU Brugmann, Brussels, Belgium
and 1 Kings College London BHF
Centre, Cardiovascular Division,
NIHR Biomedical Research Centre
at Guy's and St. Thomas' NHS
Foundation Trust

Emmanuel Tran-Ngoc MD
Cardiology Department, Brugmann
Hospital, Place Van Gehuchten 4, 1020
Brussels, Belgium

Fraz Ahmed MPhil PhD
Department of Biosciences
Barkatullah University
Bhopal (MP), India

Gabriella Vivian Flores MD
Cardiology Department, Brugmann Hospital, Place Van Gehuchten 4, 1020 Brussels, Belgium

Gennaro Izzo MD
Department of Experimental Medicine, Section of Human Physiology, and Clinical Dietetic Service, Second University of Naples via Costantinopoli, 16, 80138-Naples Italy

Giovanni Messina MD PhD
Department of Experimental Medicine, Section of Human Physiology, and Clinical Dietetic Service, Second University of Naples via Costantinopoli 16, 80138-Naples Italy

H Torrado MD
Hospital Universitari de Bellvitge Barcelona, Spain

JL Ventura MD PhD
Hospital Universitari de Bellvitge Barcelona, Spain

José Castro-Rodriguez MD
Cardiology Department, Brugmann Hospital, Place Van Gehuchten 4, 1020 Brussels, Belgium

Khawaja Husnain Haider MPharm PhD
Department of Pathology and Laboratory of Medicine, 231-Albert Sabin Way, University of Cincinnati Ohio-45267-0529, USA

L Carrió MD
Hospital Universitari de Bellvitge, Barcelona, Spain

Mahira Parveen MPhil PhD
Professor, Department of Zoology Government PG College, Bina (MP), India

Marc Cohen MD
Department of Medicine, Newark Beth Israel Medical Center, Newark NJ, USA

Marcellino Monda MD
Department of Experimental Medicine Section of Human Physiology, and Clinical Dietetic Service, Second University of Naples, via Costantinopoli 16, 80138-Naples, Italy

Marielle Morissens MD
Cardiology Department, Brugmann Hospital, Place Van Gehuchten 4, 1020 Brussels, Belgium

Mario Vassalle MD
Department of Physiology and Pharmacology, Box 31, State University of New York, Downstate Medical Center, 450 Clarkson Avenue Brooklyn, NY 11203, USA

Matthew Wright MRCP PhD
Cardiac Electrophysiology, Academic Clinical Lecturer, Rayne Institute, Department of Cardiology, St. Thomas' Hospital, Westminster Bridge Road, London, SE1 7EH, United Kingdom CHU Brugmann, Brussels, Belgium and 1 Kings College London BHF Centre, Cardiovascular Division NIHR Biomedical Research Centre at Guy's and St. Thomas' NHS Foundation Trust

Muhammad Ashraf PhD
Department of Pathology and Laboratory of Medicine, 231-Albert Sabin Way, University of Cincinnati Ohio-45267-0529, USA

Nathalie Ngo Mandag MD
Cardiology Department, Brugmann Hospital, Place Van Gehuchten 4, 1020 Brussels, Belgium

Pierre Decoodt MD
Cardiology Department, Brugmann Hospital, Place Van Gehuchten 4, 1020 Brussels, Belgium

Sebastien Knecht MD
Cardiac Electrophysiology, Academic Clinical Lecturer, Rayne Institute Department of Cardiology, St. Thomas' Hospital, Westminster Bridge Road London, SE1 7EH, United Kingdom

Sébastien Knecht MD
Cardiology Department, Brugmann Hospital, Place Van Gehuchten 4, 1020 Brussels, Belgium

Snigdha Ancha MBBS
Department of Medicine, Jawaharlal Institute of Postgraduate Medical Education and Research, Pondicherry India

Thierry Verbeet MD
Cardiology Department, Brugmann Hospital, Place Van Gehuchten 4, 1020 Brussels, Belgium

Turker Yardan MD
Department of Emergency Medicine Ondokuz Mayis University, Faculty of Medicine, Samsun, Turkey

Valentin Tatnga MD
Cardiology Department, Brugmann Hospital, Place Van Gehuchten 4, 1020 Brussels, Belgium

Vamsee Yaganti MD
Department of Medicine, Newark Beth Israel Medical Center, Newark, NJ, USA

Vien Khach Lai PhD
Department of Pathology and Laboratory of Medicine, 231-Albert Sabin Way, University of Cincinnati Ohio-45267-0529, USA

Vincenzo De Luca MD PhD
Department of Experimental Medicine, Section of Human Physiology, and Clinical Dietetic Service, Second University of Naples via Costantinopoli, 16, 80138-Naples Italy

Preface

This book covers many topics of current interest to cardiologists and physiologists ranging from cardiac conducting system to recent therapeutic approaches and researches made in the area of heart treatment. This book includes chapters on cardiac conducting system, sinoatrial node, cardiac Purkinje fibers, His system, its electrovector-cardiographic demonstration and sympathetic innervations in human heart including their autonomic regulation.

Another major highlight of this book is chapters on ablation of atrial fibrillation and ventricular fibrillation, cardiac dysfunctions, blood cholinesterase levels and QTc interval in patients with organophosphate poisoning. Besides these, sex-related differences in serum troponin in cardiac surgery have also been discussed.

Lastly, there are some chapters on myocardial repair by angiomyogenesis, suitable therapies for pathophysiology, diagnosis, medical management and nonpharmacological management of therapeutic schemes and future directions which have also been analyzed.

This book attempts to provide a valuable source of information on many highly significant aspects of cardiac structures, innervation, dysfunctioning, pathophysiology, electrocardiographs and proposed therapeutic tools. The medical practitioners, medical graduate and postgraduate students, researchers and scientific professionals in cardiology, pharmacology and physiology will find this book useful. It may also be of interest to medical planners and pharmacological laboratories engaged in manufacturing the cardioprotective drugs.

In order to create a combined collection of study material to understand outcome of recent cardiac researchers at a glance, this book is an effort. The chapters in the book have been written by the renowned and internationally established cardiologists. I sincerely thank all the contributors for accepting to write the chapters and submitting the chapters in a timely manner in spite of their heavily engaged schedules.

Mahira Parveen

Contents

Chapter

1

The Mammalian Sinoatrial Node: Functioning and Autonomic Regulation

Denis Abramochkin

Abstract. Mechanisms of cardiac automaticity exhibited in the mammalian sinoatrial node and different types of its regulation have been extensively studied during the last century using electrophysiological and biochemical methods. According to the novel conceptions, automaticity is a result of complex interactions between the membrane ion channels and the system of intracellular calcium turnover. Besides this, interactions between the cells forming the sinoatrial node are of great importance for understanding the functioning of that structure. Sinoatrial automaticity is regulated mainly by acetylcholine and noradrenaline, released from parasympathetic and sympathetic nerve fibers respectively. These neurotransmitters take antagonistic action on cAMP second messenger system via G-protein coupled receptors. Moreover, acetylcholine activates special potassium current suppressing automaticity.

Keywords. Sinoatrial node, ion currents, acetylcholine, noradrenaline.

INTRODUCTION

For many years mechanisms of heart automaticity were extensively studied by physiologists. In the end of XIX century myogenic nature of automatic activity was proven for hearts of the vertebrate animals. The organization of the heart pacemaker, a structure providing rhythmic generation of excitation, varies greatly among the classes of vertebrates. The sinoatrial node (SAN) is the primary pacemaker of the mammalian heart. It is a specialized structure, situated in the intercaval region of right atrium, where superior and inferior vena cava flow into the right atrium. Revealing mechanisms of mammalian SAN functioning is very important for treatment of heart rhythm disorders, caused by disfunction of the SAN, such as "sick sinus syndrome". Therefore, the most advanced methods of electrophysiology, biochemistry and molecular biology are applied to research automatic activity of the SAN and its neural and humoral regulation. In the present chapter findings concerning morphology of the mammalian SAN, ion mechanisms of the SAN cells automaticity and molecular mechanisms of cholinergic and adrenergic regulation of the SAN function are reviewed.

STRUCTURE OF THE SAN

The intercaval region, where SAN is situated in the majority of mammalian species, is located between the orifice of superior and inferior vena cava (Figure 1.1A). The terminal crest of right atrium (crista terminalis) separates the intercaval region from the working myocardium of the right auricle (Figure 1.1B). On the other side the intercaval region borders upon the interatrial septum (Figure 1.1B). The SAN is a spindle-shaped structure, oblonged along the crista terminalis. The size of the SAN varies from 1.5 × 0.5 mm in the mouse heart up to 40 × 15 mm in the sperm-whale (James et al 1995, Opthof 1988). In the human heart it is approximately 7-15 mm in length and 2-5 mm in width (James 1977, 2002). The dimensions depend on age and size of the individual.

The thickness of the intercaval region wall, containing the SAN, varies from 0.1 mm in rat to 1.5 mm in human. In small mammals including rabbits and small rodents the SAN is situated between the epicardium and endocardium and occupies the full thickness of the atrial wall (Opthof 1988). In large animals the SAN is completely separated from the epi- and endocardium with several layers of working

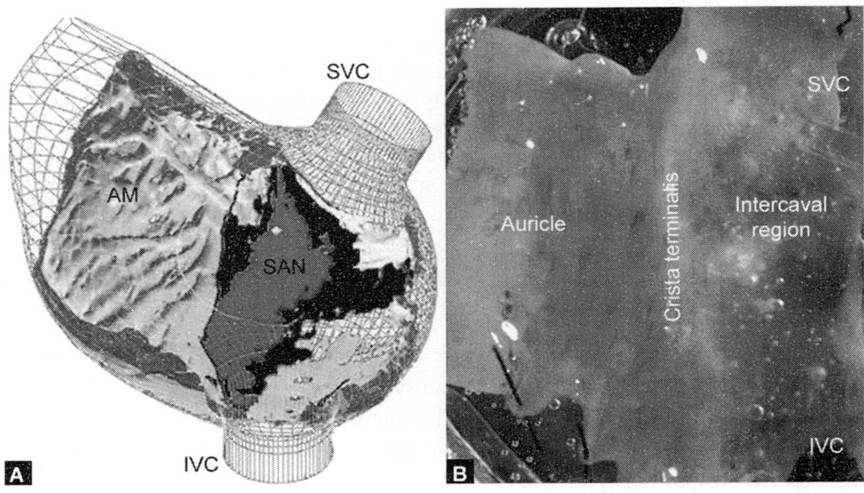

Figures 1.1A and B: A—Location of the SAN in the right atrium of rabbit—computer 3-dimensional model. B—preparation of isolated right atrium of rabbit. AM—atrial muscle, SVC— superior vena cava, IVC—inferior vena cava [A—From Boyett et al (2005) with permission from Elsevier].

myocardium, fat and connective tissue (Figure 1.2) (James 1977, 2002, Opthof et al 1986, 1987). The nutrition of the SAN in small mammals is provided mainly by diffusion and in the lesser extent by the small arterioles. In large mammals the sinoatrial node artery (SNA) is crucial for support with nutrients and oxygen (Opthof et al 1986, Opthof 1988). Therefore, the SAN preparations of dog, cat, pig and human survives only in conditions of perfusion through the SNA. It hampers the experiments with SAN of the large mammals, that is why the rabbit SAN have been used in the majority of physiological studies.

The SAN tissue contains cardiomyocytes, fibroblasts, collagen fibers and also nerve elements: Parasympathetic ganglions, preganglionic and postganglionic fibers, sympathetic postganglionic fibers. The amount of connective tissue varies from 50 to 80% depending on the animal species (Opthof et al 1985, 1986, 1987, Opthof 1988, Pavlovich and Chervova 1983). Larger mammals have respectively more collagen in their SAN. The connective tissue acts as a block of the impulse propagation in the lateral direction (Boyett et al 2000, 2003).

The SAN cardiomyocytes are divided into two groups: The typical SAN cells, which are also called pale cells, and transitional cells (James 1977, 2002). In the large mammals the SAN consists of small clusters of pale cells, each cluster contains 3-4 cells. These clusters are separated from each other with thin layers of connective tissue and connected with transitional cells. Pale cells have a large distinctive round central nucleus but only a few sparse contractive myofibrils. On the contrary, transitional cells are the muscle fibers with well-developed contractile apparatus. These cells represent a transitional form between the working

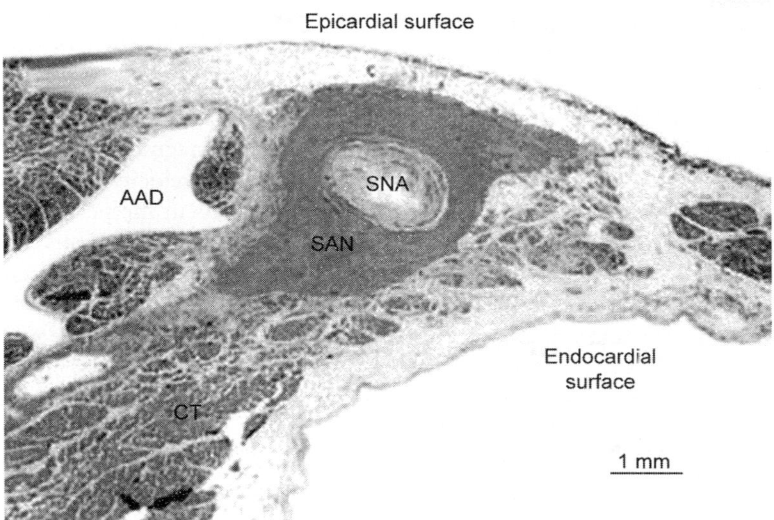

Figure 1.2: The human intercaval region – transverse section. The sinoatrial tissue is marked by grey. SNA – sinoatrial node artery, CT – crista terminalis, AAD – antrum atrii dextri [From James (2002) with permission from Elsevier].

myocardium atrial fibers and the pale cells. In the large animals transitional cells are present throughout the SAN connecting the clusters of the pale cells, their amount is larger at the periphery of the SAN (James et al 1995, James 2002, Stoletzki et al 2001). In the SAN of rabbit and rodents more simple organization of the SAN tissue was observed. The transitional cells are located only at the periphery of the SAN, while the central part is occupied with pale cells (Liu et al 2007, Masson-Pevet et al 1984, Verheijk et al 1998). Thus, the histological methods of the SAN examination show the difference between its central part, consisting mainly of typical sinoatrial cardiomyocytes and the peripheral part, where the transitional cells prevail. We will show further, that the center and periphery differ also in the expression of the various ion channels, receptors, connexins, as well as in the innervation and other important functional parameters.

BIOELECTRIC ACTIVITY OF THE SAN CELLS

Characteristics of Electric Activity in the Mammalian SAN

The first intracellular registration of the SAN electric activity was performed in the 1955 using the microelectrode technique (West 1955). The great difference between the parameters of electric activity in the SAN cells and the working myocardial fibers was clearly defined in this pioneering study. In the working cardiomyocyte the stable membrane potential (MP) of about 80 mV is usually observed. However, stable MP is absent in the typical SAN cell, the gradual decrease of MP, slow diastolic depolarization (DD), occurs during the interval between the end of AP repolarization and the depolarization phase of the next AP. During the slow DD MP decreases from the maximal level, maximal diastolic potential (MDP), to the level, which is threshold for the launch of the next AP. In the rabbit SAN MDP is about 55-60 mV (West 1955).

After reaching the threshold potential the depolarization phase of the next AP begins. In contrast to the working myocardium, the magnitude of overshoot in the SAN is no more than 1-2 mV. The depolarization velocity (dp/dt) varies from 2-3 mV/ms in the center of the SAN to 50 mV/ms in the periphery, it is much less than dp/dt in the working myocardium (150-200 mV/ms). These peculiarities of the AP depolarization phase in the SAN are due to the absence of the fast sodium channels in the central SAN. Depolarization is maintained by the slow calcium current I_{CaL}, which forms the plateau phase of AP in the working cardiomyocytes. Repolarization in the SAN consists of one phase because of the absence of overshoot. The very similar configuration of electric activity may be observed in the isolated nodal cells, although MPD and overshoot may be of greater amplitude (Figure 1.3).

Each phase of the electric activity cycle of the SAN cell depends on the different ion currents. It was supposed earlier that pacemaker activity is formed by two currents: Depolarizing calcium and repolarizing potassium current, while DD appears due to the decrease of potassium current after the repolarization of AP (Dudel and Trautwein 1958). It is now understood that more than 10 currents determine the pacemaker pattern of electric activity in the SAN cells. The beginning

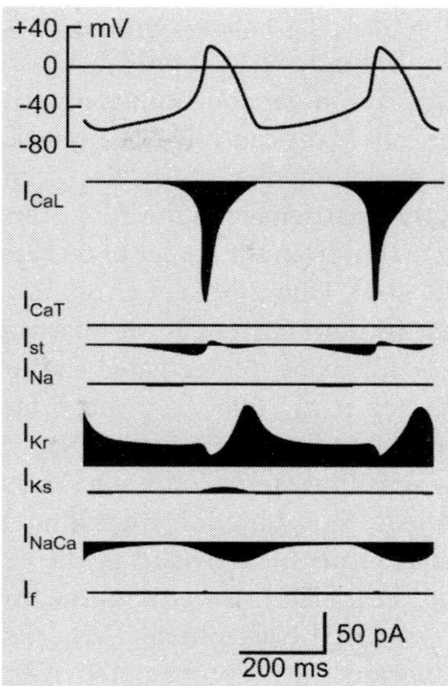

Figure 1.3: Electric activity and the main ion currents in the rabbit SAN cell [From Ono et al., 2003].

of slow DD is maintained by activation of the sodium hyperpolarization-activated pacemaker current I_f and suppression of the potassium currents (Mangoni and Nargeot 2008). The transient calcium current I_{CaT} and Na-Ca exchanger current participate in the final phase of slow DD. These currents bring the MP to the threshold level, and activation of I_{CaL} channels leading to the AP initiation occurs subsequently. Here we will describe ion mechanisms of the SAN automaticity in detail.

Currents Supporting the AP Depolarization Phase

The slow calcium current I_{CaL} is the most important current required for generation of AP in the rabbit SAN cells (Mangoni and Nargeot 2008). In contrast to working cardiomyocytes, where depolarization phase is formed by the fast sodium current, I_{CaL} is responsible for depolarization in the cells of central SAN. This fact may be clearly demonstrated using selective blockers of ion channels. Tetrodotoxin doesn't significantly alter configuration of AP in the isolated cells of primary pacemaker, but nifedipine (I_{CaL} blocker) suppresses the electric activity up to the full cessation (Kodama et al 1997, Boyett et al 2000). $Ca_v1.3$ isoform of slow calcium channels prevails in the central psrt of the SAN. This isoform differs from $Ca_v1.2$, which is predominant in the working myocardium, with lower threshold potential of activation, making the generation of AP in the pacemaker cells easier (Inada et al 2005, Tellez et al 2006).

It is believed that fast sodium current I_{Na} is absent in the cells of the SAN central part. However, 3 isoforms of voltage-gated sodium channels were found in the SAN of rabbit (Tellez et al 2006), rat and mouse (Maier et al 2003), tetrodotoxin-sensitive

$Na_v1.1$ and $Na_v1.3$ as well as $Na_v1.5$, which is common for myocardium and has low sensitivity to tetrodotoxin. But only $Na_v1.1$ and $Na_v1.3$ are present in the central SAN, their function are still not understood completely. It should be noticed that I_{Na} can't be activated in the cells of the central SAN, because the level of MP in these cells is lower than the threshold potential of I_{Na}. $Na_v1.5$ channels are expressed in the peripheral SAN cells, they participate in the AP generation and are important for the propagation of excitation from the center of SAN to the atrial myocardium (Boyett et al 2000, Lei et al 2005, Dobrzynski et al 2007).

It is believed that fast sodium current I_{Na} is absent in the cells of the SAN central part. However, 3 isoforms of voltage-gated sodium channels were found in the SAN of rabbit (Tellez et al 2006), rat and mouse (Maier et al 2003): Tetrodotoxin-sensitive $Na_v1.1$ and $Na_v1.3$ as well as $Na_v1.5$, which is common for myocardium and has low sensitivity to tetrodotoxin. But only $Na_v1.1$ and $Na_v1.3$ are present in the central SAN, their function are still not understood completely. It should be noticed that I_{Na} can't be activated in the cells of the central SAN, because the level of MP in these cells is lower than the threshold potential of I_{Na}. $Na_v1.5$ channels are expressed in the peripheral SAN cells, they participate in the AP generation and are important for the propagation of excitation from the center of SAN to the atrial myocardium (Boyett et al 2000, Lei et al 2005, Dobrzynski et al 2007).

Thus, activation of I_{CaL} is crucial for depolarization in the central region of SAN, while both I_{CaL} and I_{Na} participate in the depolarization development at the periphery os SAN.

Currents Responsible for the AP Repolarization

Activation of several delayed rectifier potassium currents supports the repolarization phase of AP in the SAN cells. In small mammals the fast delayed rectifier current $I_{K,r}$ plays the most important role in the repolarization of cellular membrane (Figure 1.3) (Anumonwo et al 1992, Ito and Ono 1995, Cho et al 2003), while the slow potassium current $I_{K,s}$ prevails in the large animals (Ono et al 2003). The presence of the ultrarapid potassium current $I_{K,ur}$, which is of great importance in the working atrial myocardium, was not detected using the methods of electrophysiology, although the respective channels were found (Dobrzynski et al 2007). The net potassium current gets smaller in the end of the repolarization phase, facilitating the initiation of DD. The $I_{K,r}$ blocker E-4031 provokes gradual depression of the MDP, decrease of the AP amplitude and finally, cessation of electric activity in the leading pacemaker of the rabbit SAN (Baruscotti and DiFrancesco 2004) or two-fold slowing of rhythm in the mouse SAN (Nikmaram et al 2008). Thus, delayed rectifier potassium currents maintain the automatic activity of the SAN.

The transient potassium current I_{to} is two-fold weaker in the rabbit SAN versus atrial myocardium. It flows through the $K_v4.2$ channels ($K_v1.4$ in the working myocardium) (Uese et al 1999, Boyett et al 2006). It is hypothesized that the smaller density of this current provides larger duration of AP in the central SAN versus atrial myocardium.

The inward rectifier potassium current $I_{K,1}$ is very important for the maintainance of the MP in the woking cardiomyocytes, but it is not found in the SAN cells (Irisawa et al 1993).

Currents Supporting the Slow DD

According to the early hypothesis, the decay of the hyperpolarizing potassium currents is the main factor supporting the development of the slow DD in the SAN cells. It was soon understood that another factor necessary for the initiation of DD is activation of the inward depolarizing current (Mangoni and Nargeot, 2008). Therefore, several research groups tried to find such current, crucial for the pacemaker functioning. The I_f current, known also as "funny" current was discovered in 1979 (Brown et al 1979). This current flows through HCN cyclic nucleotidegated channels. HCN channels are permeable for both sodium and potassium ions, but the certain depolarizing inward I_f current is carried by sodium ions. (DiFrancesco 1981). I_f is activated by hyperpolarization of membrane, it appears if MP is more negative than -60 mV, the half-maximal activation is observed at -85-90 mV (DiFancesco and Tromba 1988, Wu et al 2001, Mangoni and Nargeot 2008). Among the different HCN channels, HCN1, HCN2 and HCN4 are present in the SAN, the latter isoform prevails (Shi et al 1999, Yamamoto et al 2006). It was believed for a long time that I_f is the "pacemaker" current, the most important for automaticity in the SAN cells. However, selective I_f blockers zatebradine and ivabradine doesn't suppress the automatic activity in the rabbit SAN, just slowing the sinus rhythm less than 2-fold. (Nikmaram et al 1997). Similar data were obtained in the human SAN (Verkerk et al 2007). In the porcine SAN the slowing of rhythm is even smaller – 10% of control. Interestingly, in the mouse SAN I_f blocker ZD7288 prolongs the cycle duration on 13%, while in the isolated atrioventricular node its effect is much greater – 75% prolongation (Liu et al 2008). By analogy, in the SAN periphery the negative chronotropic effect of ZD7288 is several times larger versus the center of SAN (Nikmaram et al., 1997), although the HCN channels density in the central part of SAN is much greater in comparison to the SAN periphery and atrioventricular node (Tellez et al 2006, Liu et al 2007). It was proposed that in the SAN center other currents compensate the the slowing of DD caused by the block of I_f. Thus, I_f contributes to the SAN automaticity, although several researchers cast doubt on its crucial role (Baruscotti and Difrancesco 2004).

The transient calcium current I_{CaT}, which flows through $Ca_v3.1$ and $Ca_v3.2$ channels, may be also important for normal automatic activity. Selective blocking of I_{CaT} with nickel ions slows down the rhythm of rabbit isolated SAN cells via the inhibition of the second half of DD (Hagiwara et al 1988). Therefore, it was supposed that I_{CaT} activates in the end of DD together with I_{NaCa}, providing the smooth transition from the DD to the upstroke AP. The quantity of RNA of $Ca_v3.1$ and $Ca_v3.2$ channels detected in the SAN was a significantly larger than in the atrial myocardium (Tellez et al 2006).

Another current important for the SAN automatic activity was found in 1995. It was called sustained inward current – I_{st} (Musa et al 2002). This current is similar to the I_{CaL} in its pharmacological properties: It can be blocked by verapamil, nicardipine and activated by Bay-K8644, I_{CaL} activator. However I_{st} is carried by sodium ions. I_{st} was found in the SAN cells of rabbit (Guo et al 1995), rat (Shinagawa et al 2000) and guinea pig (Guo et al 1997). This current is depolarization-activated, threshold potential is -65 mV. Therefore, I_{st} may be also contributed to the generation of DD. This current is found only in the cells of SAN and atrioventricular node. The molecular determinants of I_{st} have not yet been identified.

Besides I_f, I_{CaT} and I_{st}, the current of sodium-calcium exchanger is also very important for generation of slow DD. The special hypothesis of "calcium clock" arose from the research of the I_{NaCa} function.

The Na-Ca Exchanger Current and the Hypothesis of "Calcium Clock"

The Na-Ca exchanger has two modes of functioning. While working in the direct mode the molecule of exchanger transports one calcium ion outside the cell and three sodium ions inside, therefore the exchanger is electrogenic. During the direct mode the inward depolarizing current I_{NaCa} appears. Blocking of exchanger with a fast replacing of Na^+ by Li^+ in the perfusing solution leads to the cessation of automatic activity in the isolated SAN cells of rabbit (Bogdanov et al 2001). Selective blocker of Na-Ca exchanger KB-R7943 also quitenes the cells (Sanders et al 2007).

In which phase of the cardiac cycle activation of I_{NaCa} occurs? It is clear that the current arises in response to the increase of the intracellular calcium concentration. Experiments with fluorescent calcium imaging revealed the small releases of calcium from the sarcoplasmic reticulum stores, coincided with the final stage of DD, besides the total depletion of calcium stores in response to the AP. Such releases of calcium are local, that is appearing in relatively small region of the cell, and spontaneous, independent from the membrane potential (Vinogradova et al 2004, Bogdanov et al 2006). According to the authors terminology we will call these phenomenom the local calcium release (LCR). As far as the ryanodine receptors, releasing calcium from the sarcoplasmic reticulum, and the molecules of Na-Ca exchanger are colocalized in the SAN cells (Lyashkov et al 2007), LCRs lead to the activation of I_{NaCa}. This results in the acceleration of DD in its last third and transition from linear to exponential DD. The latter allows the MP to reach the threshold potential of I_{CaL} activation faster, enhancing generation of AP (Maltsev and Lakatta 2008). Then I_{CaL} launches the total activation of ryanodine receptors with subsequent depletion of sarcoplasmic reticulum calcium stores. Thereupon calcium ATPase SERCA2a pumps calcium from cytosol to reticulum until the calcium concentration in the reticulum reaches the threshold level, sufficient for the spontaneous initiation of LCR (Lakatta et al 2008). The whole cycle is shown at the Fig. 1.4. Thus, according to the "calcium clock" hypothesis I_{NaCa} serves as a link between the intracellular calcium cycling and the depolarization of sarcoplasmic membrane. Suppression of LCRs by ryanodine eliminates the exponential phase of DD, leading to the marked slowing of the sinus rhythm (Bogdanov et al 2001).

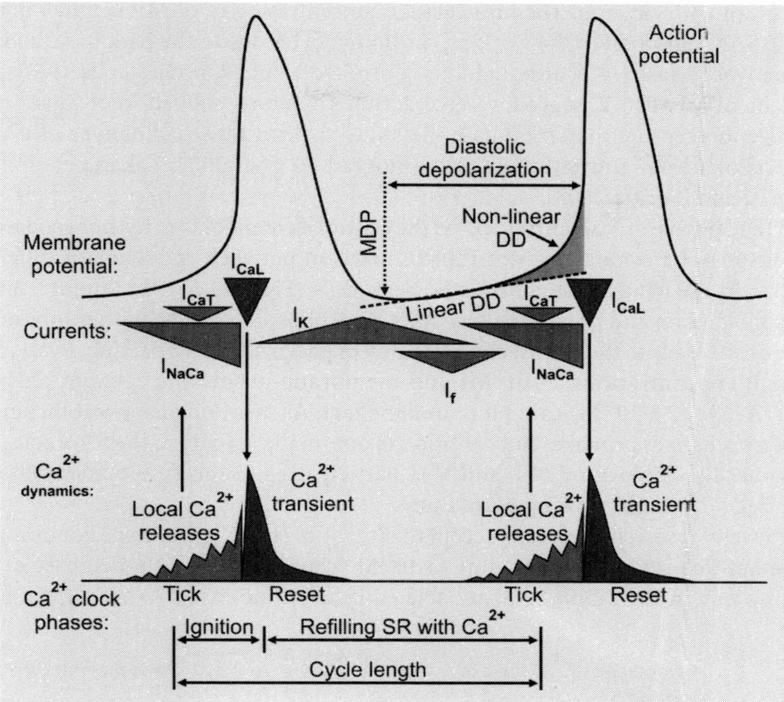

Figure 1.4: A schematic illustration of the fine structure of the DD and spontaneous AP in rabbit SAN cell shown together with inward ion currents and related Ca^{2+} signals [From Maltsev and Lakatta (2007) with permission from Elsevier].

According to the "calcium clock" hypothesis, the central role in the initiation of excitation belongs not to single ion current or group of currents, but to the rhythmic spontaneous LCRs independent of sarcoplasmic membrane potential. In the voltage clamp experiments, conducted on the rabbit SAN cells, small (3-10 pA) ryanodine-sensitive oscillations of MP with a frequency of 4.9 Hz were observed (Vinogradova et al 2004, 2006). It was proposed that these oscillations are caused by the LCRs. It was shown in fluorescent calcium imaging experiments that LCRs persist after the clamp of membrane potential (Lakatta et al 2006). The rate of LCRs depends principally on the velocity of sarcoplasmic reticulum filling with calcium and the threshold level of calcium concentration, sufficient for the initiation of LCR (Lakatta et al 2008). Therefore there are two mechanisms of LCRs rate\control: Phosphorylation of the phospholamban, the SERCA2 regulating protein, that leads to the enhancement of calcium pumping into the sarcoplasmic reticulum and phosphorylation of ryanodine receptors, lowering the threshold level of calcium concentration. Both mechanisms are regulated by proteinkinase A (PKA). Activity of this enzyme depends on the intracellular cAMP level (Vinogradova et al 2006). Moreover, PKA phosphorylates channels of I_{CaL} and increases this current, additionally enhancing the filling of sarcoplasmic reticulum with calcium. The intracellular concentration of cAMP is much higher in the SAN cells than in the working cardiomyocytes due to the high basal activity of adenylylcyclase (AC), although it is controlled by phosphodiesterases with also high basal activity (Vinogradova et al 2008). Therefore, activation of muscarinic or adrenoreceptors may modulate the sinus rhythm rate via changes of cAMP intracellular level and rate of LCRs (Vinogradova et al 2002, Lakatta et al 2008, Maltsev and Lakatta 2008).

The key role of "calcium clock" as the central element of the rhythm generation system may be evaluated from the comparison between influence of different factors on the beating rate of isolated SAN cells (Figure 1.5). The suppression of phospholamban and ryanodine receptors PKA phosphorylation with inhibitors of PKA or AC leads to the almost complete stop of pacemaker cells beating. Ryanodine in high concentrations ($3{\cdot}10^{-5}$M) and membrane-permeable calcium chelator BAPTA-AM ($2.5{\cdot}10^{-5}$M) cause the similar effect. As mentioned above, blocking of Na-Ca exchanger provokes full cessation of automatic activity in the SAN cells. On the other hand, blocking of I_f and I_{CaT}, participating in the development of slow DD, leads to a slight slowing of rhythm.

Several researchers doesn't accept the "calcium clock" hypothesis. For example, some authors state that ryanodine ($3{\cdot}10^{-5}$M) causes just 19-21% decrease of the beating rate in the rabbit SAN an isolated cells (Hono et al., 2003) and rat SAN

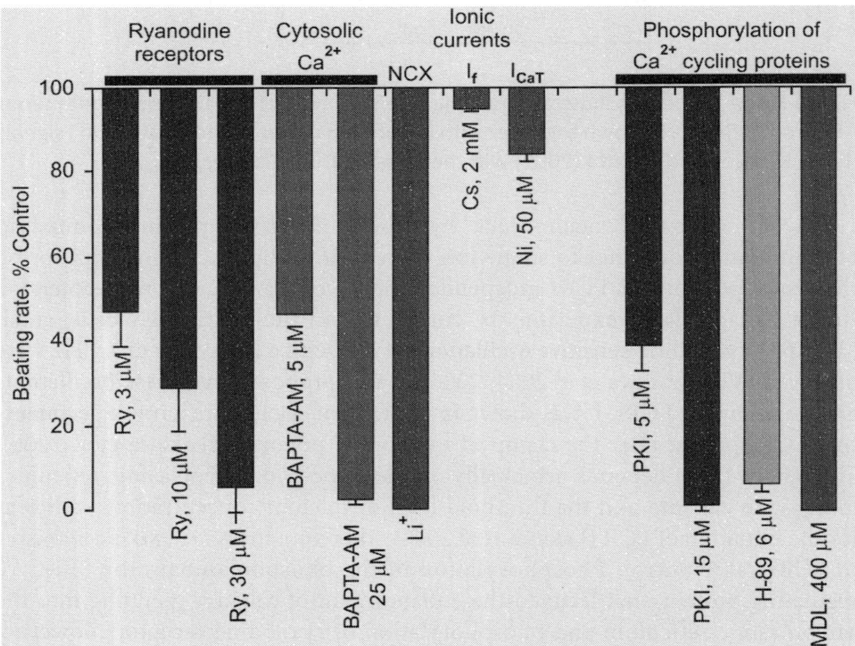

Figure 1.5: Decrease in the beating rate (% control) induced by different drugs that affect Ca^{2+} cycling or ion currents. PKI and H-89 are PKA inhibitors and MDL is an adenylyl cyclase inhibitor [From Maltsev and Lakatta (2007) with permission from Elsevier].

(Nikmaram et al 2008). These data contradicts the main postulates of the "calcium clock" hypothesis. Other authors propose that LCRs appear not spontaneously, but in response to the I_{CaT} (Huser et al 2000). Some investigators note that specific activator of HCN channels Rp-cAMP significantly accelerates the sinus rhythm even in the presence of ryanodine. Thereby the authors conclude the key role of I_f current in rhythm generation (Bucchi et al. 2003, 2007). Thus, subsequent investigation focused mainly on the intact SAN is needed to absolve arising controversies.

We can now summarize the stated findings and describe the ion mechanism of the SAN cell automaticity (Figure 1.4). Repolarization phase of the AP is maintained by the delayed rectifier potassium currents, $I_{K,s}$ and $I_{K,r}$. Fading of these currents makes possible the initiation of the DD. The hyperpolarization-activated I_f current produces the first half of DD, linear depolarization. The Na-Ca exchanger current I_{NaCa} and transient calcium current I_{CaT} transform the linear DD to exponential. Then the MP reaches the threshold level of I_{CaL} activation and the AP arises. Moreover, the sodium I_{st} current takes part in the development of DD. This mechanism is supplemented with the "calcium clock" hypothesis, explaining that I_{NaCa}, which is crucial for the transition from the DD to the AP upstroke, appears in response to the spontaneous LCRs depending only on the intracellular calcium turnover.

THE ACTIVATION SEQUENCE OF THE SAN REGION

Although the isolated SAN cells are capable of automatic generation of excitation, the heart rhythm is determined by the whole SAN as a complex structure. Functioning of the SAN depends not only on the single cells properties, but on the interactions between the cells. That is why we should discuss the process of excitation propagation within the SAN region.

The activation sequence of the SAN was studied using different methods of preparation mapping: The mapping, based on consecutive microelectrode impalements in the different points of the preparation (Bleeker et al 1980), electric mapping with array of extracellular electrodes (Shibata et al 2001) and, finally, the most precise method of optical mapping (Abramochkin et al 2008, Fedorov et al 2006). The microelectrode mapping was sufficient to determine the SAN activation sequence in normal conditions (Bleeker et al 1980) and further studies have approved these early findings. On the other hand, the continuous monitoring of beat-to-beat SAN activation sequence changes could be conducted only using the optical mapping technique, based on the application of the voltage-sensitive fluorescent dye di-4-ANNEPS.

Analysis of the excitation chronotopography of the SAN shows that there is a small region where the first excitation appears and then spreads throughout the SAN. This region is called the primary (dominant) pacemaker of the SAN region. In the rabbit heart this primary pacemaker site is located in the central part of the SAN during normal conditions. As mentioned above, the SAN is elongated along the crista terminalis. The velocity of excitation wave in the longitudinal direction is about 4.5-5 sm/s versus 3 sm/s in the transversal direction: The excitation wave spreads anisotropically (Figure 1.6) (Boyett et al 2000, Yamamoto et al 1998). The large block zone, formed by the inexcitable tissue, is situated right to the SAN, it prevents the excitation from the direct propagation to the interatrial septum. (Sano et al 1965, Boyett et al 2000). In the periphery of the SAN the conduction velocity is much higher than in the center: 50 sm/s along the CT and 36 sm/s in the perpendicular direction (Yamamoto et al 1998). This pattern of the SAN region excitation was obtained in the experiments with rabbit. In the large mammals the mapping of the SAN is much more difficult due to the epicardial and endocardial layers. In the experiments on dogs quite similar results were obtained after the cut-off the subepicardial tissue layer (Bromberg et al 1995).

It is believed that the low excitation propagation velocity in the central part of the SAN is due to absence of the high-permeable connexins Cx43 and 45, Only low-permeable connexin Cx40 is expressed in the center of SAN (Coppen et al

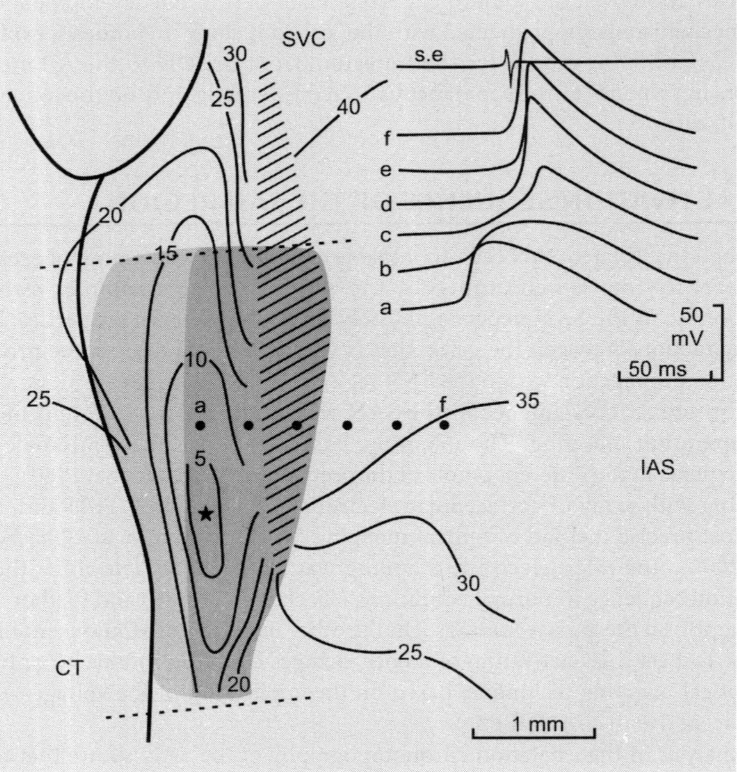

Figure 1.6: The isochronic map of activation of the rabbit intercaval region, obtained with consecutive microelectrode registrations. SVC – superior vena cava, CT – crista terminalis, IAS – interatrial septum. Curved lines with numbers are isochrones, numbers indicate the time of excitation [From Bleeker et al (1982) with permission from Elsevier].

1999, Hescheler et al 1986). At the rabbit SAN periphery special transitional cells, expressing Cx43 and 45, prevail, therefore the conduction velocity is higher at the periphery (Boyett et al 2000). The predominant longitudinal orientation of the SAN cells determines anisotropic propagation of excitation (Bleeker et al 1980, Masson-Pevet 1984).

Thus, we have discussed the mechanisms of automaticity in the separate SAN cells and the activation of the whole SAN. Autonomic regulation of automaticity may be studied also at both cellular and multicellular levels of organization.

MECHANISMS OF NEGATIVE CHRONOTROPIC EFFECT OF ACETYLCHOLINE

Acetylcholine (ACh) is the main neurotransmitter of the parasympathetic nervous system. In the heart it is released from the postganglionic parasympathetic nerve endings and affects the cardiomyocytes via muscarinic (M) cholinoreceptors. Five subtypes of M-cholinoreceptors were found (M1-M5), but only 4 of them are present in the heart (M1-M4) (Dhein et al 2001). M-cholinoreceptors are metabotropic and G-protein associated. Effects arising due to the activation of certain subtype of M-receptors depend on which type of G-protein is associated with this receptor subtype. Therefore, two classes of M-receptors are usually segregated: Odd-numbered receptors (M1, M3, M5) and even-numbered (M2, M4). Even-numbered receptors are associated with G_i-proteins, the main effect of activation of these receptors is inhibition of adenylylcyclase (AC) and consecutive reduction of cAMP intracellular concentration leading to alterations in activity of different enzymes and ion channels. Odd-numbered receptors are associated with G_q-proteins. Therefore, stimulation of these receptors cause activation of phospholipase C with consecutive calcium release from sarcoplasmic reticulum-mediated via inositoltriphosphate receptors and activation of proteinkinase C (Felder 1995, Dhein et al 2001).

The quantity of M2-receptors is about 90% of overall M-receptors quantity in the myocardium, so their role in the mediation of cholinergic cardiotropic effects is the most important. However, the physiological role of M3-receptors in the myocardium was also shown during the last decade (Wang et al 2007, Abramochkin et al 2009). In the SAN presence of M3-receptors is not shown, therefore here we will discuss mechanisms of negative chronotropic effect mediation via the M2-receptors (Figure 1.7).

Stimulation of M2-receptors causes replacement of GDP with GTP in the nucleotide-binding site of G_i-protein and dissociation of G_i-protein into α and βγ-subunits. Next these subunits perform their specific functions until the hydrolysis of bound GTP and subsequent reassociation of G_i-protein occurs (Dhein et al 2001).

The main function of G_i-protein βγ-subunit is activation of potassium ACh-dependent channels of I_{KACh} current. The molecule of potassium ACh-dependent channel is tetrameric, consisting of two GIRK1 and two GIRK4 subunits. The lag period of ACh-dependent channels activation is about 30-70 ms. It is slower than activation of ionotropic receptors, but much faster than activation via the

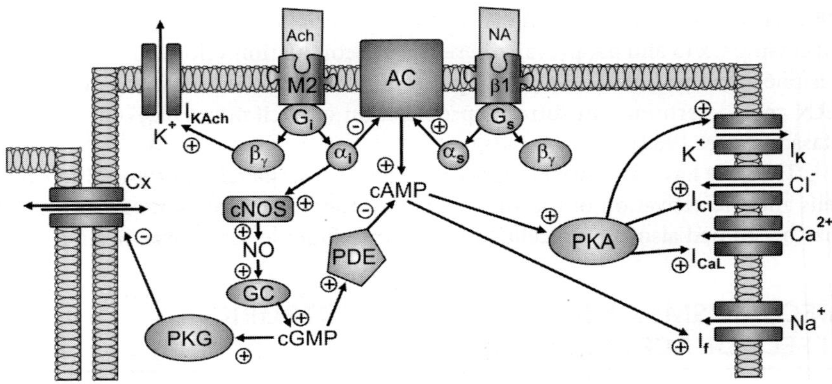

Figure 1.7: Mechanisms of antagonistic regulation of the sinus rhythm by ACh and NA. See comments in the text. PDE – phosphodiesterase (type 2), GC – guanylyl cyclase, PKG – proteinkinase G.

second messenger system (Brodde and Michel 1999). The outward potassium current I_{KACh} causes membrane hyperpolarization. It is negligible in the working cardiomyocytes, because the MP is high there and is close to the potassium equilibrium potential. However, in the nodal cells the hyperpolarization may reach 25-30 mV. The hyperpolarization increases the MDP and the time needed for MP to reach the threshold level of I_{CaL} activation, therefore, the slowing of sinus rhythm occurs. Besides hyperpolarization, activation of I_{KACh} provokes the decrease of AP duration due to the acceleration of repolarization phase. In the pacemaker cells this effect is less pronounced than in the working myocardium. Ba^{2+}, which blocks I_{KACh} channels (Osterrieder et al 1982, Boyett et al 1995), reduces the negative chronotropic effect of ACh and vagal stimulation manifold. Therefore, I_{KACh} plays important role in mediation of cholinergic bradycardia (Boyett et al 1995, Kodama et al 1996). Note, that knockout of GIRK4 gene seriously impairs the cholinergic regulation of heart (Wickman et al 1998).

α-subunit of G_i-protein suppresses activity of AC 5/6 isoforms, predominant in the myocardium (Sunahara et al 1996), and decreases the cAMP level. The molecules of cAMP bind with special cyclonucleotide binding sites within the molecule of HCN4 channel and shift the I_f activation curve to less negative potentials (DiFrancesco and Tromba, 1988, DiFrancesco and Tortora 1991), enhancing the linear phase of slow DD in the SAN cells (Bucchi et al 2007). Therefore, ACh provokes the opposite effect by reducing the cAMP intracellular concentration: It suppresses I_f and prolongs the DD. Note, that the concentration of ACh sufficient for inhibition of I_f current is ten-fold lower than the concentration capable of I_{KACh} activation (DiFrancesco and Tromba 1988). There is also an additional mechanism of I_f modulation: Direct binding of $α_i$-subunit with HCN-channel molecule (Yatani et al 1990).

It has been recently shown that ACh inhibits I_{st} current, which also maintains the automatic activity, via the reduction of cAMP concentration

(Toyoda et al 2005). It is still not clear if this effect is mediated via the reduction of PKA activity or it is based on the direct action of cAMP.

Thus, the second mechanism of negative chronotropic effect of ACh includes the suppression of pacemaker currents and reduction of the slow DD velocity.

On the other hand the reduction of cAMP intracellular concentration inhibits PKA activity. PKA phosphorylates and activates calcium L-type channels (Bean et al 1984, Hescheler et al 1986, Kameyama et al 1985, Trautwein et al 1987), chloride cAMP-activated channels (Harvey et al 1989, 1990), fast sodium channels of I_{Na} current (Cho et al 2002, Ono et al 1993) and delayed rectifier potassium channels (Harvey and Hume 1989, Marx et al 2002). Therefore, ACh provokes the reduction of these currents via PKA inhibiton.

The well-known suppression of I_{CaL} by ACh was first described in the atrial bullfrog myocardium (Giles and Noble 1976) and then demonstrated in the rabbit SAN cells (Petit-Jacques et al 1993, Zaza et al 1996). The computer simulation studies show that ACh may reduce the AP amplitude in the SAN central part via the I_{CaL} inhibition (Aliev et al 2004). However, other researches argue that ACh doesn't affect the magnitude of I_{CaL} in normal conditions without preliminary adrenergic activation of this current (Honjo et al 1992).

Which current is the most important for the mediation of negative chronotropic cholinergic effect? It seems that in different concentrations ACh affects different ion currents supporting the automatic activity of the SAN cells (DiFrancesco et al 1989). Experiments conducted on the isolated rabbit heart and designed to determine the respective contribution of I_{KACh} and I_f to the mediation of ACh negative chronotropic effect confirm this hypothesis (Yamada 2002). In this study the new selective peptide blocker of potassium ACh-dependent channels tertiapin, obtained from the honey-bee venom (Jin and Lu 1998), and conventional I_f blocker CsCl were used. Muscarinic agonist carbacholine in low concentrations ($\leq 10^{-7}$M) caused slowing of the sinus rhythm insensitive to tertiapin. After the block of I_f with CsCl the sinus rhythm decreased, low concentrations of carbacholine failed to cause bradycardia in the presence of CsCl. High concentrations of carbacholine ($\geq 3 \cdot 10^{-7}$M) provoked more prominent rhythm deceleration, but in the presence of tertiapin this effect was not higher than effect of low carbacholine concentrations. In the presence of CsCl the negative chronotropic effect of high carbacholine concentrations was completely abolished by tertiapin. Thus, the low concentrations of carbacholine cause tertiapin-insensitive rhythm deceleration via the inhibition of I_f, the bradycardia induced by high concentrations is sensitive to tertiapin and mediated by both inhibition of I_f and activation of I_{KACh}.

The hypothesis of "calcium clock" reveals the new mechanism of cholinergic sinus rhythm slowing. ACh decreases the intracellular cAMP concentration and PKA activity, therefore cholinergic influence suppresses phosphorylation of phospholamban and ryanodine receptors in the SAN cells. As noted above, this leads to the decrease of the LCRs rate and consecutive slowing of the SAN cells rhythmic excitation (Vinogradova et al 2006). Thus, according to the "calcium clock" hypothesis, the negative chronotropic effect of ACh is mediated predominantly via the AC inhibition and decrease of cAMP intracellular concentration.

MECHANISMS OF POSITIVE CHRONOTROPIC EFFECT OF CATECHOLAMINES

There are two main types of sympathetic influence on the heart function. First, neurotransmitter noradrenaline is released in the myocardium from the intramural sympathetic postganglionic fibers. Second, hormone adrenaline secreted from the adrenal glands circulates in the blood and also affects the myocardium.

Nine subtypes of adrenoreceptors are known: $\alpha_{1A, 1B, 1D}$, $\alpha_{2A, 2B, 2C}$, β_1, β_2, β_3. Only α_{1A}, β_1 and β_2-adrenoreceptors are expressed in the cardiomyocytes and mediate the adrenergic regulation of the myocardium (Brodde et al 2006). In addition, α_2-adrenoreceptors inhibit the release of noradrenaline from the sympathetic endings (Rump et al 1995). Like muscarinic receptors, adrenoreceptors are 7-domain transmembrane glycoproteins, associated with G-proteins. α_1-receptors are associated with G_q-proteins, therefore their stimulation leads to activation of phospoinositide signaling cascade (Terzic et al 1993). β_1 and β_2-adrenoreceptors associate withG_s-proteins, stimulation of these receptors causes activation of AC and increase of cAMP concentration (Brodde et al 1999, 2006). Note that β_2-receptors are also associated with G_i-proteins, so the effect of G_s-activation is attenuated during the β_2-receptors stimulation (Xiao et al 1999, 2003).

In the mammalian SAN catecholamines produce the prominent positive chronotropic effect based on the β-adrenoreceptors stimulation (Mangoni and Nargeot 2008). The role of α-adrenoreceptors seems to be inessential in the SAN. According to the universally recognized conception, the acceleration of the sinus rhythm appears from modulation of different ion currents by catecholamines via the increase of cAMP concentration in pacemaker cells.

The largest number of evidence is collected concerning the participation of I_f current in the mediation of adrenergic effects (DiFrancesco and Tortora, 1991, DiFrancesco 1993). Just a slight increase of the cAMP concentration caused by adrenergic stimulation leads to increase of HCN-channels opening probability. cAMP shifts the activation curve of I_f current to the less negative potentials, therefore enhancing the linear DD. Low concentrations of β-adrenoreceptors agonist isoproterenol produce substantial acceleration of slow DD, but don't affect the AP configuration. Therefore, activation of I_f seems to be the most important mechanism of adrenergic acceleration of rhythm (DiFrancesco 1993). Membrane-permeable cAMP analogs are capable of slow DD acceleration and I_f enhancement as well (Bucchi et al 2003, 2007). In the embryonic heart of mice with HCN4 knockout the increase of cAMP concentration doesn't produce the rhythm acceleration (Stieber et al 2003). On the other hand, several authors report that blocking of I_f with Cs^+ doesn't alter the positive chronotropic effect of adrenergic stimulation in the rabbit SAN cells (Nikmaram et al 1997, Vinogradova et al 2002), although zatebradin (I_f blocker) suppresses the effect of β-stimulation in experiments on pigs *in vivo* (Guth and Diete 2000).

Calcium current I_{CaL} is also highly sensitive to the β-adrenoreceptors stimulation by isoproterenol (Zaza et al 1996). Note that the blocking of I_{CaL} with dihydropyridines reduces the positive chronotropic effect of stellate ganglion stimulation in mice (Choate and Feldman 2003). In isolated heart of mice with

$Ca_v1.3$ knockout the positive chronotropic effect of isoproterenol is less pronounced than in the wild type (Matthes et al 2000). Under this findings several researchers suppose the participation of I_{CaL} together with I_f in the mediation of adrenergic regulation of sinoatrial automaticity (Mangoni and Nargeot 2008).

Besides these, several other currents may be involved in the mediation of sympathetic effects. For example, the magnitude of I_{st} doubles under the action of 10^{-7}M isoprenaline (Guo et al 1997). The net delayed rectifier potassium current is also enhanced during the activation of β-adrenoreceptors with isoprenaline (Lei et al 2000), this effect is PKA-mediated. The activation curve of the current shifts to more negative potentials. However, all these effects are less pronounced and may be concerned as subsidiary in comparison with I_f and I_{CaL} activation. The chloride cAMP-dependent current, that is activated in the working myocardium during adrenergic stimulation, was not found in the SAN cells (Takano and Noma 1992).

The "calcium clock" hypothesis widens our knowledge about the mechanisms of adrenergic sinus rhythm acceleration. According to it, the positive chronotropic effect of adrenoreceptors stimulation is determined by the increase of the LCRs rate. The increase of cAMP leads to the PKA activation, phosphorylation of phospholamban and ryanodine receptors (Vinogradova et al 2006). This enhances the filling of sarcoplasmic reticulum with calcium and lowers the threshold concentration of calcium sufficient for the initiation of the LCR. Therefore, the LCRs rate increases and the sinus rhythm accelerates. The partial block of ryanodine receptors by ryanodine causes complete abolishment of the positive chronotropic effect of isoproterenol in the isolated rabbit SAN cells and the dog heart in situ (Vinogradova et al 2002, 2006). Note that some authors present the opposite data that isoproterenol accelerates the rhythm on 52% of control in the presence of $3 \cdot 10^{-5}$M ryanodine (Honjo et al 2003).

THE PACEMAKER SHIFT WITHIN THE SAN REGION

The described mechanisms of the sinus rhythm regulation by autonomic neurotransmitters are based generally on the modulation of the slow DD slope via alteration of different ion currents or the frequency of LCRs. These mechanisms work in the single SAN cells as well as in the whole SAN. Nevertheless, the rhythm regulation is a more complex process and the phenomenon of pacemaker shift is likely to be important for its implementation.

The repositioning of the leading pacemaker site within the SAN, called the pacemaker shift, was first shown in the pioneering studies, where microelectrode mapping was used to reveal the SAN activation sequence. The pacemaker shift occurs under cholinergic or adrenergic influence (Mackaay et al 1980a), changes in the concentration of potassium (Lu 1970), calcium (Mackaay et al 1980b), sodium (Opthof 1988) and chloride (Opthof et al 1986). The method based on consecutive microelectrode recordings from different points of preparation doesn't allow to analyze the pacemaker shift dynamics during the effect of the different factors. Therefore, Shibata et al (2001) used multiple extracellular potential recordings to determine beat-to-beat changes of the SAN activation sequence during vagal nerve stimulation. The high-resolution optical mapping technique allowed to perform this task more precisely.

In our recent studies (Abramochkin et al 2009a,b) we demonstrated using optical mapping, that acetylcholine (10 μM) and strong intramural parasympathetic nerve stimulation cause a pacemaker shift as well as rhythmic slowing and the formation of an inexcitable region in the central part of SAN. In this region the generation of action potentials was suppressed. The slowing of the sinus rhythm (which exceeded 12.8+/-3.1% of the rhythm control rate) always accompanies the pacemaker shift. Isoproterenol (10, 100 nM, 1 μM) and sympathetic postganglionic nerve stimulation also evoke a pacemaker shift but without formation of an inexcitable zone. The acceleration of the sinus rhythm over 10.5+/-1.3% of the control rate, always accompany the shift. Thus, modest changes in the sinus rhythm do not coincide with the pacemaker shift, while the greater changes always accompany the shift.

But what is a physiological role of the pacemaker shift? In 1960 Hoffman and Cranefield proposed that the pacemaker shift may act as a sinus rhythm modulation mechanism (Hoffman and Cranefield 1960). Bouman et al (1968) have further developed this conception. It is well known that different parts of the SAN have different automatic ability, some regions can produce faster rhythm than others (Noma and Irisawa 1976, Mackaay et al 1980). Therefore, if the region that is capable of generating only a slow rhythm becomes a dominant pacemaker due to the acetylcholine (ACh) action, then the overall sinus rhythm will decrease. Thus, the pacemaker shift may act as an additional mechanism of the autonomic regulation of the overall sinus rhythm side by side with the modulation of the slow DD velocity. This phenomenon may be widely distributed *in vivo* because despite modest sinus rhythm changes do not coincide with the pacemaker shift, larger changes always accompany the shift (Abramochkin et al 2009a) and may be caused by the shift according to the hypothesis of Hoffman and Cranefield.

What are the mechanisms of the intranodal pacemaker shift? The ACh-induced suppression of excitability in the initial leading pacemaker site, shown in several microelectrode (Vinogradova et al 1998) and optical mapping studies (Fedorov et al 2006, Abramochkin et al 2009a,b) is likely to be one of the mechanisms of the pacemaker shift, caused by cholinergic factors. Recently, we have demonstrated that cholinergic suppression of electric activity in the SAN center is caused by the activation of I_{KACh} (unpublished data). Obviously, if the leading pacemaker shuts down, then the subsidiary pacemaker should become dominant; otherwise the heart will stop beating. However, the pacemaker shift provoked by noncholinergic factors seems to have another mechanisms. Most authors argue that the heterogeneity of the SAN and multiple differences between the center and the periphery of SAN should be concerned as the basis of the pacemaker shift phenomenon.

THE FUNCTIONAL AND MOLECULAR DETERMINANTS OF THE SAN HETEROGENEITY

The center and periphery of the SAN differ in the density of autonomic innervations, sensitivity to the neurotransmitters and composition of ion currents

(Bouman et al 1968, Mackaay et al 1980a, Opthof 1988, Boyett et al 2000). These differences depends on expression of ion channels, receptors, connexins and other functionally important proteins (Table 1.1).

The gap junctions (connexons) providing the electrical coupling of cardiomyocytes consist of specialized proteins called connexins. Cx43 forms the gap junctions of medium conductance. It is the main connexin of the working myocardium, but it is not expressed in the central part of the SAN. Cx45 forms low conductance gap junctions, it is present in the SAN, but absent in the working myocardium (Coppen et al 1999). Cx40 forms high conductance connexons, it is found in the working atrial myocardium (Verheule et al 1997), but not in the center of SAN (Boyett et al 2006, Dobrzynski et al. 2006). It is supposed that poor electrical coupling in the SAN caused by the absence of high-conductance connexins prevents the hyperpolarizing influence of the atrial myocardium to the central part of SAN (Joyner and Capelle 1986, Boyett et al 2000). On the other hand the presence of all three main connexins in the SAN periphery supports effective transduction of excitation to the atrial myocardium (Winslow and Jongsma 1995, Dobrzynski et al 2007).

Table 1.1: Ion channels, receptors, connexins and other proteins expressed in the central SAN, periphery of the SAN and working atrial myocardium

Protein	SAN center	SAN periphery	Atrial myocardium
Connexins:			
Cx43	-	+	++
Cx45	+	+	-?
Cx40	-	+	+
Calcium channels:			
$Ca_v1.3(I_{CaL})$	++	+	-
$Ca_v1.2(I_{CaL})$	-	+	++
$Ca_v3.1(I_{CaT})$	+	+	-
$Ca_v3.2(I_{CaT})$	+	+	-
Sodium channels:			
$Na_v1.5$	-	+	++
$Na_v1.1$	+	+	-
HCN	++	+	-
Potassium channels:			
$K_{ir}2.1$, $K_{ir}2.2$ ($I_{K,1}$)	-	-	+
Calcium cycling proteins:			
Na-Ca exchanger	++	+	++
RYR2	+	++	+++
RYR3	+++	++	+
β-adrenoreceptors	++	+	+
Muscarinic receptors	+++	++	+
Neurofilament NF-M	++	+	-
Atrial natriuretic peptide	-	+	+++

The L-type calcium channels are present in all cells of the SAN region. $Ca_V1.3$ isoform prevails in the central part of SAN, while $Ca_V1.2$ is predominant in the atrial myocardium (Inada et al 2005, Marionneau et al 2005). The cardiac $Na_V1.5$ isoform of the fast sodium channels, which is low sensitive to tetrodotoxin, is absent in the SAN center, but present in the periphery and atrial myocardium (Lei et al 2004, Maier et al 2003). HCN4-channels of I_f current are more abundant in the center of rabbit and murine SAN than in the periphery and are almost absent in the atrial myocardium (Tellez et al 2006, Liu et al 2007).

The proteins maintaining the "calcium clock" functioning are also differentially expressed in the SAN and the working myocardium. The Na-Ca exchanger mRNA is less abundant in the periphery of the SAN than in the SAN center and atrial myocardium (Tellez et al 2006). Ryanodine receptors of the second type (RYR2) are predominant in the atrial myocardium, but scarce in the SAN central part, the opposite is for RYR3 (Musa et al 2002, Masumiya et al 2003). These data indicate, that serious functional differences in the "calcium clock" system between the center, periphery of SAN and the atrial myocardium should be revealed further (Lakatta et al 2008).

Two proteins are used together with the Cx43 connexin as markers to differ the SAN tissue from the surrounding atrial myocardium: Middle (160/165 kDa) neurofilament (NF-M) and the famous hormone, atrial natriuretic peptide (ANP). NF-M is a cytoskeleton protein, in rabbit heart it is expressed only in the SAN, atrioventricular node and the cardiac conduction system (Gorza et al 1988, Maier et al 2003). The central part of SAN demonstrates the highest expression of NF-M, the less prominent expression is found in the SAN periphery, while in the working myocardium NF-M is absent (Dobrzynski et al 2005). In contrast to NF-M, ANP is produced mainly in the working atrial cardiomyocytes, traces of ANP are found in the SAN periphery, but not in the central part (Dobrzynski et al 2005).

The distribution of muscarinic and adrenoreceptors in the SAN and atrial myocardium is studied scarcely. In the dog SAN the density of muscarinic and adrenoreceptors was estimated using the autoradiography with radioactive ligands of both types of receptor. The central part of the SAN demonstrated the highest density of both receptors, the density was slightly lower in the periphery and much lower in the working myocardium (Beau et al 1995). Similar results were obtained in the human intercaval region (Rodefeld et al 1996). Radioligand analysis of the membrane homogenates showed that the density of both muscarinic and adrenoreceptors is much higher in the SAN versus atrial myocardium (Kurogouchi et al 2002).

The density of autonomic innervation is also higher in the SAN in comparison with surrounding myocardium. In the SAN center autonomic nerve endings form especially dense "basket"-like network that underlies the cardiomyocytes of the SAN center (Roberts et al 1989).

Thus, the difference between the SAN and atrial myocardium in the level of expression of functionally important protein is quite obvious. The peripheral part of the SAN combine the specific features of both the SAN center and working atrial myocardium, therefore it can be also clearly distinguished from the central part of SAN. Many authors consider the inhomogeneity of autonomic innervations and expression of receptors and ion channels (CaL, HCN) as the main reason of pacemaker shift (Roberts et al 1989, Beau et al 1995, Boyett et al 2000, Kurogouchi et al 2002, Shinagawa et al 2000), although the certain electrophysiological mechanisms of this phenomenon are still not understood.

CONCLUSION

We have reviewed the basic conceptions of sinoatrial automaticity and discussed the mechanisms of SAN autonomic regulation. The automatic activity of the single SAN cells results from the complex interactions of several ion currents and the system of calcium turnover. The functioning of whole SAN depends also on the intercellular interactions forming the specific pattern of the SAN activation. The autonomic regulation of pacemaker function is based mainly on the modulation of the slow DD slope via various ion currents and calcium cycling proteins. However, the pacemaker shift resulting from the heterogeneity of the SAN may serve as an additional mechanism of rhythm modulation under autonomic influence.

BIBLIOGRAPHY

1. Abramochkin DV, Kuzmin VS, Sukhova GS, Rosenshtraukh LV. Changes of activation sequence in a rabbit sinoatrial node induced by cholinergic influences. Kardiologiia. 2009;49(3):57-9.
2. Abramochkin DV, Kuzmin VS, Sukhova GS, Rosenshtraukh LV. Modulation of rabbit sinoatrial node activation sequence by acetylcholine and isoproterenol investigated with optical mapping technique. Acta Physiologica (Oxf). 2009;196(4):385-94.
3. Abramochkin DV, Sukhova GS. M3-cholinoreceptors in mammalian heart. Usp Fiziol Nauk. 2009;40(1):16-27.
4. Aliev RR, Fedorov VV, Rozenshtraukh LV. Study of the effect of acetylcholine on ion currents in single cells of true and latent pacemakers of rabbit sinus node using computer simulation. Dokl Biol Sci. 2004;397:288-91.
5. Anumonwo JM, Freeman LC, Kwok WM, Kass RS. Delayed rectification in single cells isolated from guinea pig sinoatrial node. Am J Physiol. 1992;262:921-5.
6. Baruscotti M, DiFrancesco D. Pacemaker channels. Ann NY Acad Sci. 2004;1015:111-21.
7. Bean BP, Nowycky MC, Tsien RW. Beta-adrenergic modulation of calcium channels in frog ventricular heart cells. Nature. 1984;307:371-5.
8. Beau SL, Hand DE, Schuessler RB, et al. Relative densities of muscarinic cholinergic and β-adrenergic receptors in the canine sinoatrial node and their relation to sites of pacemaker activity. Circ Res. 1995;77:957-63.
9. Benvenuti LA, Aiello VD, Higuchi ML, Palomino SA. Immunohistochemical expression of atrial natriuretic peptide (ANP) in the conducting system and internodal atrial myocardium of human hearts. Acta Histochem. 1997;99:187-93.
10. Bleeker WK, Mackaay AJ, Masson-Pevet M, et al. Functional and morphological organization of the rabbit sinus node. Circ Res. 1980;46:11-22.
11. Bleeker WK, Mackaay AJC, Masson-Pevet M, Opthof T, Jongsma HJ, Bouman LN. Assymmetry of the sinoatrial conduction in the rabbit heart. J Mol Cell Cardiol. 1982;14:633-43.

12. Bogdanov KY, Maltsev VA, Vinogradova TM, et al. Membrane potential fluctuations resulting from submembrane Ca^{2+} releases in rabbit sinoatrial nodal cells impart an exponential phase to the late diastolic depolarization that controls their chronotropic state. Circ Res. 2006;99:979-87.
13. Bogdanov KY, Vinogradova TM, Lakatta EG. Sinoatrial nodal cell ryanodine receptor and Na-Ca exchanger: molecular partners in pacemaker regulation. Circ Res. 2001;88:1254-8.
14. Bouman LN, Gerlings ED, Biersteker PA, Bonke FIM. Pacemaker shift in the sinoatrial node during vagal stimulation. Pflugers Arch. 1968;302:255-67.
15. Boyett MR, Dobrzynski H, Lancaster MK, et al. Sophisticated architecture is required for the sinoatrial node to perform its normal pacemaker function. J Cardiovasc Electrophysiol. 2003;14:104-6.
16. Boyett MR, Honjo H, Kodama I. The sinoatrial node, a heterogeneous pacemaker structure. Cardiovasc. Res. 2000;47:658-87.
17. Boyett MR, Inada S, Yoo S, et al. Connexins in the sinoatrial and atrioventricular nodes. Adv. Cardiol. 2006;42:175-97.
18. Boyett MR, Kodama I, Honjo H, et al. Ionic basis of the chronotropic effect of acetylcholine on the rabbit sinoatrial node. Cardiovasc Res. 1995;29:867-78.
19. Boyett MR, Li J, Inada S, Dobrzynski H, Schneider JE, Holden AV, Zhang H. Imaging the heart: Computer 3-dimensional anatomic models of the heart. J Electrocardiol. 2005;38:113-20.
20. Brodde O-E, Bruck H, Leineweber K. Cardiac adrenoreceptors: physiological and pathophysiological relevance. J Pharmacol Sci. 2006;100:323-37.
21. Brodde O-E, Michel MC. Adrenergic and muscarinic receptors in the human heart. Pharmacol Rev. 1999;51(4):651-89.
22. Bromberg BI, Hand DE, Schuessler RB, Boineau JP. Primary negativity does not predict dominant pacemaker location: implications for sinoatrial conduction. Am J Physiol. 1995;269:877-87.
23. Brown HF, DiFrancesco D, Noble SJ. How does adrenaline accelerate the heart? Nature. 1979;280:235-6.
24. Bucchi A, Baruscotti M, Robinson RB, DiFrancesco D. Modulation of rate by autonomic agonists in SAN cells involves changes in diastolic depolarization and the pacemaker current. J Mol Cell Cardiol. 2007;43:39-48.
25. Bucchi A, Baruscotti M, Robinson RB. I_f-dependent modulation of pacemaker rate mediated by cAMP in the presence of ryanodine in rabbit sionoatrial node cells. J Mol Cell Cardiol. 2003;35 905-13.
26. Choate JK, Feldman R. Neuronal control of heart rate in isolated mouse atria. Am J Physiol Heart Circ Physiol. 2003;285:1340-6.
27. Cho H, Hwang JY, Kim D, et al. Acetylcholine-induced phosphatidylinositol 4,5-bisphosphate depletion does not cause short-term desensitization of G protein-gated inwardly rectifying K+ current in mouse atrial myocytes. J Biol Chem. 2002;277:27742-7.
28. Cho HS, Takano M, Noma A. The electrophysiological properties of spontaneously beating pacemaker cells isolated from mouse sinoatrial node. J Physiol. 2003;550:169-80.
29. Coppen SR, Kodama I, Boyett MR. Connexin45, a major connexin of the rabbit sinoatrial node, is co-expressed with connexin43 in a restricted zone at the nodal-crista terminalis border. J Histochem Cytochem. 1999;47:907-18.
30. Dhein S, Van Koppen CJ, Brodde O. Muscarinic receptors in the mammalian heart. Pharmacol Res. 2001;44(3):161-82.
31. DiFrancesco D, Tortora P. Direct activation of cardiac pacemaker channels by intracellular cyclic AMP. Nature. 1991;351:145-7.
32. DiFrancesco D, Tromba C. Muscarinic control of the hyperpolarizing-activated current, i_f, in rabbit sinoatrial node myocytes. J Physiol. 1988;405:493-510.

33. DiFrancesco D, Ducouret P, Robinson RB. Muscarinic modulation of cardiac rate at low acetylcholine concentrations. Science. 1989;243:669-71.
34. DiFrancesco D. A study of the ionic nature of the pacemaker current in calf Purkinje fibers. J Physiol. 1981;314:377-93.
35. DiFrancesco D. Pacemaker mechanisms in cardiac tissue. Annu Rev Physiol. 1993;55:455-72.
36. Dobrzynski H, Billeter R, Greener ID, et al. Expression of Kir2.1 and Kir6.2 transgenes under the control of the α-MHC promoter in the sinoatrial and atrioventricular nodes in transgenic mice. J Mol Cell Cardiol. 2006;41:855-67.
37. Dobrzynski H, Boyett MR, Anderson RH. New insights into pacemaker activity: promoting understanding of sick sinus syndrome. Circulation. 2007;115:1921-32.
38. Dobrzynski H, Li J, Tellez J, et al. Computer three-dimensional reconstruction of the sinoatrial node. Circulation. 2005;111:846-54.
39. Dudel J, Traitwein W. The mechanism of formation of automatic rhythmical impulses in heart muscle. Pflugers Arch. 1958;267:553-65.
40. Fedorov VV, Hucker WJ, Dobrzynski H, et al. Postganglionic nerve stimulation induces temporal inhibition of excitability in rabbit sinoatrial node. Am J Physiol Heart Circ Physiol. 2006;291:612-23.
41. Felder CC. Muscarinic acetylcholine receptors: signal transduction through multiple effectors. Faseb J. 1995;9:619-25.
42. Fischmeister R, Hartzell HC. Mechanism of action of acetylcholine on calcium current in single cells from frog ventricle. J Physiol. 1986;376:183-202.
43. Giles W, Noble SJ. Changes in membrane currents in bullfrog atrium produced by acetylcholine. J Physiol. 1976;261:103-23.
44. Gorza L, Schiaffino S, Vitadello M. Heart conduction system: a neural crest derivative? Brain Res. 1988;457:360-6.
45. Guo J, Mitsuiye T, Noma A. The sustained inward current in sinoatrial node cells of guineapig heart. Pflugers Arch. 1997;433:390-6.
46. Guo J, Ono K, Noma A. A sustained inward current activated at the diastolic potential range in rabbit sinoatrial node cells. J Physiol (Lond.). 1995;483:1-13.
47. Guth BD, Diete T. I_f current mediates β-adrenergic enhancement of heart rate but not contractivility in vivo. Basic Res Cardiol. 2000;90:192-202.
48. Hagiwara N, Irisawa H, Kameyama M. Contribution of two types of calcium currents to the pacemaker potentials of rabbit sinoatrial node cells. J Physiol. 1988;395:233-53.
49. Harvey RD, Clark CD, Hume, JR. Chloride current in mammalian cardiac myocytes. Novel mechanism for autonomic regulation of action potential duration and resting membrane potential. J Gen Physiol. 1990;95:1077-102.
50. Harvey RD, Hume JR. Autonomic regulation of delayed rectifier K+ current in mammalian heart involves G proteins. Am J Physiol. 1989;257:818-23.
51. Harvey RD, Hume JR. Autonomic regulation of a chloride current in heart. Science. 1989;244:983-5.
52. Hescheler J, Kameyama M, Trautwein W. On the mechanism of muscarinic inhibition of the cardiac Ca current. Pflugers Arch. 1986;407:182-9.
53. Hoffman BF, Cranefield P. Electrophysiology of the Heart. NY: McGraw-Hill Book Co. 1960.
54. Honjo H, Boyett MR, Coppen SR, et al. Heterogeneous expression of connexins in rabbit sinoatrial node cells: correlation between connexin isotype and cell size. Cardiovasc Res. 2002;53:89-96.
55. Honjo H, Inada S, Lancaster MK, et al. Sarcoplasmic reticulum Ca^{2+} release is not a dominating factor in sinoatrial node pacemaker activity. Circ Res. 2003;92(e):41-4.
56. Honjo H, Kodama I, Zang W-J, Boyett MR. Desensitization to acetylcholine in single sinoatrial node cells isolated from the rabbit heart. Am J Physiol. 1992;263:1779-89.

57. Huser J, Blatter LA, Lipsius SL. Intracellular Ca^{2+} release contributes to automaticity in cat atrial pacemaker cells. J Physiol. 2000;524:415-22.
58. Inada S, Mitsui K, Honjo H, Boyett MR. Why is Cav1.3 expressed in the sinoatrial node. Biophys J. 2005.
59. Irisawa H, Brown HF, Giles W. Cardiac pacemaking in the sinoatrial node. Physiol Rev. 1993;73:197-227.
60. Ito H., Ono K. A rapidly activating delayed rectifier K+ current in rabbit sinoatrial node cells. Am J Physiol. 1995;269:443-52.
61. James TN, Kawamura K, Meijler FL, et al. Anatomy of the sinus node, AV node, and His bundle of the heart of the sperm whale (Physeter macrocephalus), with a note on the absence of an os cordis. Anat Rec. 1995;242:355-73.
62. James TN. The sinus node. Am J Cardiol. 1977;40:965-86.
63. James TN. Structure and function of the sinus node, AV node and His bundle of the human heart: part I — structure. Prog Cardiovasc Dis. 2002;45(3):235-67.
64. Jin W, Lu Z. A novel high-affinity inhibitor for inward-rectifier K^+ channels. Biochemistry. 1998;37:13291-9.
65. Joyner RW, van Capelle FJL. Propagation through electrically coupled cells: how a small SA node drives a large atrium. Biophys J. 1986;50:1157-64.
66. Kameyama M, Hofmann F, Trautwein W. On the mechanism of β-adrenergic regulation of the Ca channel in the guinea-pig heart. Pflugers Arch. 1985;405:285-93.
67. Kodama I, Boyett MR, Suzuki R, et al. Regional differencies in the response of the isolated sinoatrial node to vagal stimulation. J Physiol. 1996;495:785-801.
68. Kodama I, Nikmaram MR, Boyett MR, et al. Regional differences in the role of the Ca^{2+} and Na^+ currents in pacemaker activity in the sinoatrial node. Am J Physiol. 1997;272:2793-806.
69. Kurogouchi F, Nakane T, Furukawa Y, et al. Heterogeneous distribution of β-adrenoreceptors and muscarinic receptors in the sinoatrial node and right atrium of the dog. Clin Exp Pharmacol Physiol. 2002;29:666-72.
70. Lakatta EG, Vinogradova T, Lyashkov A, et al. The integration of spontaneous intracellular Ca^{2+} cycling and surface membrane ion channel activation entrains normal automaticity in cells of the heart's pacemaker. Ann NY Acad Sci. 2006;1080:178-206.
71. Lakatta EG, Vinogradova TM, Maltsev VA. The missing link in the mystery of normal automaticity of cardiac pacemaker cells. Ann NY Acad Sci. 2008;1123:41-57.
72. Lei M, Brown HF, Terrar DA. Modulation of delayed rectifier potassium current, i_K, by isoprenaline in rabbit isolated pacemaker cells. Exp Physiol. 2000;85(1):27-35.
73. Lei M, Goddard C, Liu J, et al. Sinus node dysfunction following targeted disruption of the murine cardiac sodium channel gene. J Physiol. 2005;567:387-400.
74. Lei M, Jones SA, Liu J, et al. Requirements of neuronal- and cardiac-type sodium channels for murine sinoatrial node pacemaking. J Physiol. 2004;559(3):835-48.
75. Liu J, Dobrzynski H, Yanni J, et al. Organisation of the mouse sinoatrial node: structure and expression of HCN channels. Cardiovasc Res. 2007;73:729-38.
76. Liu J, Noble PJ, Xiao G, et al. Role of pacemaking current in cardiac nodes: Insights from a comparative study of sinoatrial node and atrioventricular node. Progr Bioph Mol Biol. 2008;96:294-304.
77. Lu HH. Sinoatrial region of cat and rabbit hearts resulting from increase of extracellular potassium. Circ Res. 1970;26:339-46.
78. Lyashkov AE, Juhaszova M, Dobrzynski H, et al. Calcium cycling protein density and functional importance to automaticity of isolated sinoatrial nodal cells are independent of cell size. Circ Res. 2007;100:1723-31.
79. Mackaay AJC, Opthof T, Bleeker WK. et al. Interaction of adrenaline and acetylcholine on cardiac pacemaker function. Functional inhomogeneity of the rabbit sinus node. J Pharmacol Exp Ther. 214:417-22.

80. Mackaay AJC, Bleeker WK, Opthof T, Bouman LN. Temperature dependence of the chronotropic action of calcium: functional inhomogeneity of the rabbit sinus node. J Mol Cell Cardiol. 1980;12:433-43.
81. Maier SKG, Westenbroek RE, Yamanushi TT, et al. An unexpected requirement for brain-type sodium channels for control of heart rate in the mouse sinoatrial node. PNAS. 2003;100(6):3507-12.
82. Maltsev VA, Lakatta EG. Cardiac pacemaker cell failure with preserved I_f, I_{CaL}, and I_{Kr}: a lesson about pacemaker function learned from ischemia-induced bradycardia. J Mol Cell Cardiol. 2007;42:289-94.
83. Maltsev VA, Lakatta EG. Dynamic interactions of an intracellular Ca^{2+} clock and membrane ion channel clock underlie robust initiation and regulation of cardiac pacemaker function. Cardiovasc Res. 2008;77:274-84.
84. Mangoni ME, Nargeot J. Genesis and regulation of the heart automaticity. Physiol Rev. 2008;88:919-82.
85. Marionneau C, Couette B, Liu J, et al. Specific pattern of ionic channel gene expression associated with pacemaker activity in the mouse heart. J Physiol. 2005;562:223-34.
86. Marx SO, Kurokawa J, Reiken S, et al. Requirement of a macromolecular signaling complex for beta adrenergic receptor modulation of the KCNQ1-KCNE1 potassium channel. Science. 2002;295:496-9.
87. Masson-Pevet MA, Bleeker WK, Besselsen E, et al. Pacemaker cell types in the rabbit sinus node: a correlative ultrastructural and electrophysiological study. J Mol Cell Cardiol. 1984;16:53-63.
88. Masumiya H, Yamamoto H, Hemberger M, et al. The mouse sinoatrial node expresses both the type 2 and type 3 Ca^{2+} release channels/ryanodine receptors. FEBS Lett. 2003;553:141-4.
89. Matthes J, Huber I, Haaf O, et al. Pharmacodynamic interaction between mibefradil and other calcium channel blockers. Naunyn-Schmiedebergs Arch Pharmacol. 2000;361:578-83.
90. Mitsuiye T, Shinagawa Y, Noma A. Sustained inward current during pacemaker depolarization in mammalian sinoatrial node cells. Circ Res. 2000;87:88-91.
91. Musa H, Lei M, Honjo H, et al. Heterogeneous expression of Ca^{2+} handling proteins in sinoatrial node. J Histochem Cytochem. 2002;50:311-24.
92. Nikmaram MR, Boyett MR, Kodama I, et al. Variation in the effects of Cs^{+}, UL-FS49 and ZD7288 within the sinoatrial node. Am J Physiol. 1997;272:2782-92.
93. Nikmaram MR, Liu J, Abdelrahman M, et al. Characterization of the effects of ryanodine, TTX, E-4031 and 4-AP on the sinoatrial and atrioventricular nodes. Progr Bioph Mol Biol. 2008;96:452-64.
94. Noma A, Irisawa H. Membrane currents in the rabbit sinoatrial node cell as studied by the double microelectrode method. Pflugers Arch. 1976;384:45-52.
95. Ono K, Fozzard HA, Hanck DA, Mechanism of cAMP-dependent modulation of cardiac sodium channel current kinetics. Circ Res. 1993;72:807-15.
96. Ono K, Shibata S, Ijima T. Pacemaker mechanism of porcine sinoatrial node cells. J Smooth Muscle Res. 2003;39(5):195-204.
97. Opthof T, de Jonge B, Jongsma HJ, Bouman LN. Functional morphology of the mammalian sinuatrial node. Eur Heart J. 1987;8:1249-59.
98. Opthof T, de Jonge B, Jongsma HJ, Bouman LN. Functional morphology of the pig sinoatrial node. J Mol Cell Cardiol. 1987;19:1221-36.
99. Opthof T, de Jonge B, Masson-Pevet M, et al. Functional and morphological organization of the cat sinoatrial node. J Mol Cell Cardiol. 1986;18:1015-31.
100. Opthof T, Duivenvoorden JJ, Van Ginneken ACG, et al. Electrophysiological effects of alinidine (St 567) on sinoatrial node fibers in the rabbit heart. Cardiovasc Res. 1986;20:727-39.
101. Opthof T. The mammalian sinoatrial node. Cardiovasc Drug Ther. 1988;1:573-97.

102. Optof T, de Jonge B, Mackaay AJC, et al. Functional and morphological organization of the guinea-pig sinoatrial node compared with the rabbit sinoatrial node. J Mol Cell Cardiol. 1985;17:549-64.
103. Osterrieder W, Yang Q-F, Trautwein W. Effects of barium on the membrane currents in the rabbit s-a node. Pflugers Arch. 1982;394:78-84.
104. Pavlovich ER, Chervova IA. Morphometric examination of the sinoatrial region of the heart. Cor et Vasa. 1983;25(2):138-46.
105. Petit-Jacques J, Bois P, Bescond J, Lenfant J. Mechanism of muscarinic control of the high-threshold calcium current in rabbit sinoatrial node myocytes. Pflugers Arch. 1993;423:21-7.
106. Roberts IA, Slocum GR, Riley DA. Morphological study of the innervation pattern of the rabbit sinoatrial node. Am J Anat. 1989;185:74-88.
107. Rodefeld MD, Beau SL, Schuessler RB, et al. β-Adrenergic and muscarinic cholinergic receptor densities in the human sinoatrial node: Identification of a high β2-receptor density. J Cardiovasc Electrophysiol. 1996;7:1039-49.
108. Rump LC, Bohmann C, Schaible U, et al. α2C-Adrenoceptor-modulated release of noradrenaline in human right atrium. Br J Pharmacol. 1995;116:2617-24.
109. Sanders L, Rakovic S, Lowe M, et al. Fundamental importance of Na^+–Ca^{2+} exchange for the pacemaking mechanism in guinea-pig sinoatrial node. J Physiol. 2006;571(3):639-49.
110. Sano T, Yamagishi S. Spread of excitation from the sinus node. Circ Res. 1965;16:423-30.
111. Shibata N, Inada S, Mitsui K, et al. Pacemaker shift in the rabbit sinoatrial node in response to vagal nerve stimulation. Exp Physiol. 2001;86:177-84.
112. Shinagawa Y, Satoh H, Noma A. The sustained inward current and inward rectifier K1 current in pacemaker cells dissociated from rat sinoatrial node. J Physiol. 2000;523:593-605.
113. Shi W, Wymore R, Yu H, et al. Distribution and prevalence of hyperpolarization-activated cation channel (HCN) mRNA expression in cardiac tissues. Circ Res. 1999;85(e):1-6.
114. Stieber J, Herrmann S, Feil S, et al. The hyperpolarization-activated channel HCN4 is required for the generation of pacemaker action potentials in the embryonic heart. PNAS. 2003;100:15235-40.
115. Stoletzki S, Schmiedl A, Richter J. Intercalated clear cells or pale cells in the sinus node of canine hearts? An ultrastructural study. Anat Rec. 2001;260:33-41.
116. Sunahara RK, Dessauer CW, Gilman AG. Complexity and diversity of mammalian adenylyl cyclases. Annu Rev Pharmacol Toxicol. 1996;36:461-80.
117. Takano M, Noma A. Distribution of the isoprenaline-induced chloride current in the rabbit heart. Pflugers Arch. 1992;420:223-6.
118. Tellez JO, Dobrzynski H, Greener ID, et al. Differential expression of ion channel transcripts in atrial muscle and sinoatrial node in rabbit. Circ Res. 2006;99:1384-93.
119. Terzic A, Puceat M, Vassort G, Vogel SM. Cardiac α1-adrenoceptors: an overview. Pharmacol Rev. 1993;45:147-75.
120. Toyoda F, Ding W, Matsuura H. Responses of the sustained inward current to autonomic agonists in guinea-pig sinoatrial node pacemaker cells. Brit J Pharmacol. 2005;144:660-8.
121. Trautwein W, Cavalie A, Flockerzi V, et al. Modulation of calcium channel function by phosphorylation in guinea pig ventricular cells and phospholipid bilayer membranes. Circ Res. 1987;61(Suppl I):17-23.
122. Uese K, Hagiwara N, Miyawaki T, Kasanuki H. Properties of the transient outward current in rabbit sinoatrial node cells. J Mol Cell Cardiol. 1999;31:1975-84.
123. Verheijck EE., Wessels A, van Ginneken ACG, et al. Distribution of atrial and nodal cells within rabbit sinoatrial node: models of sinoatrial transition. Circulation. 1998;97:1623-31.
124. Verheule S, van Kempen MJ, te Welscher PH, et al. Characterization of gap junction channels in adult rabbit atrial and ventricular myocardium. Circ Res. 1997;80:673-81.
125. Verkerk AO, Wilders R, Borren MM, et al. Pacemaker current (I_f) in the human sinoatrial node. Eur Heart J. 2007;28:2472-8.

126. Vinogradova TM, Bogdanov KY, Lakatta EG. β-adrenergic stimulation modulates ryanodine receptor Ca^{2+} release during diastolic depolarization to accelerate pacemaker activity in rabbit sinoatrial nodal cells. Circ Res. 2002;90:73-9.
127. Vinogradova TM, Fedorov VV, Yuzyuk TN, et al. Local cholinergic suppression of pacemaker activity in the rabbit sinoatrial node. J Cardiovasc Pharmacol. 1998;32:413-24.
128. Vinogradova TM, Lyashkov AE, Zhu W, et al. High basal protein kinase A-dependent phosphorylation drives rhythmic internal Ca^{2+} store oscillations and spontaneous beating of cardiac pacemaker cells. Circ Res. 2006;98:505-14.
129. Vinogradova TM, Sirenko S, Lyashkov AE, et al. Constitutive phosphodiesterase activity restricts spontaneous beating rate of cardiac pacemaker cells by suppressing local Ca^{2+} releases. Circ Res. 2008;102:761-9.
130. Vinogradova TM, Zhou YY, Maltsev V, et al. Rhythmic ryanodine receptor Ca^{2+} releases during diastolic depolarization of sinoatrial pacemaker cells do not require membrane depolarization. Circ Res. 2004;94:802-9.
131. Wang H, Lu Y, Wang Z. Function of cardiac M3 receptors. Auton Autac Pharmacol. 2007;27:1-11.
132. West TC. Ultramicroelectrode recording from the cardiac pacemaker. J Pharmacol Exp Ther. 1955;115(3):283-90.
133. Wickman K, Nemec J, Gendler SJ, Clapham DE. Abnormal heart rate regulation in GIRK4 knockout mice. Neuron. 1998;20:103-14.
134. Winslow RL, Jongsma HJ. Role of tissue geometry and spatial localization of gap junctions in generation of the pacemaker potential. J Physiol. 1995;487:126-7.
135. Wu J, Schuessler RB, Rodefeld MD, et al. Morphological and membrane characteristics of spider and spindle cells isolated from rabbit sinus node. Am J Physiol Heart Circ Physiol. 2001;280:1232-40.
136. Xiao RP, Avdonin P, Zhou YY, et al. Coupling of β2-adrenoceptor to G_i proteins and its physiological relevance in murine cardiac myocytes. Circ Res. 1999;84:43-52.
137. Xiao RP, Zhang SJ, Chakir K, et al. Enhanced G_i signaling selectively negates β2-adrenergic receptor (AR), but not β1-AR-mediated positive inotropic effect in myocytes from failing rat hearts. Circulation. 2003;108:1633-9.
138. Yamada M. The role of muscarinic K^+ channels in the negative chronotropic effect of a muscarinic agonist. J Pharmacol Exp Ther. 2002;300:681-7.
139. Yamamoto M, Dobrzynski H, Tellez J, et al. Extended atrial conduction system characterized by the expression of the HCN4 channel and connexin45. Cardiovasc Res. 2006;72:271-81.
140. Yamamoto M, Honjo H, Niwa R, Kodama I, Low frequency extracellular potentials recorded from the sinoatrial node. Circ Res. 1998;39:360-72.
141. Yatani A, Okabe K, Codina J, et al. The sinoatrial nodal pacemaker current (I_f) is directly regulated by G-proteins. Biophys J. 1990;57.
142. Zaza A, Robinson RB, DiFrancesco D. Basal responses of the L-type Ca^{2+} and hyperpolarization-activated currents to autonomic agonists in the rabbit sinoatrial node. J Physiol. 1996;491:347-55.

Chapter

2

The Trifascicular Nature of the Human Left Intraventricular His System and its Electrovectorcardiographic Demonstration

Andrés Ricardo Perez Riera

Abstract. Several publications considering anatomical, histological, pathological, electrocardiographic, vectorcardiographic, and electrophysiologic studies have shown that the left bundle branch splits into three fascicles or in a "fan-like interconnected network" in the vast majority of human hearts. The left His system is trifascicular with a left anterior, a left posterior, and a left septal fascicle. Consequently, the classic term "hemiblock", to describe the block of one of the fascicles, established several decades ago by the Rosembaum's school, should be updated. Electrovectorcardiographic changes resulting from conduction abnormalities of the left anterior and left posterior fascicles are commonly diagnosed, mainly by their changes in the frontal plane. However, the existence of conduction defects of the left septal fascicle remains controversial. The ECG/VCG hallmark of left septal fascicular block is prominent anterior QRS forces (PAF) on the horizontal plane. This ECG/VCG phenomena should be distinguished from other conditions that also produce anterior QRS shift in the HP as: Normal variants, right ventricular enlargement, misplaced precordial leads, lateral myocardial infarction, right bundle branch block, Wolff-Parkinson-White, obstructive and nonobstructive forms of hypertrophic cardiomyopahty, diastolic left ventricular enlargement, endomiocardial fibrosis, Duchenne muscular dystrophy and dextroposition.

The two highly frequent etiologies of LSFB are coronary artery disease (CAD) with critical proximal obstruction of the left anterior descending coronary artery and, in Latin America, Chagas' cardiomyopathy.

The aims of this review are to revise the evidence of the existence of a trifascicular left Hissian system and to help in the ECG/VCG recognition of the LSFB.

Keywords. Heart conduction system, fascicular block, bundle of His, electrocardiography.

INTRODUCTION

The three left fascicles of the left bundle branch (LBB) along with the right bundle branch (RBB), constitute the quadrifascicular structure of the intraventricular conduction system of the heart, coined by Dr Uhley (Uhley 1972, 1973).

ANATOMICAL CONSIDERATIONS OF THE LEFT INTRAVENTRICULAR CONDUCTION SYSTEM

Anatomopathological studies showed that the left septal fascicle (LSF) has diverse morphologies and considerable variability in its structure. Thereby, six basic anatomical variations can be described (Kulbertus 1973, 1975, Kulbertus and Demolium 1976, Demolium and Kulbertus 1972, 1973):

- **Type I:** The LSF arises independently from the main LBB (65% of the cases).
- **Type II:** The LSF originates from the left anterior fascicle (LAF) of the LBB.
- **Type III:** The LSF originates from the left posterior fascicle (LPF). This type represents about 2.4% of all cases.
- **Type IV:** The LSF originates concomitantly with the other two fascicles (LAF and LPF).
- **Type V:** The LSF is represented as a "fan-like interconnecting network".
- **Type VI:** The LSF is absent; consequently, the left Hissian intraventricular system has only two fascicles: LAF and LPF. It occurs in approximately 15% to 40% of the cases (Kulbertus 1973).

Blood Supply (modified from Frink and James 1973)

The blood supply of the human his bundle and its proximal branches have a dual origin, with anastomoses within the His bundle. The conduction system is irrigated as follows:

1. His bundle: It has a dual supply by the AV node artery from the right coronary artery (RCA) and the first septal branch of the left anterior descending artery (LAD) in 90% of the cases, and entirely supplied by the AV node artery in 10% of the cases
2. Proximal right bundle branch: It is supplied by both the AV node artery and the septal branch in 50% of the cases, and only by the septal branch in 40% of the cases. The AV node artery as a single supply occurs in about 10% of the cases
3. Left bundle branch: It is supplied by the AV node artery (ramus septi fibrosi) from the RCA (in 90% of the cases) and ramus septi ventriculorum superior and ramus critae, branches of the LAD
4. Left branch fascicles or divisions branches irrigation: See Table 2.1.

The LSF is irrigated exclusively by the septal perforating branches of the LAD (Hosseinpour et al 2001). Critical lesions of the LAD before the first septal perforating branch are the main cause of LSFB in developed countries, and it is a major determinant of prominent R-wave amplitude (PAF) from V1 to V3 during

Table 2.1: Blood supply of the left branch fascicles or divisions

Responsible system	LAF	LPF	LSF
LAD branches	40%	10%	100%
Double irrigation (LAD and RCA)	50%	40%	0%
RCA branches	10%	50%	0%

LAD – Left Anterior Descending Artery; RCA – Right Coronary Artery

acute myocardial ischemia (Riera et al 2008). In Brazil, where Chagas' disease is very common, coronary artery disease represents only 18% of all LSFB.

LSFB can be also induced by exercise. (Uchida et al 2006), sometimes originating giant R-waves in the precordial leads (Moffa et al 1996, 1997, Tranchesi et al 1979, 2001).

Sudden development of LSFB in critical LAD lesions indicates a proximal location of the lesion, and therefore, a worse prognosis.

Electrophysiology of the Left Intraventricular Conduction System

The electrophysiologic demonstration of the activation of the middle third of the left septal surface 5 ms before the anterosuperior and posteroinferior regions was made in 1970 by Durrer et al (Durrer et al 1970). They demonstrated in 870 intramural terminals of isolated human hearts, that three endocardial areas were synchronously excited from 0 to 5 ms after the initiation of the left ventricle (LV) activity potential. To demonstrate the time course and instantaneous distribution of the excitatory process of the normal human heart, the authors studied isolated human hearts from seven individuals who died from neurologic disease with no history of cardiac disease. The first LV areas excited were located in the following regions:

1. High on the anterior paraseptal wall just below the insertion of the anterolateral papillary muscle (ALPM) where the LAF ends.
2. Central on the left surface of the intraventricular septum (IVS), where the LSF ends. Septal activation started in the middle third of the left side of the IVS, in the anterior and lower third at the junction of the IVS and posterior wall.
   The LSF, the left middle septum surface, and the inferior two-thirds of the septum originate the first vector, also called vector 1 or first anteromedial (1AM) vector and left inferior two-thirds of the IVS (second vector or vector of the inferior 2/3 of IVS) (Alboni et al 1977).
3. Posterior paraseptal, about one third of the distance from the apex to the base, near the insertion of the posteromedial papillary muscle (PMPM), where the LPF ends. The posterobasal area is the last part of the LV to activate.

Rosenbaum et al (Rosenbaum et al 1967, 1971) postulated that the activation of the middle-septal region occurs in most cases, from the anterior "false tendons" that originate from the LPF. His group considered that the LPF in its final portion opens as a fan, and the anterior "pseudo-tendons" are those responsible for the activation of the middle-septal region. We think that in fact, only one of the anatomical variations of the LSF (type III) is precisely the one that originates on the LPF (2.4% of cases).

Another evidence of the trifascicular nature of the left Hissian system is the electric or electrovectorcardiographic recording of the anterior shift of the ventricular depolarization, sometimes intermittent or transient, manifested in the surface ECG as high voltage R-waves in the precordial leads V3 and V4. The VCG manifestation of the same phenomenon is anterior and leftward shift of the QRS loop in the horizontal plane (HP); as seen in some cases of critical proximal LAD lesion, before the origin of the first septal branch. Other causes of prominent anterior forces (PAF) such as lateral infarction, RVH, cardiomyopathies, RBBB, WPW and others should be carefully ruled out before arriving to the diagnosis of LSFB.

Angiographic studies of patients with PAF and absence of other diseases capable of generating this ECG manifestation showed that coronary artery lesions were mainly located in the proximal LAD; and ventricular dysfunction confined only to the LV anterior wall. PAF were observed intermittently along with LAFB. These observations, in addition to the lessons from post surgery studies, strongly suggested that the mechanism of PAF in these cases was the consequence of conduction delay in the LSF.

Another consideration should be done for the electrophysiologic explanation of the so called "atypical LBBB". There are cases of divisional or fascicular LBBB (LAFB + LPFB) that depict a Q-wave in the left leads, turning the electrocardiographic pattern of LBBB "atypical". Alboni et al 1977 called them "LBBB with normal septal activation".

Rosenbaum et al 1971 called the same phenomenon "left intraventricular blocks without changes in the initial portion of the QRS". His group did not provide an explanation for these cases, and stated in their traditional book, that they were "difficult to explain".

Three years later, Medrano et al 1970 proposed that in these atypical LBBB cases, the fibers of the LSF would originate prior to the site or area of the block in the LPF and LAF, so the middle-septal activation is preserved (1AM vector), originating the Q-waves of leads V5-V6, and turning the LBBB into an atypical one.

Gambeta and Childers 1973 also proposed the trifascicular nature of the left Hissian system. The authors observed the development of transient abnormal Q-waves during exercise as the heart rate increased. This phenomenon was attributed to transient tachycardia-dependent ischemic block in the LSF. The initial activation is conducted by the non blocked divisions (LAF and LPF). Since these fascicles have opposite directions and LPF activation predominates over LAF, produces the appearance of initial Q-wave in intermediate precordial leads.

The same phenomenon was observed during the acute phase of myocardial infarction with the same electrophysiological explanation (Athanassopoulos 1979, Madias et al 2005).

Another strong argument for the existence of LSFB, was provided by several electrophysiological animal models (dogs) and human models. They showed the development of PAF (anterior shift of QRS loop) as a manifestation of intraventricular block, a consequence of intermittent intraventricular dromotropic disorder in the LSF region, during atrial extrastimuli (Cohen et al 1967, 1968, Iwamura et al 1976, Lazzara et al 1976, Kulbertus et al 1976, Hoffman et al 1976, Dhala et al 1996).

A delay in the LSF may explain certain type of ventricular aberration pattern observed by introducing premature atrial beats. This pattern consists of PAF with no or minimal QRS duration prolongation (≤ 20 ms) and without incomplete RBBB. Such delay is manifested as a narrow QRS with anterior shift in the HP, but no axis shift in the FP. It is important to recognize this aberration, because it may mimic the ECG findings of lateral MI (true posterior MI of the "old nomenclature") or RVH (Reiffel and Bigger 1978).

In another study, aberrant ventricular conduction was induced in 44 subjects by introduction of atrial premature beats. The distribution of the patterns were RBBB (28); LAFB combined with RBBB (21); LAFB (17); LPFB combined with RBBB (12); LPFB (10); complete LBBB (10) and incomplete LBBB (N=6).

Other configurations could not be classified into the usual categories of intraventricular blocks. In 7 of them, the alterations only consisted on trivial modifications of the QRS contour. In the other 5, aberrant conduction manifested itself by conspicuous PAF of the QRS loop on the HP. The latter observation is worthy of notice, as it indicates that, in the differential diagnosis of the VCG pattern characterized by PAF, conduction disturbances should be considered a possible etiological factor in addition to RVH, and true posterior MI (Kulbertus et al 1976, Hoffman et al 1976, Dhala et al 1996).

About the historical controversy about the bifascicular or trifascicular nature of the human left His system, we conclude that in most cases, the left His system is trifascicular. Consequently, the term "hemiblock", to refer to the block of the fascicles, should be avoided (De Pádua et al,1976, De Pádua 1977,1977).

TERMINOLOGY: CRITICAL ANALYSIS AND SEMANTIC DISCUSSIONS

There is a large variety of nomenclatures to name the LSF. This indicates the need of a consensus to unify terminology. This discussion should take place in an International or Worldwide Conference on Electrocardiology. The authors of this review strongly advocate for such a consensus.

In Brazil, a committee of experts in Resting Electrocardiology met in 2003 and developed the "Brazilian Guidelines for Interpretation of Resting Electrocardiogram". In this consensus, the diagnostic criteria of LSFB were determined and published (Pastore et al 2003). However, it is important to remember different terminologies used in the literature:

1. Left septal fascicular block (LSFB) (Dabrowska et al 1978, Nakaya et al 1978, Mori et al 1992, Sakai 1996, Sanches et al 2001, MacAlpin 2002, 2003, Moffa et al 1996). This is the currently accepted terminology and frequently used in more recent publications. The terminology fascicular could be inappropriate because the LSF does not always display the morphology of a fascicle (a small bundle). In occasions, it has the aspect of an interconnected network that

opens as fan ("fan-like interconnected network") or depends on two fascicles that originate in another two fascicles or divisions: the LAF and the LPF
2. Septal fascicle of the left bundle branch (Dabrowska 1979)
3. Focal septal block (Athanassopoulos 1979)
4. Septal focal block (Gambeta and Childers 1973)
5. Left parietal septal block (De Micheli 1976, Alboni 1980)
6. Septal fascicular conduction disorders of the left branch (Magnacca et al 1988)
7. Left septal Purkinje network block (Iwamura et al 1978, Nakaya et al 1981) this name highlights the cellular type of the fibers that constitute the LSF (Purkinje cells). Unlike the two other divisions, the LSF is constituted by Purkinje cells with faster conduction. The LAF and LPF are constituted by bundle cells, which have slightly different electrophysiologic properties, with slower conduction velocity. The term "network" (a complex and interconnected group or system) seems inappropriate, because the LSF is more often a fascicle than a network or interconnected system
8. Left anterior septal block (Moffa et al 1982)
9. Anterior fascicular block (Alboni et al 1979)
10. Left septal subdivision block of the left bundle branch (Nakaya and Hiraga 1981, Hassapoyannes and Nelson 1991, Reiffel and Bigger 1978)
11. Left median hemiblock (De Padua et al 1978, De Padua 1978)
12. Middle subdivision block of the left bundle branch (Inoue et al 1983): The term «subdivision block» seems appropriate, since the term subdivision means division of something previously divided. As the His bundle initially divides into the RBB and the LBB, the authors support this terminology
13. Middle fascicle block (Alboni et al 1977): This term may be controversial. The middle division does not always have the features of a fascicle, since it may be constituted by a fan-like network or originating from both divisions
14. Block of the anteromedial division of the left bundle branch of His (Tranchesi et al 1979)
15. Anteromedial divisional block (AMDB) (Moffa et al 1997)
16. Block of the anterior median branch of the bundle of his: The last three definitions seem appropriate because provide a clear idea of its location (anteromedial) and it does not involve the morphological aspects of the division
17. Blocking of the anteriormedial Ramulus (Georgiev 1986): This nomenclature should be considered partially appropriate. It provides a complete idea about the location (anteromedial) of the fascicle and, in addition, the Latin term "ramulus" literally means "one of the terminal divisions of a branch", small branch or thread-like. In some cases, the division has a network configuration, different from the aspect of a thread
18. Anterior conduction delay (Hoffman et al 1976, Reiffel and Bigger 1978, Hassapoyannes and Nelson 1991): This terminology only indicates the existence of slow conduction or dromotropic delay in the activation of the anterior region
19. Intraventricular aberrant conduction (Iwamura et al 1976; Iwamura 1978): This term only indicates the existence of ventricular aberrant conduction, which does not help to clarify the origin of the conduction delay.

We conclude that the various denominations only reflect the disparity of opinions on the existence of an anatomic structure defined as LSF. There are still some reasonable doubts on its electrophysiological properties and the effect of its disturbances (delay, block) on the surface ECG.

This group of authors does not consider themselves the "owners of the truth", and advocate for an international consensus to find a single terminology, based on a common interpretation of the literature. This will help to recognize this frequently misdiagnosed disorder and will help researchers to organize and focus their opinions on this issue.

LEFT SEPTAL FASCICULAR BLOCK: ALL POSSIBLE ETIOLOGIES

The following list identifies all possible causes of LSFB recognized in the literature:

1. Coronary Artery Disease (CAD): Critical lesion of proximal LAD and/or its septal branches before the first septal perforating (Uchida et al 2006)
2. Chronic Chagas' Cardiomyopathy: Main cause of LSFB in Latin America (Moffa et al 1982)
3. Nonobstructive hypertrophic cardiomyopathy (NO-HCM);(Maron et al 1983)
4. Hypertrophic obstructive cardiomyopathy (HOCM); (Yamaguchi et al 1983, Comella et al 2004)
5. Diabetes mellitus(Magnacca et al 1988)
6. Papillary muscle dysfunction
7. Kearns-Sayre syndrome (Riera et al 2008).

LEFT SEPTAL FASCICULAR BLOCK: ELECTROCARDIOGRAPHIC CRITERIA (DABROWSKA ET AL 1978, MORI ET AL 1992, SANCHES ET AL 2001, MACALPIN 2002, 2003, MADIAS 1993)

1. Normal QRS duration or minimal widening (up to 110 ms). If LSFB is associated with other fascicular or bundle blocks, the QRS could be wider than 120 ms
2. Frontal plane leads with normal QRS duration and amplitude
3. Increased ventricular activation time or intrinsic deflection in leads V1 and V2 $\geq$ 35 ms
4. R-wave voltage of lead V1 $\geq$ than 5 mm
5. R/S ratio in lead V1 > 2
6. R/S ratio in lead V2 > 2
7. S-wave depth in lead V1 < 5 mm
8. Small Q-wave in leads V2, V3 or V1 and V2
9. R-wave of lead V2 > 15 mm
10. RS or Rs pattern in leads V2 and V3 (frequent rS in V1) with R-wave "in crescendo" from V1 through V3 and decreasing from V5 to V6
11. Absence of Q-wave in left precordial leads V5, V6 and I (by absence of vector 1AM)

12. Intermittent PAF during hyperacute phase of myocardial infarction (Madias 1993), exercise stress testing in patients with severe myocardial ischemia (Uchida et al 2006, Moffa et al 1997) and during early atrial extrastimuli (Hoffman et al 1976)
13. Intermittent rate-dependent Q-wave in leads V1 and V2 (Gambeta and Childers 1973).

The authors propose to classify the above ECG diagnostic criteria in major and minor criteria according to their frequency in:

I. Major Criterion

Intermittent PAF: Intermittent or transient increment in the R-wave voltage in intermediary precordial leads and intermittent or transient anterior displacement of the QRS loop on HP.

II. Minor Criteria

All the other criteria mentioned above.

The diagnosis of LSFB could be done with 1 major criterion or with 2 minor criteria.

The Brazilian Guidelines for Interpretation of Resting Electrocardiogram (Pastore et al 2003) defined the following ECG criteria for diagnosis of LSFB:

1. QRS duration <120 ms, (closer to 100 ms). The development of LFB does not increase QRS duration by more than 25 ms, due to multiple interconnections between the fascicles of the LBB ("passage way zone" as defined by Rosenbaum). The QRS complex is slightly prolonged (between 100 ms to 115 ms). Thus, LSFB pattern with a prolonged QRS duration indicates the presence of additional conduction disturbances such as other fascicular blocks, RBBB, MI, focal block, or a combination of any of them
2. R-wave in leads V1 or V2 and V3 of 15 mm
3. Increased R-wave voltage in all intermediary precordial leads and decreased voltage in leads V5 and V6
4. Early transition from lead V1 to V2
5. Absence of SAQRS shift
6. Predominantly negative T-waves in the right precordial leads.

All the above mentioned criteria are valid in the absence of RVH, septal hypertrophy or lateral dorsal MI, and other causes of PAF.

LEFT SEPTAL FASCICULAR BLOCK VECTORCARDIOGRAPHIC CRITERIA (ALL IN THE HP) (TRANCHESI ET AL 1979, DE PÁDUA ET AL 1976, 1978)

QRS loop in the HP with an area predominantly located in the left anterior quadrant (> 2/3 of the loop facing the orthogonal X lead: 0° to ±180°);

1. Absence of normal convexity to the right, of the initial 20 ms of the QRS loop
2. Discrete dextroorientation with moderate delay of the vector from 20 to 30 ms
3. Anterior location of the vector from 40 to 50 ms
4. Posterior location with a reduced magnitude of the vector from 60 to 70 ms;
5. Maximal vector of the QRS loop located to the right of +30°
6. Intermittent or transient anterior displacement of the QRS loop
7. T loop with posterior orientation tendency (useful for the differential diagnosis with posterior MI)
8. The QRS loop rotation may be.
   a. Counterclockwise: incomplete LSFB
   b. Clockwise: advanced or complete LSFB or in association with complete RBBB, LAFB, or LPFB.

Typical examples of LSFB are shown in Figures 2.1A to C, 2.2A to C. Figures 2.3 and 2.4 show examples of intermittent or transient exercise-related LSFB.

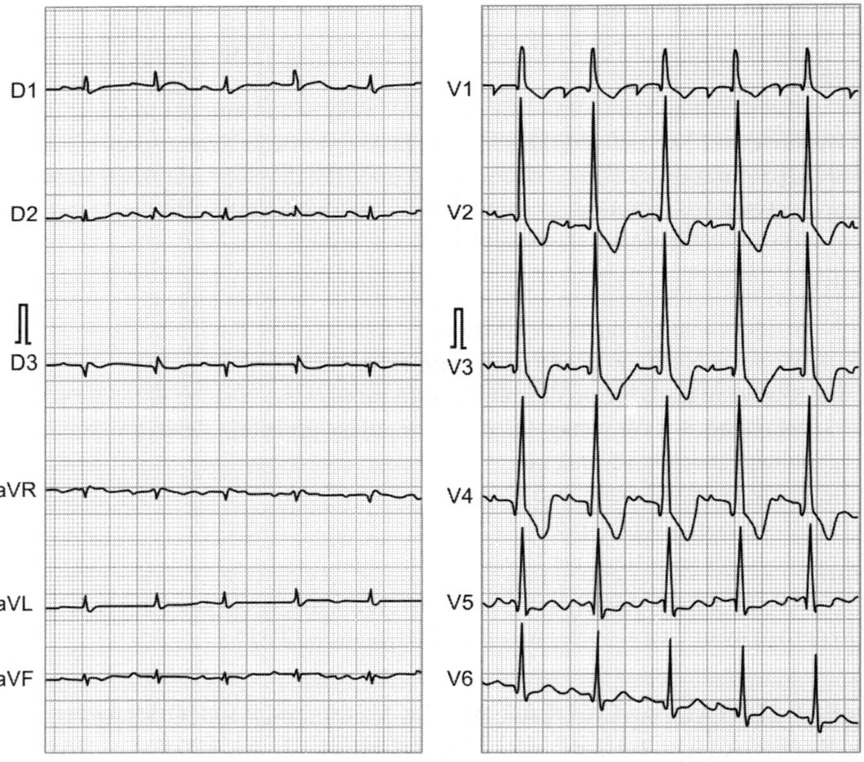

Figure 2.1A: Electrocardiogram: This ECG belongs to an 75 years old male with severe congestive heart failure and severe CAD. LAD: 100%; left circumflex: 100%, RCA: 90% obstructed. It depicts first degree AV block + LSFB + Anterior MI. Low QRS voltage only in the FP leads.

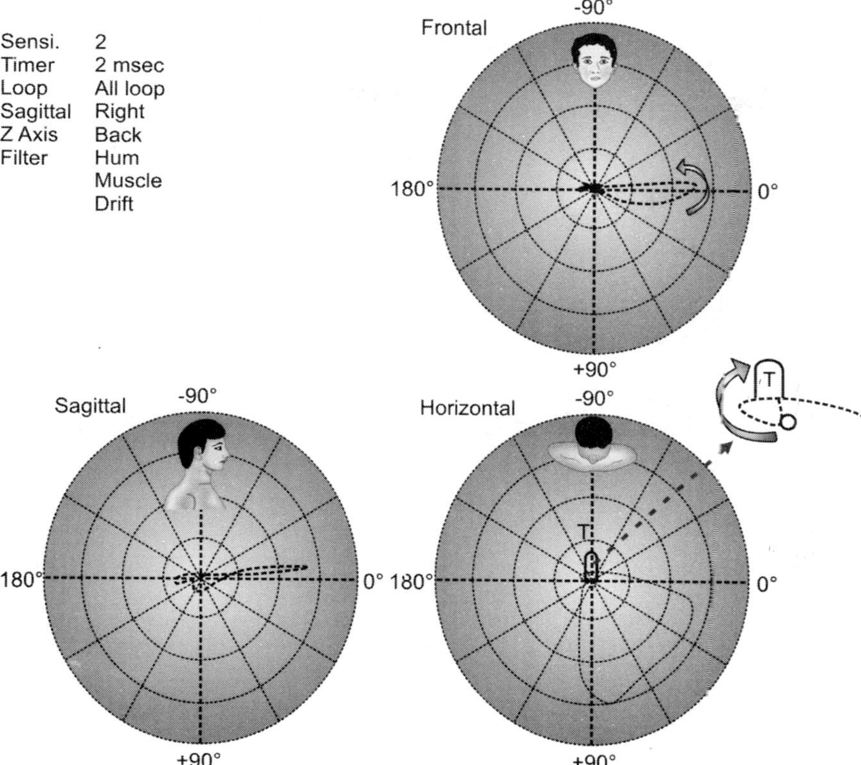

Figure 2.1B: Vectorcardiogram of LSFB

- Frontal Plane: QRS loop with counterclockwise (CWW) rotation directed to left
- Horizontal Plane: QRS loop with initial forces directed posteriorly, the remained of QRS loop dislocated to the front and leftward (predominantly located on left anterior quadrant) and CCW rotation: LSFB
- Right Sagittal Plane: QRS loop directed to front: PAF.

DIAGNOSIS OF LSFB

The differential diagnoses of LSFB include all possible etiologies of PAF.

The electrocardiographic diagnosis of PAF can be made when the R-wave voltage in any anterior or anteroseptal precordial leads from V1 (+115°) through V4 (+47°) is greater than the normal upper limit for gender and age. Electrovectorcardiographic criteria of PAF should be age and gender-related.

The accepted gender and age variations for the amplitude of the precordial leads are:

- Between 30 to 40 years old, R-wave voltage in lead V1 > 5.4 mm in woman and > 5.8 mm in men is considered a criterion for PAF

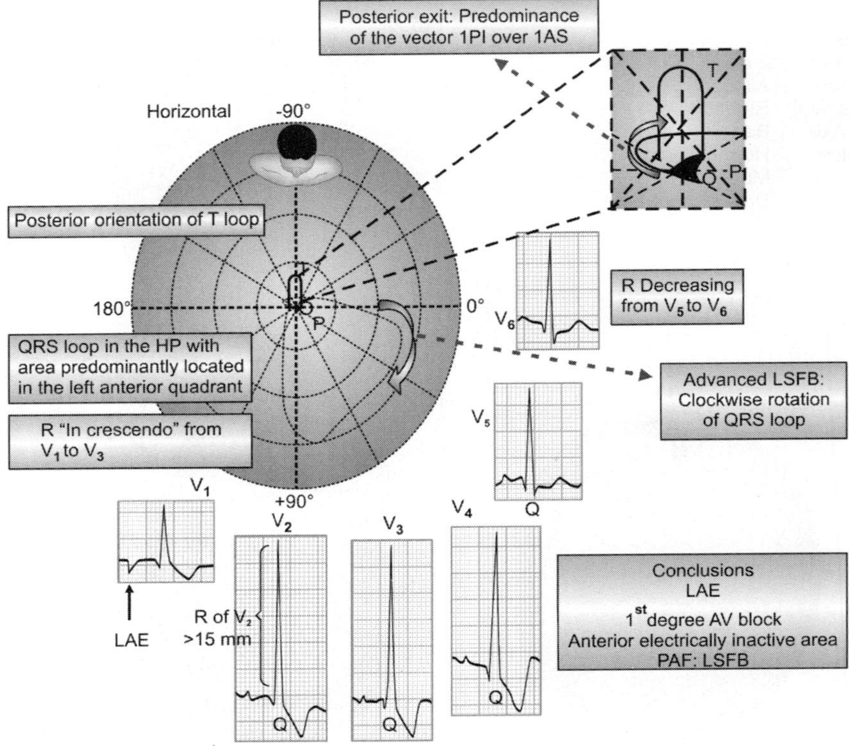

Figure 2.1C: ECG/VCG correlation in the horizontal plane. ECG/VCG diagnosis
- Deep negative component of the P-wave in lead V1: Left atrial enlargement (LAE)
- First degree AV block
- Initial Q-wave in the anterior leads: Anterior MI
- PAF: V2 R-wave voltage > 15mm, R-waves "in crescendo" from leads V1 to V3 and decreasing from leads V4 to V6: LSFB
- Initial 10 to 20ms vectors directed posteriorly
- CW rotation of the QRS loop
- QRS loop dislocated to front and leftward quadrant.

- Between 40 to 60 years old, R-wave voltage in lead V1 > 4.9 mm in woman and > 4.0 mm in men is considered a criterion for PAF.

Table 2.2 shows normal average and range of R-wave amplitude in lead V1 (Mattu et al 2001).

Another criterion used by some authors to consider the presence of PAF regards the R/S ratio in V1. Thus, an R/S ratio in V1 ≥1 is considered abnormal in adults. Tall R-wave in lead V1 is defined as an R/S ratio equal to or greater than 1. From our point of view, this criterion cannot be considered universally valid, given that in about 1% of normal individuals this ratio (R/S ratio in V1 ≥1) can

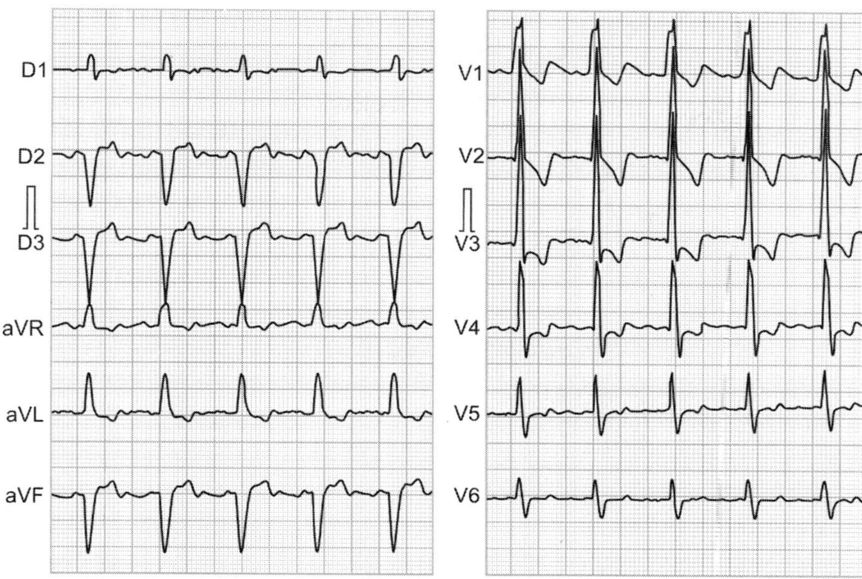

Figure 2.2A: This ECG depicts extreme left QRS axis deviation (-85°). SIII > SII, final S-wave in left leads V5 and V6; all ECG features compatible with LAFB.

PAF, R-wave voltage "in crescendo" from leads V1 to V3 and decreasing from leads V4 to V6, small initial Q-wave in leads V1 toV3, absence of initial Q-wave in leads V5 and V6; all ECG features compatible with LSFB. The diagnosis is Left bifascicular block: LAFB + LSFB.

be found as a normal variant. In lead V2, approximately 25% of men and 12% of women the R/S ratio is 1.

Normal R-wave amplitude in lead V2, V3 and V4 can be seen in Tables 2.3 to 2.5.

Table 2.2: Normal R-wave amplitude in lead V1

Age (years-old)	Woman (mean)	Man (mean)	Woman (range)	Man (range)
20-30	3.3	1.6	0.3-8.9	0-5.3
30-40	2.2	1.6	0.2-5.4	0-5.8
40-60	1.7	1.4	0.1-4.9	0.1-4.0

Table 2.3: Normal R-wave amplitude in lead V_2

Age (years-old)	Woman (mean)	Man (mean)	Woman (range)	Man (range)
20-30	7.4	4.6	1.7-13.9	1.1-9.2
30-40	5.4	3.7	0.6-12.1	0-4.10.1
40-60	4.6	3.6	0.6-12.0	0.2-9.1

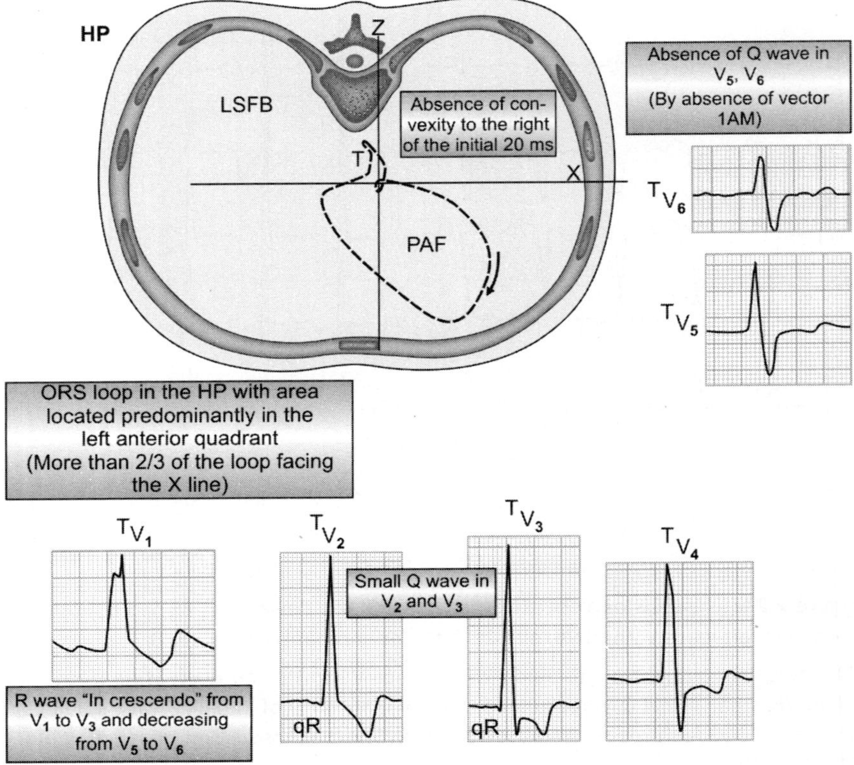

Figure 2.2B: ECG/VCG correlation in the horizontal plane. ECG/VCG diagnosis:

- **ECG:** R-wave voltage "in crescendo" from leads V1 to V3 and decreasing from ledas V4 to V6, small initial Q-wave from leads V1 toV3, absence of initial Q-wave in leads V5 and V6; all ECG features compatible with LSFB.
- **VCG:** QRS loop with initial QRS 10ms vector directed posteriorly and leftward, CW rotation and localized predominantly on left anterior quadrant: PAF. T loop directed to back.

Table 2.4: Normal R-wave amplitude in lead V_3

Age (years-old)	Woman (mean)	Man (mean)	Woman (range)	Man (range)
20-30	11.6	8.2	2.2- 26.6	2.3 -17.5
30-40	9.4	7.1	2.2-22.5	0-8.23.3
40-60	8.4	7.1	1.4-11.6	1.0-17.7

Table 2.5: Normal R-wave amplitude in lead V_4

Age (years-old)	Woman (mean)	Man (mean)	Woman (range)	Man (range)
20-30	16.6	11.5	6.1- 27.7	5.0 -19.6
30-40	14.8	11.8	5.2-29.2	4.1-25.9
40-60	14.2	12.4	5.2-25.6	3.7-23.6

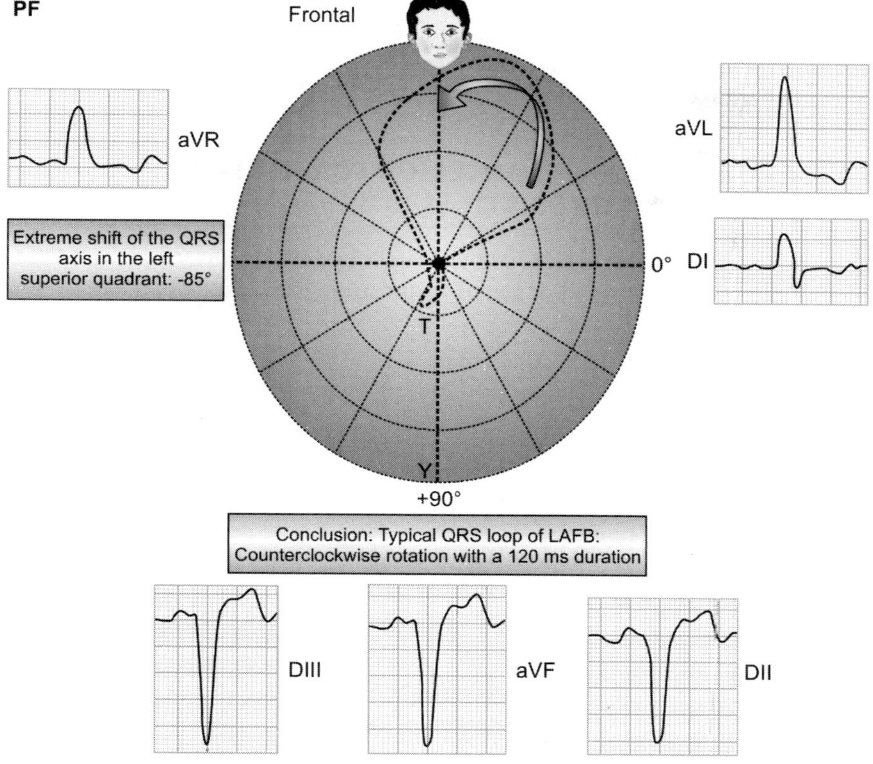

Figure 2.2C: ECG/VCG correlation in the frontal plane.

- **ECG:** Extreme QRS left axis deviation (-85°) SIII > SII; all features compatible with LAFB.
- **VCG:** QRS loop with CCW rotation and localized predominantly on left superior quadrant: LAFB

- Between 20 to 30 years old, R-wave in lead V2 > 13.9 mm in women and > 9.2 mm in men is considered a criterion for PAF.
- Between 30 to 40 years old, R-wave in lead V2 > 12.1 mm in women and > 10.1 mm in men is considered a criterion for PAF.
- Between 40 to 60 years old, R-wave in lead V2> 12.0 mm in women and > 9.1 mm in men is considered a criterion for PAF.
- Between 20 to 30 years old, R-wave in lead V3> 11.6 mm in women and > 8.2 mm in men is considered a criterion for PAF.
- Between 30 to 40 years old, R-wave in lead V3> 9.4 mm in women and > 7.1 mm in men is considered a criterion for PAF.
- Between 40 to 60 years old, R-wave in lead V3> 8.4 mm in women and > 7.1 mm in men is considered a criterion for PAF.
- Between 20 to 30 years old, R-wave in lead V4 > 27.7 mm in women and > 19.6 mm in men is considered a criterion for PAF.

- Between 30 to 40 years old, R-wave in lead V4> 29.2 mm in women and > 25.9 mm in men is considered a criterion for PAF.
- Between 40 to 60 years old, R-wave in lead V4> 25.6 mm in women and > 23.6 mm in men is considered a criterion for PAF.

CAUSES OF PROMINENT ANTERIOR FORCES (PAF) DIFFERENTIAL DIAGNOSIS OF LSFB

In the presence of PAF in the right and/or middle precordial leads V1 through V3 or V4, the following clinical and/or electrovectorcardiographic differential diagnosis should be accounted:

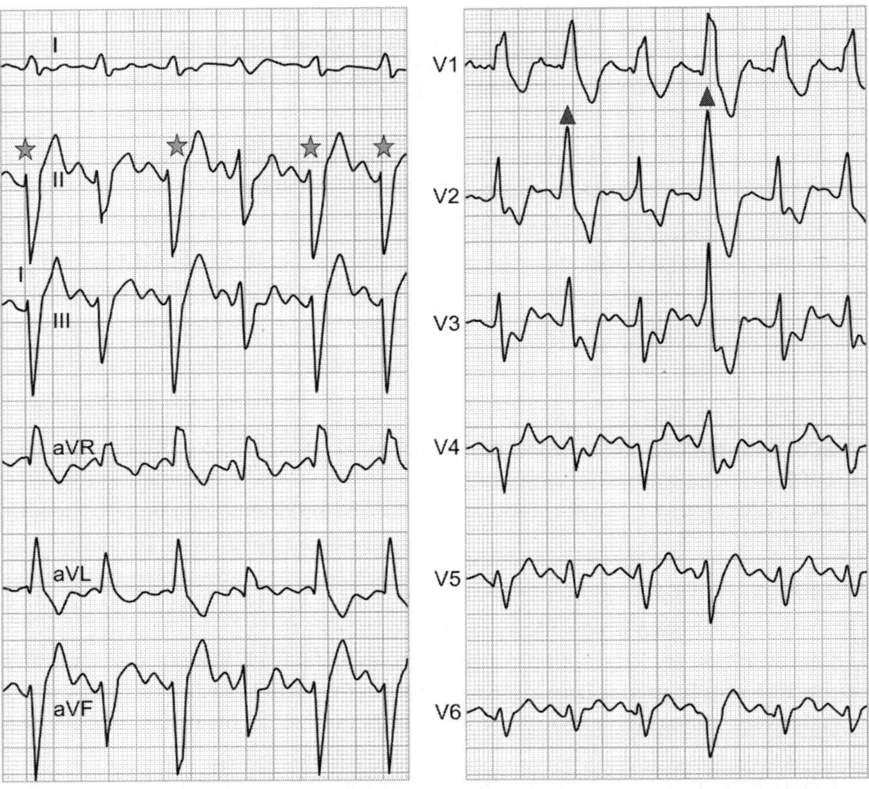

Figure 2.3: ECG. Name: LCV; Gender: Female; Age: 52 y.o; Ethnic group: White; Weight: 78 kg; Height: 1.80 m; Biotype: Mesomorphic. This is a case of a 59 years old female with Chagas' cardiomyopathy; depressed left ventricular ejection Fraction (35%), LV end diastolic diameter of 74 mm. The 12-lead ECG shows complete RBBB, LAFB, and LSFB.
FP: First, third, fifth and sixth beats (asterisks) show higher degree of LAFB.
HP: Second and fourth beats (triangles asterisk); LSFB is associated with RBBB.
Conclusions. 1. Variable degree LAFB; 2. RBB; 3. Intermittent LSFB 4. Intermittent trifascicular block.

1. Normal variant: PAF are observed in about 1% of normal subjects (Mattu et al 2001). Two main types can be distinguished: Normal variant with counterclockwise (CCW) rotation of the heart around the longitudinal axis and athlete's heart, described predominantly in black athletes (Basavarajaiah et al 2008)
2. LSFB (see above)
3. Misplaced precordial leads (MacKenzie 2004)
4. Strictly posterior, posterobasal, high posterobasal, dorsal, posterolateral, posteroinferior, and postero-lateral-inferior MI (from the "old" nomenclature) (Zema 1990) or lateral (from the "new"nomenclature) (Bayés de Luna and Zareba 2007)
5. Right ventricular hypertrophy (RVH): Vectocardiographic types A and B (Suzuki and Toyama 1978)
6. Diastolic LVH, volumetric or eccentric LVH, secondary to septal hypertrophy (magnitude of increased vector 1AM) and CCW heart rotation around the longitudinal axis (Budhwani et al 2005)
7. Complete RBBB, Kennedy type III, vectocardiographic type C, Kennedy type II, or Grishman type and Kennedy type I, or Cabrera type
8. Ventricular preexcitation (Wolff-Parkinson-White syndrome), with accessory pathway (Kent fiber) located in the posterior region (Type A). Left-sided accessory pathways are manifested as prominent R-waves in the right precordial leads mimicking right ventricular hypertrophy (Khan and Shaw 2000)

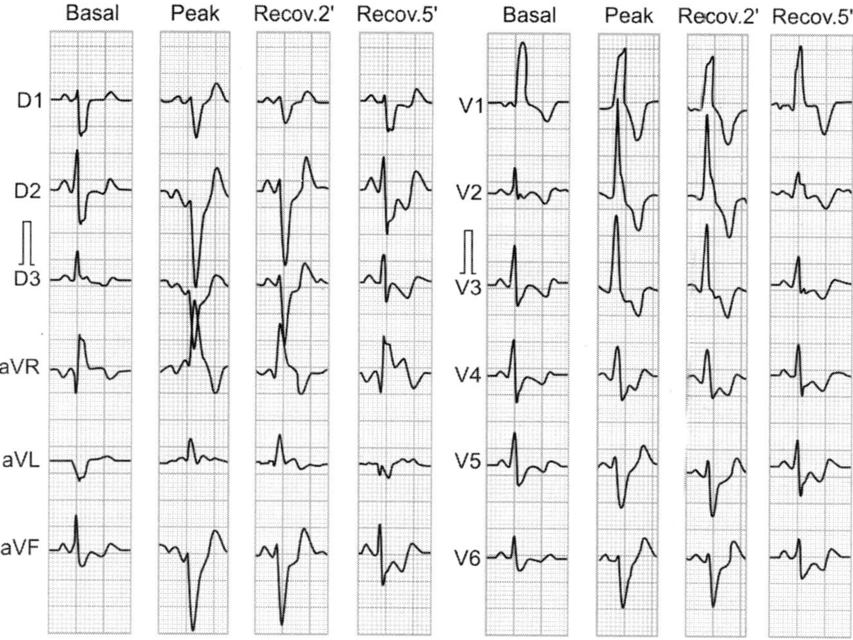

Figure 2.4: Exercise-induced LSFB. Transient ischemic bifascicular block. Exercise induced transient LAFB, LSFB, and complete RBBB. This case (stress test) belongs to a 60-year-old man, with prior MI for evaluation of stable chronic angina.

9. Hypertroph ic cardiomyopathy: HOCM and NO-HCM forms (Kukla et al 2009)
10. Progressive childhood muscular dystrophy, Duchenne muscular dystrophy/ cardiomyopathy, X-linked muscular dystrophy, or pseudohypertrophic muscular dystrophy (Thrush et al 2009)
11. Endomyocardial fibrosis (Tobias et al 1992)
12. Dextroposition. It is important to carefully differentiate dextroposition from true dextrocardia and dextroversion. An electrocardiographic clue of dextroposition is the presence of PAF, as usually seen in postpneumonectomy surgery (Cíhalík 2002).

CONCLUSION

There is conclusive evidence of a left human trifascicular His system. The isolated left septal fascicular block has been described by several authors using different terminology inducing confusion in clinicians and researchers. Traditional teaching does not include the concept of a trifascicular left system. The authors provided with the current acceptable terminology and definitions for electrovectorcardiographic diagnosis of left septal fascicular block. Additionally, a call is made to the international societies to generate a position paper or consensus to unify nomenclature and definitions.

BIBLIOGRAPHY

1. Alboni P, Malacarne C, Baggioni G, et al. Left bifascicular block with normally conducting middle fascicle. J Electrocardiol. 1977;10401.
2. Alboni P, Malacarne C, De Lorenzi E, et al. Right precordial q waves due to anterior fascicular block. Clinical and vectorcardiographic study. J Electrocardiol. 1979;12:41-8.
3. Alboni P. Left parietal septal block. A physiopathological hypothesis or new diagnostic element? G Ital Cardiol. 1980;10:365-71.
4. Athanassopoulos CB. Transient focal septal block. Chest. 1979;75:728-30.
5. Basavarajaiah S, Boraita A, Whyte G, et al. Ethnic differences in left ventricular remodeling in highly-trained athletes relevance to differentiating physiologic left ventricular hypertrophy from hypertrophic cardiomyopathy. J Am Coll Cardiol. 2008;51:2256-62.
6. Bayés de Luna A, Zareba W. New terminology of the cardiac walls and new classification of Q-wave M infarction based on cardiac magnetic resonance correlations. Ann Noninvasive Electrocardiol. 2007;12:1-4.
7. Budhwani N, Patel S, Dwyer EM Jr. Electrocardiographic diagnosis of left ventricular hypertrophy: The effect of left ventricular wall thickness, size, and mass on the specific criteria for left ventricular hypertrophy. Am Heart J. 2005;149:709-14.
8. Cohen SI, Lau SH, Haft JI, et al. Experimental production of aberrant ventricular conduction in man. Circulation. 1967;36:673-85.
9. Cohen SI, Lau SH, Steiner E, et al. Variations of aberrant ventricular conduction in man: Evidence of isolated and combined block within the specialized conduction system. Circulation. 1968;38:899-916.
10. Comella A, Magnacca M, Gistri R, Lombardi M, Neglia D, Poddighe R, et al. Right ventricular involvement in hypertrophic cardiomyopathy. A case report and brief review of the literature. Ital Heart J. 2004;5:154-9.

11. Cíhalík C. Evaluation of the ECG recording in abnormal positions of the heart in the thorax. Vnitr Lek. 2002;48 Suppl 1:90-4.
12. Dabrowska B, Ruka M, Walczak E. The electrocardiographic diagnosis of left septal fascicular block. Eur J Cardiol. 1978;6:347-57.
13. Dabrowska B. Role of the septal fascicle of the left bundle branch in the system of intraventricular conduction. Kardiol Pol. 1979;22:497-501.
14. De Micheli A. Diagnosis of fascicular or left partial block. G Ital Cardiol. 1976;6:1148-9.
15. Demolium JC, Kubertus HE. Histopathological examination of concept of left hemiblock. Br Heart J. 1972;34:807-14.
16. Demoulin JC, Kulbertus HE. Left hemiblocks revisited from the histopathological view point. Am Heart J. 1973;86:712-23.
17. De Padua F, dos Reis DD, Lopes VM, et al. Left median hemiblock- a chimera? Adv Cardiol. 1978;21:242-8.
18. De Pádua F, Lopes VM, Reis DD, et al. O hemibloqueio esquerdo mediano. Uma entidade discutível. Bol Soc Port Cardiol. 1976.
19. De Pádua F, Reis DD, Lopes VM, et al. Left median hemiblock - a chimera? In: Rijlant P; Kornreich F, editors. 3rd Int. Congr. Electrocardiology. 17th Int. Symp. Vectorcardiography. Brussels. 1976.
20. De Pádua F. Bloqueios fasciculares - Os hemibloqueios em questão. Rev Port Clin Terapeutica. 1977;3:199.
21. De Pádua F. Methodology and basic problems of ECG and VCG research. Hemiblocks Adv Cardiol. 1977;19:105-14.
22. Dhala A, Gonzalez Zuelgaray J, Deshapande S, et al. Unmasking the trifascicular left intraventricular conduction system by ablation of the right bundle block. Am J Cardiol. 1996;77:706-12.
23. Durrer D, van Dam RT, Freud GE, et al. Total excitation of the isolated human heart. Circulation. 1970;44:899-912.
24. Frink RJ, James TN. Normal blood supply to the human His bundle and proximal branches. Circulation. 1973;47:8-18.
25. Gambeta M, Childers RW. Rate-dependent right precordial Q waves: "Septal focal block". Am J Cardiol. 1973;32:196-201.
26. Georgiev N. Block of the anterior median branch of the bundle of His Vutr Boles. 1986;25:112-5.
27. Hassapoyannes CA, Nelson WP. Myocardial ischemia-induced transient anterior conduction delay. Am Heart J. 1991;67:659-60.
28. Hoffman I, Mehta J, Hilsenrath J, et al. Anterior conduction delay: A possible cause for proeminent anterior QRS forces. J Electrocardiol. 1976;9:15-21.
29. Hosseinpour AR, Anderson RH, Ho SY. The anatomy of the septal perforating arteries in normal and congenitally malformed hearts. J Thorac Cardiovasc Surg. 2001;121:1046-52.
30. Inoue H, Nakaya Y, Niki T, et al. Vectorcardiographic and epicardial activation studies on experimentally –induced subdivision block of the left bundle branch. Jpn Circ J. 1983;47:1179-89.
31. Iwamura N, Kodama I, Shimizu T, et al. Functional properties of the left septal Purkinje network in premature activation of the ventricular conduction system. Am Heart J. 1978;95:60-9.
32. Iwamura N, Shimizu T, Kodama I, et al. *In vitro* study on the cause of intraventricular aberrant conduction: Comparison of the functional refractory period between the canine right and left bundle branch systems. Jpn Circ J. 1976;40:461.
33. Iwamura N. Experimental study on the cause of ventricular aberrant conduction. Jpn Circ J. 1978;42: 489-99

34. Khan IA, Shaw IS. Pseudo ventricular hypertrophy and pseudo myocardial infarction in Wolff-Parkinson-White syndrome. Am J Emerg Med. 2000;18:807-9.
35. Kukla P, Petkow-Dimitrow P, Jastrzebski M, et al. Malignant form of familial hypertrophic cardiomyopathy complicated with ventricular fibrillation in siblings. Electrocardiogram in hypertrophic cardiomyopathy - a review. Kardiol Pol. 2009;67:774-80.
36. Kulbertus HE, de-Leval-Rutten F, Casters P. Vectorcardiographic study of aberrant conduction. Anterior displacement of QRS: another form of intraventricular block. Br Heart J. 1976;38:549-57.
37. Kulbertus HE, Demoulin J. Pathological basis of concept of left hemiblock. The Conduction System of the Heart. Wellens HJJ, Lie KI, Janse MJ, HE Stenfert Krpses (eds), Leiden, Philadelphia. Lea and Febiger. 1976; p287.
38. Kulbertus HE. Significance of segmental blocks of the left branch of the bundle of His. Bull Acad R Med Belg. 1973;128:481-93.
39. Kulbertus HE. Concept of left hemiblocks revisited. A histopathological and experimental study. Advances in Cardiol. 1975;14:126-35.
40. Lazzara R, El-Sherif N, Befeler B, et al. Regional Refractoriness within the Ventricular Conduction System. Circ Res. 1976;39:254-62.
41. MacAlpin RN. In search of left septal fascicular block. Am Heart J. 2002;144:948-56.
42. MacAlpin RN. Left Septal Fascicular Block: Myth Or Reality? Indian Pacing Electrophysiol J. 2003;3:157-77.
43. MacKenzie R. Tall R wave in lead V1. J Insur Med. 2004;36:255-9.
44. Madias JE, Ashtiani R, Agarwal H, et al. Diagnosis of ventricular aneurysm and other severe segmental LV dysfunction consequent to a myocardial infarction in the presence of right bundle branch block: ECG correlates of a positive diagnosis made via echocardiography and/or contrast ventriculography. Ann Noninvasive Electrocardiol. 2005;10:53-9.
45. Madias JE. The "giant R waves" ECG pattern of hyperacute phase of myocardial infarction. J Electrocardiol. 1993;26:77-80.
46. Magnacca M, Valesano G, Rizzo G, et al. Diagnostic value of electrocardiogram in septal fascicular conduction disorders of the left branch in diabetics Minerva Cardioangiolica. 1988;36:361-3.
47. Maron BJ, Wolfson JK, Ciro E, et al. Relation of electrocardiographic abnormalities and patterns of left ventricular hypertrophy identified by 2-dimensional echocardiography in patients with hypertrophic cardiomyopathy. Am J Cardiol. 1983;51:189-94.
48. Mattu A, Brady WJ, Perron AD, et al. Prominent R wave in lead V1: electrocardiographic differential diagnosis. Am J Emerg Med. 2001;19:504-13.
49. Medrano GA, Brenes C, De Michelis A, et al. Simultaneous block of the anterior and posterior subdivisions of the left branch of the bundle of His (biphasic block), and its association with the right branch block (triphasic block). Experimental and clinical electrocardiographic study. Arch Inst Cardiol Mex. 1970;40:752-70.
50. Moffa PJ, Del Nero E, Tobias NM, et al. The left anterior septal block in Chagas' disease. Jap Heart J. 1982;23:163-5.
51. Moffa PJ, Ferreira BM, Sanches PC, et al. Intermittent ântero-medial divisional block in patients with coronary disease. Arq Bras Cardiol. 1997;68:293-6
52. Moffa PJ, Pastore CA, Sanches PCR. The left-middle (septal) fascicular block and coronary heart disease. In Liebman J (ed). Electrocardiology' 96 – From the cell to body surface. Cleveland Ohio Word Scientific. 1996;547-50.
53. Mori H, Kobayashi S, Mohri S. Electrocardiographic criteria for the diagnosis of the left septal fascicular block and its frequency among primarily elderly hospitalized patients. Nippon Ronen Igakkai Zasshi. 1992;29:293-7.
54. Nakaya Y, Hiasa Y, Murayama Y, et al. Prominent anterior QRS force as a manifestation of left septal fascicular block J Electrocardiol. 1978;11:39-6.

55. Nakaya Y, Hiraga T. Reassessment of the subdivision block of the Left Bundle Branch. Jpn Circ J. 1981;45:503-16.
56. Nakaya Y, Inoue H, Hiasa Y, et al. Functional importance of the left septal Purkinje network in the left ventricular conduction system. Jpn Heart J. 1981;22:363-76.
57. Pastore CA, et al. Guidelines for Interpreting Rest Electrocardiogram. Arq Bras Cardiol. 2003;80:1-17.
58. Reiffel JA, Bigger Jr T. Pure anterior conduction delay: a variant "fascicular" defect. J Electrocardiol. 1978;11:315-19.
59. Riera AR, Ferreira C, Ferreira Filho C, et al. Wellens syndrome associated with prominent anterior QRS forces: an expression of left septal fascicular block? J Electrocardiol. 2008;41:671-4.
60. Riera AR, Kaiser E, Levine P, et al. Kearns-Sayre syndrome: electro-vectorcardiographic evolution for left septal fascicular block of the his bundle. J Electrocardiol. 2008;41:675-8.
61. Rosenbaum MB, Elizari M, Lazzari JO. The Hemiblocks: New Concepts of Intraventricular Conduction Based on Human Anatomical, Physiological and Clinical Studies. Oldsmar, FL. Tampa Tracings. 1971.
62. Rosenbaum MB, Elizari MV, Lazzari JO. Los Hemibloqueos, Editorial Paidos. SAICF. Buenos Aires. Spanish. 1967;p72.
63. Sakai T. Left anterior fascicular block, left posterior fascicular block, left septal fascicular block. Ryoikibetsu Shokogun Shirizu. 1996;12:282-4.
64. Sanches PCR, Moffa PJ, Sosa E, et al. Electrical Endocardial Mapping Of Five Patients With Typical Ecg Of Left-Middle (Septal) Fascicular Block. In Proceeeding of the XXVIII International Congress on Electrocardiology Guarujá SP Brazil. Pastore CA (ed), Heart Institute of the University of São Paulo School of Medicine São Paulo Brazil Atheneu. 2001;pp89-95.
65. Suzuki K, Toyama S. Vectorcardiographic criteria of high posterior infarction: differentiation from normal subjects, right ventricular hypertrophy and primary myocardial disease. J Electrocardiol. 1978;11:159-63.
66. Thrush PT, Allen HD, Viollet L, et al. Reexamination of the electrocardiogram in boys with Duchenne muscular dystrophy and correlation with its dilated cardiomyopathy. Am J Cardiol. 2009;103:262-5.
67. Tobias NM, Moffa PJ, Pastore CA, et al. The electrocardiogram in endomyocardial fibrosis Arq Bras Cardiol. 1992;59:249-53.
68. Tranchesi, J. Moffa, PJ. Electrocardiograma Normal e Patológico. Moffa, PJ & Sanches, PCR, editors. Sao Paulo: Roca Chap. 2001;19:413-61.
69. Tranchesi J, Moffa PJ, Pastore CA, et al. Block of the antero-medial division of the left bundle branch of His in coronary diseases. Vectrocardiographic characterization. Arq Bras Cardiol. 1979;32:355-60.
70. Uchida AH, Moffa PJ, Pérez Riera AR, et al. Exercise-induced Left septal Fascicular Block: An Expression of Severe Myocardial Ischemia. Indian Pacing and Electrophysiology Journal. 2006;6:135-8.
71. Uhley HN. Some controversy regarding the peripheral distribution of the conduction system. Am J Cardiol. 1972;30:919-20.
72. Uhley HN. The Quadrifascicular Nature of the Peripheral Conduction System, in Dreifus LS, and Likoff W, (eds.): Cardiac Arrhythmias (New York): Grune and Stratton. Inc. 1973.
73. Yamaguchi H, Nishiyama S, Nakanishi S, Nishimura S. Electrocardiographic, echocardiographic and ventriculographic characterization of hypertrophic non-obstructive cardiomyopathy. Eur Heart J. Nov; 1983;4 Suppl F:105-19.
74. Zema MJ. Electrocardiographic tall R waves in the right precordial leads. Comparison of recently proposed ECG and VCG criteria for distinguishing posterolateral myocardial infarction from prominent anterior forces in normal subjects. J Electrocardiol. 1990;23:147-56.

Chapter

3

Cardiac Purkinje Fibers: Normal Function and its Derangements

Mario Vassalle

Abstract. Under normal conditions, the function of Purkinje fibers is fast conduction of impulses originating in the sinoatrial node, in order to secure a synchronous ventricular contraction. However, when the activation from the atria fails to activate the Purkinje network, the pacemaker activity of Purkinje fibers is physiologically responsible for the initiation of the idioventricular rhythm. The functions of Purkinje fibers require a set of characteristics suitable for fast conduction and pacemaker activity, such as a large and fast upstroke and diastolic depolarization, respectively. The aim of this chapter is to present the ionic events that are responsible for the action potential and diastolic depolarization of Purkinje fibers. Furthermore, some mechanisms of recovery from excitation are considered, such as the extrusion of Na^+ by the Na^+-K^+ pump and of Ca^{2+} by the Na^+-Ca^{2+} exchange. The sympathetic and frequency-dependent control of Purkinje fiber automaticity is discussed as well. The ion fluxes associated with electrical activity in systole and diastole as well as the events involved in recovery from excitation can become deranged under a variety of conditions. Therefore, the characteristics and consequences of derangements of the events responsible for excitation and recovery from excitation of Purkinje fibers are discussed and their mechanisms analyzed. This approach intends to provide insights as to the manner by which derangements of physiological mechanisms lead to disturbances of cardiac function, often in the form of life-threatening arrhythmias.

Keywords. Cardiac Purkinje fibers; events underlying excitation and recovery; control of discharge; derangements of normal function; ionic mechanisms underlying abnormalities.

INTRODUCTION

Cardiac Purkinje fibers form an extensive subendothelial network in ventricles and have three major functions: (1) Insure the electrical continuity between the atria and ventricles through the continuity of the atrioventricular (A-V) node with the His bundle; (2) Insure a fast conduction of the impulses that originate from the sinoatrial node (SAN); and (3) Act as subsidiary ventricular pacemakers in the event of complete A-V block caused either by disease or by strong vagal stimulation.

The aim of this chapter is first to present an overview of the normal events underlying the activity of Purkinje fibers and then the derangements of normal function that leads to different abnormalities, such as different kinds of arrhythmias. This approach allows linking normal function with the derangements of physiological mechanisms, a precondition for the understanding of mechanisms underlying abnormalities and for any rational therapeutic approach.

NORMAL FUNCTIONS OF PURKINJE FIBERS

The Resting and Action Potential

The function of Purkinje fibers is related to the changes of their electrical activity both in systole and diastole. *In vitro*, at ~ 4-5 mM $[K^+]_o$, Purkinje fibers are generally quiescent, but an electrical stimulus typically initiates a sudden depolarization (the upstroke, phase 0), followed by an initial rapid repolarization (phase 1), a phase of slow repolarization (phase 2, plateau) and a final faster repolarization (phase 3). Phase 3 repolarization undershoots the previous resting potential to attain the more negative maximum diastolic potential (MDP) (Figure 3.1A).

The MDP marks the end of action potential (AP) and it is followed by a phase of slow depolarization (diastolic depolarization, phase 4) to the resting potential (Figure 1A). If $[K^+]_o$ is decreased (e.g., ~3 mM), the resting potential undergoes voltage oscillations which increase progressively in magnitude and (if they attain the threshold) initiate spontaneous discharge (Figure 3.1B) (Spiegler and Vassalle 1995, Berg and Vassalle 2000).

In comparison to ventricular myocardium, Purkinje fibers have a greater rate of rise of the upstroke (~ 500 mV/s), a larger upstroke with a positive overshoot of ~ 30 mV (Weidmann 1956), a longer AP (~500 ms in Purkinje and ~300 ms in ventricular muscle fibers; Lin and Vassalle 1978), weaker and shorter twitch (Lin and Vassalle 1978), a more negative maximum diastolic potential (~ -90 mV), larger cell diameter (~30 microns), more abundant Cx40, Kv4.3, Kir3.1, TWIK1, HCN4, ClC6 and CALM1 (Gaborit et al. 2007) as well as Cx43, which is selectively expressed in the intercalated disk membrane (Oosthoek et al 1993).

These differences have major functional significance. Thus, the faster and larger upstroke, the larger diameter and the abundant gap junctions are essential fast propagation of excitation (3-5 m/s; Weidmann 1956). The long action potential prevents reentry of excitation from myocardium and the more negative diastolic potential insures full availability of the fast sodium channels prior to excitation. In addition, diastolic depolarization (DD) is a necessary contributor to spontaneous discharge in complete A-V block. In turn, the fast conduction velocity of Purkinje fibers permits a more synchronous (and therefore more effective) ventricular contraction.

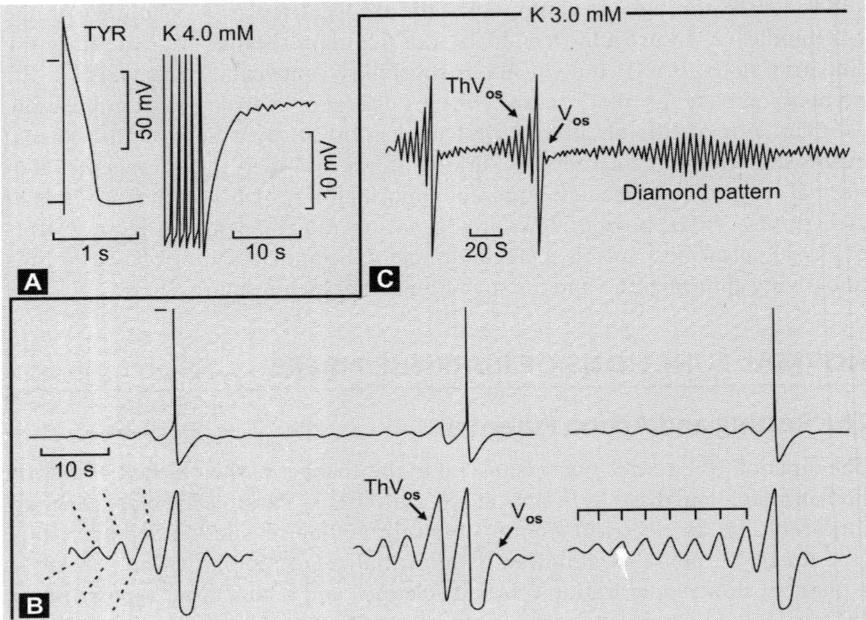

Figures 3.1A to C: Oscillatory potentials and spontaneous discharge. In panel A, the traces were recorded in Tyrode solution (4 mM K^+). The cessation of drive is shown at higher gain. In panel B, in 3 mM K^+, the arrows indicate the ThV_{os} that initiated the AP and the V_{os} that followed it. In the bottom panels, the dotted lines extrapolate the depolarizing and hyperpolarizing phases of ThV_{os} In the last B panel, the spikes on the horizontal line point to the peaks of ThV_{os} In panel C, ThV_{os} that failed to reach the threshold for the upstroke led to the diamond pattern. [Modified and reproduced by permission from Spiegler P and Vassalle M (1995) Can J Physiol Pharmacol 73: 1165-1180.]

Brief Outline of Major Ionic Events Underlying Resting and Action Potential

The resting potential is mainly due to the inward rectifier current I_{K1} (Kir2.1, Kir2.2 and Kir2.3). I_{KATP} (Kir6.1 and Kir6.2) and I_{KACh} (Kir3.1 and Kir3.4) may contribute to it if and when they are activated. $[K^+]_i$ (~150 mM) is greater than $[K^+]_o$ (4-5 mM) and I_{K1} channel conductance predominates at the resting potential. Therefore, I_{K1} perse would set the resting potential at the potassium equilibrium potential (E_K). In actuality, the resting potential is less negative than E_K, since at rest there is a small Na^+ background current. This state of affairs is essential for the pacemaker potential, since if the resting potential were identical to E_K the decay of the pacemaker current I_{Kdd} would not cause diastolic depolarization.

Thus, the resting potential is not an equilibrium potential, but a steady-state potential, since the sodium that leaks in the cells has to be extruded by the Na^+-K^+ pump ("Na-pump") against the sodium gradient. If the Na-pump is inhibited under abnormal conditions, the resting potential can not be maintained, as it happens in digitalis toxicity (Vassalle et al 1962, Vassalle and Musso 1976). Similarly, a decrease of I_{K1} (however brought about) decreases the resting potential, with the attendant modifications of other currents.

The features of the AP are related to the interplay of several voltage- and time-dependent ion currents. The currents are responsible for depolarization and repolarization of the AP and for DD. At the resting potential, the gates for the fast Na^+ current (I_{Na1}; predominantly $Na_v1.5$) are available for activation. Therefore, when the resting potential of Purkinje fibers is decreased electrotonically by a conducted AP or by an electrical stimulus to a critical potential (the threshold for the fast I_{Na1}), the sodium gates open. The consequent Na^+ entry under its electrochemical gradient drive leads to the rapid and large upstroke, which electrotonically brings the resting potential of adjacent cell to the threshold for the upstroke. On depolarization, I_{Na1} gates become inactivated and this is the main basis for the absolute refractory period.

The depolarization brought about by I_{Na1} allows the potential to attain the threshold for other currents (such as the transient outward current $I_{to,}$ the delayed rectifier current I_K, the L type calcium current I_{CaL} ($Ca_V1.2$ with the poreforming α1C subunit and $Ca_V1.3$ with the α1D subunit) and the T-type calcium current I_{CaT}, the slowly inactivating Na^+ current (I_{Na2}, Vassalle et al 2007, Bocchi and Vassalle 2008), which is possibly due to the skeletal muscle Na^+ channel isoform, $Na_v1.4$ (Qu et al 2007). Phase 1 repolarization is mainly due to the activation of I_{to}, which brings the potential within the plateau range. The importance of this is that the plateau range is more negative than the overshoot to the reversal potentials of I_{CaL} and I_{Na2}.

Several findings indicate that the longer AP of Purkinje fibers might be related to a greater Na^+ influx. Thus, the Na^+-channel blocker tetrodotoxin (TTX) (Figure 3.2A), high $[Na^+]_o$ and the Na^+-channel agonist veratridine modify the AP more in Purkinje than in myocardial fibers (Figure 3.2B; Iacono and Vassalle 1990a). Also, TTX reduces intracellular sodium activity (a^i_{Na}) more in Purkinje than in muscle fibers (Figures 3.2A and B, respectively; Iacono and Vassalle 1990a). The sodium load may be greater in Purkinje fibers because of a greater sodium influx during the plateau, which possibly could result from the slowly inactivating I_{Na2} (see below). Local anesthetics (Vassalle and Bhattacharyya 1980, Bhattacharyya and Vassalle 1981, Carmeliet and Saikawa 1982) and TTX shorten the AP of Purkinje fibers more than that of ventricular muscle fibers (Coraboeuf et al 1979, Vassalle and Bhattacharyya 1980, Bhattacharyya and Vassalle 1982).

In fact, in single Purkinje cells, there are three inward Na^+ components: fast activating and inactivating I_{Na1}, the slowly inactivating I_{Na2} in the plateau range (Figure 3.3) (Vassalle et al 2007, Bocchi and Vassalle 2008) and the slowly inactivating I_{Na3} in the diastolic depolarization range (see below) (Rota and Vassalle 2003).

In Purkinje cells, I_{Na2} occurs also in the absence of I_{Na1}, since I_{Na2} is absent at the threshold (-50 mV) of I_{Na1} (Figure 3.3). I_{Na2} is markedly reduced by TTX (Vassalle et al 2007), suggesting that it is a Na^+ currents. As shown in Figure 3.3, depolarizing steps from a holding potential (V_h) of -90 mV to -50 mV induced a fast and large inward transient which quickly inactivated (I_{Na1}). With larger

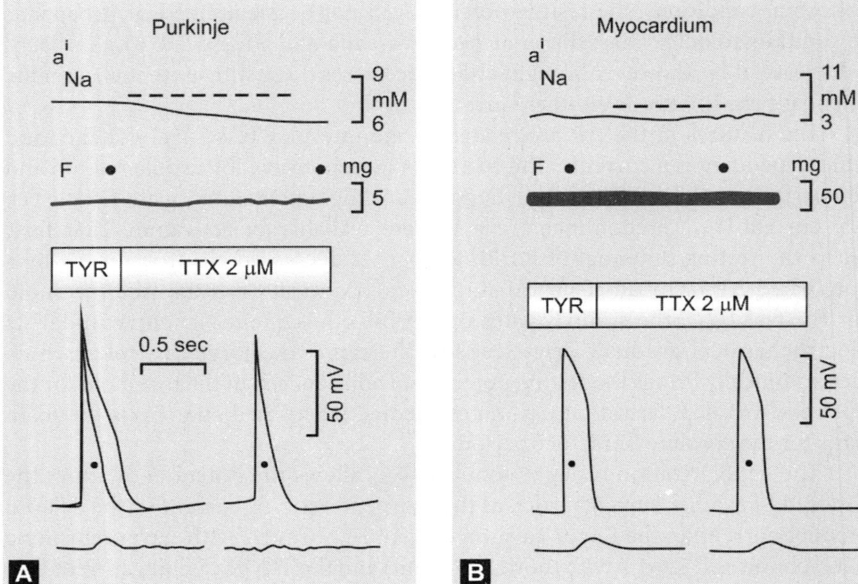

Figures 3.2A and B: Effects of tetrodotoxin (TTX) on a^i_{Na}, action potential and force in Purkinje and myocardial fibers. The trace of intracellular sodium activity (a^i_{Na}), force (F), action potential and twitch curves are shown. The traces recorded from Purkinje fibers are shown in A and those recorded from myocardial fibers in B. The preparations were exposed to TTX as indicated below the force traces. The dashed lines extrapolate the value of a^i_{Na} before TTX exposure. Modified and reproduced by permission from Iacono G and Vassalle M (1990a). J Pharmacol Exp Ther 253: 1-12.

depolarizing steps (-30,-20 and-10 mV), I_{Na1} did not decay to the original level (as at -50 mV), but instead it was followed by an inward tail (I_{Na2}) which decayed slowly during the 500 ms step. With larger depolarizations, I_{to} appeared (not shown).

I_{Na2} was no longer present on depolarization from V_h of -60 mV and was blocked by TTX, lidocaine and cadmium (but not manganese). During fast depolarizing ramps, I_{Na1} was followed by a region of negative slope, which was decreased by a less negative V_h and by TTX (Vassalle et al 2007). Thus, the shortening of the AP of Purkinje fibers by TTX, local anesthetics or lower resting potential appears mediated by a decrease of I_{Na2}.

In other experiments, I_{Na2} was separated from I_{Na1} by applying a first step to -50 mV (to quickly activate and inactivate of I_{Na1}) followed by depolarizing steps to activate I_{Na2}. I_{Na2} activated quickly and inactivated slowly with time constant of hundreds milliseconds, while its slope conductance decreased as a function of time. Progressively longer conditioning steps to –50 mV decreased the magnitude of I_{Na2} during the subsequent test steps, whereas hyperpolarizing steps which were gradually longer or gradually more negative were followed by progressively larger I_{Na2} tails on return to –30 mV (Bocchi and Vassalle 2008). Thus, I_{Na2} is a sodium current with distinctive characteristics, can be activated independently of I_{Na1} at a less negative threshold and is largest in the plateau range of potentials.

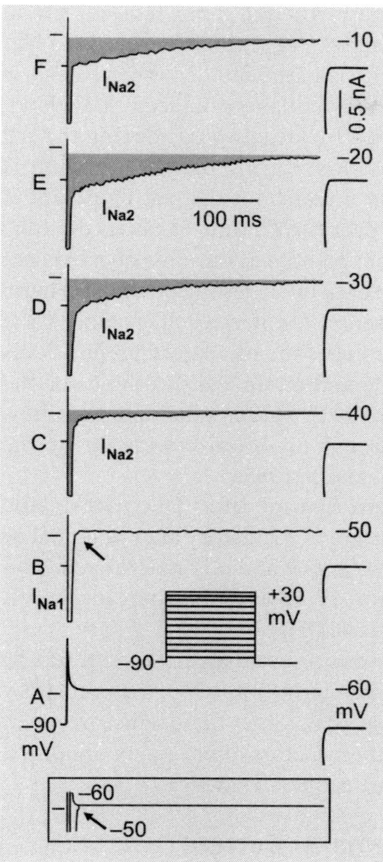

Figures 3.3A to F: I_{Na1} and I_{Na2} have different threshold and inactivation kinetics. Depolarizing steps (500 ms) were applied from V_h -90 mV to -60, -50, -40, -30, -20 and -10 mV. The current traces at various V_{test} are shown in A-F. The arrows within and without the boxed inset point to the fast inactivation of I_{Na1} at −50 mV (only part of the I_{Na1} traces is shown). The slowly inactivating component of I_{Na2} is emphasized by the shaded areas. The boxed inset shows the superimposed current traces recorded at −60 and −50 mV [Modified and reproduced by permission from Vassalle M, Bocchi L and Du F (2007) Exper Physiol 92.1:161–173.]

Outline of Major Ionic Events Underlying Diastolic Depolarization

To maintain homeostasis with continuous rhythmic activity, during diastole ion channels and ion distributions must be restored to the conditions prevailing before the AP. Furthermore, in Purkinje fibers the slow depolarization that occurs during diastole must be accounted for in term of underlying currents.

During the AP, Na^+ and Ca^{2+} enter the cell and K^+ is lost. These ions must be restored to their original environment against their electrochemical gradient. During each pump cycle, the Na-pump extrudes 3 Na ions while taking up 2 K ions, thereby creating an outward pump current (see Vassalle 1982, 1987).

Ca^{2+} entering during the AP (I_{CaL}) is extruded during diastole by the Na^+-Ca^{2+} exchange (NaCaX). The driving force for Ca^{2+} extrusion is provided by Na^+ gradient. Since one Ca ion is extruded in exchange with three Na ions, the NaCaX is electrogenic. Therefore, during diastole the NaCaX generates an inward current (I_{CaNaX}) superimposed on DD (see Vassalle and Lin 2004). Therefore, the extrusion of Ca^{2+} depends directly on NaCaX and indirectly on the Na-pump. If the Na-pump activity is inhibited, the intracellular sodium activity (a^{i}_{Na}) increases and the Na^{+} gradient across the cell membrane decreases with consequent increase in $[Ca^{2+}]_i$. If $[Ca^{2+}]_i$ increases to the point of Ca^{2+} overload, arrhythmias are induced (see below).

The ion channels activated and inactivated (or deactivated) during the AP must recover at negative voltages, but in addition, during the AP a current is modified which makes phase 3 repolarization undershoot the resting potential to attain the MDP. As this pacemaker current decays with time, it causes diastolic depolarization (DD), which therefore is an after potential. If Purkinje fibers are not spontaneously active, DD of a driven AP decays back to the resting potential (Figure 3.1A). Instead, if spontaneous discharge is present, DD enters a voltage range ("the oscillatory zone"). In this voltage range, DD initiates the oscillatory prepotentials ThV_{os} which gradually increase in magnitude and attain the threshold for the upstroke (Figure 3.1B, Spiegler and Vassalle 1995). Under suitable conditions, DD attains the threshold for the upstroke through an upward swing due to the depolarizing slope of ThV_{os} (see Figure 3.2 in Vassalle 1983).

There is another oscillatory phenomenon that modifies DD, namely, the after potential V_{os} (also referred to in the literature as oscillatory after potential or delayed after depolarization). V_{os} always follows an AP and it is superimposed on the initial diastolic depolarization (DD_1) (Figures 3.1B and C), whereas ThV_{os} is superimposed on the late diastolic depolarization (DD_2).

Therefore, during diastole there are three major events which contribute to the pacemaker mechanism, namely, diastolic depolarization (*DD*), the oscillatory afterpotential V_{os} and the oscillatory prepotential $Th\,V_{os}$. Since there is no agreement on the mechanisms or contribution of any of these factors to normal or abnormal discharge, it is necessary to review some of the pertinent evidence.

Diastolic Depolarization and the Pacemaker Current

As mentioned above, DD is an after potential (it appears after a driven AP) and is necessary but not sufficient for spontaneous discharge, since DD may decay to the resting potential (Figure 3.1A). Still, DD is an essential component of the pacemaking process, since it allows the membrane potential to decay from the MDP toward the threshold for the upstroke.

The undershoot to the MDP and the subsequent decay of the membrane potential require that during the AP a net outward current should develop that subsides during diastole, thereby causing DD. In fact, during the AP the outward K^{+} current I_{Kdd} is activated, which subsequently decays during diastole (Vassalle 1966; Vassalle et al, 1995). However, it has been also proposed that during the AP an inward current would be deactivated (the hyperpolarizationactivated I_f), which would then reactivate during diastole, thereby causing DD. This disagreement necessitates a critical evaluation of the evidence presented (for more details, see Vassalle et al 1999; Vassalle 2003; Vassalle 2007).

In the experiments of Vassalle (1966), voltage-clamping the membrane of spontaneous Purkinje fiber at the MDP resulted in a time-dependent net inward current. The pacemaker current was associated with a decrease in slope

59. Lin C-I, Vassalle M. Calcium overload and strophanthidin-induced mechanical toxicity in cardiac Purkinje fibers. Can J Physiol Pharmacol. 1983;61:1329-39.
60. Lin C-I, Kotake H, Vassalle M. On the mechanism underlying the oscillatory current in cardiac Purkinje fibers. J Cardiovasc Pharmacol. 1986;8:906-14.
61. Liu B, Golyan F, McCullough GR, Vassalle M. Electrophysiological and antiarrhythmic effects of the K-channel opener, BRL 34915, in cardiac Purkinje fibers. Drug Develop Res. 1988;14:123-39.
62. Liu YM, Yu H, Li CZ, Cohen IS, Vassalle M. Cs^+ effects on i_f and i_K in rabbit sinoatrial node myocytes: Implications for SA node automaticity. J Cardiovasc Pharmacol. 1998;32:783-90.
63. Lu HH, Lange G, Brooks C McC. Factors controlling pacemaker action in cells of the sinoatrial node. Circ Res. 1965;17:460-71.
64. Maguy A, Le Bouter S, Comtois P, Chartier D, Villeneuve L, Wakili R, Nishida K, Nattel S. Ion channel subunit expression changes in cardiac Purkinje fibers: a potential role in conduction abnormalities associated with congestive heart failure. Circ Res. 2009;104:1113-22.
65. Makielski JC, Limberis J, Fan Z, Kyle JW. Intrinsic lidocaine affinity for Na channels expressed in Xenopus oocytes depends on alpha (hH1 vs. rSkM1) and beta 1 subunits, Cardiovasc Re. 1999;42:503-9.
66. Masson-Pévet M, Bleeker WK, Mackaay AJC, Gros D, Bouman LN. Ultrastructural and functional aspects of the rabbit sinoatrial node. In: The Sinus Node: Structure, Function and Clinical Relevance. (Ed. FIM Bonke), 195-211, Martinus Nijhoff Publisher, The Hague. 1978.
67. Mevorach D, Elchalal U, Rein AJ. Prevention of complete heart block in children of mothers with anti-SSA/Ro and anti-SSB/La autoantibodies: detection and treatment of first-degree atrioventricular block. Curr Opin Rheumatol. 2009;21:478-82.
68. Michael G, Xiao L, Qi XY, Dobrev D, Nattel S. Remodelling of cardiac repolarization: How homeostatic responses can lead to arrhythmogenesis. Cardiovasc Res. 2009;81:491-99.
69. Musso E, Vassalle M. The role of calcium in overdrive suppression of canine cardiac Purkinje fibers. Circ Res. 1982;51:167-80.
70. Nattel S, Maguy A, Le Bouter S, Yeh YH. Arrhythmogenic ion-channel remodeling in the heart: heart failure, myocardial infarction, and atrial fibrillation. Physiol Rev. 2007;87:425-56.
71. Nett MP, Vassalle M. Obligatory role of diastolic voltage oscillations in sino-atrial node discharge. J Mol Cell Cardiol. 2003;35:1257-76.
72. Noble D. The surprising heart: A review of recent progress in cardiac electrophysiology. J Physiol (Lond.). 1984;353:1-50.
73. Noble D and Tsien RW. The kinetics, rectifier properties of the slow potassium current in cardiac Purkinje fibres. J Physiol (London). 1968;195:185-214.
74. Oosthoek PW, Viragh S, Lamers WH, Moorman JR. Immunohistochemical delineation of the conduction system. II The atrioventricular node and Purkinje system. Circ Res. 1993;73:482-91.
75. Otsuka M. Die Wirkung von Adrenalin auf Purkinje-Fasern von Saugertierherzen. Pflügers Arch. 1958;266:512-17.
76. Parveen M, Kumar S. Acetylcholinesterase, acetylcholine in cardiac tissues and cardiomyopathy. In: Recent trends in the acetylcholinesterase system (Ed. M Parveen and S Kumar) 1-10. IOS Press, Netherland. 2005.
77. Paspa P, Vassalle M. Mechanism of caffeine-induced arrhythmias in canine cardiac Purkinje fibers. Am J Cardiol. 1984;53:313-9.
78. Peper K, Trautwein W. A note on the pacemaker current in Purkinje fibres. Pflügers Arch. 1969;309:356-61.
79. Pliam, MB, Krellenstein DJ, Brooks C McC, Vassalle M. Norepinephrine, potassium and overdrive suppression. Basic Res Cardiol. 1977;72:34-45.

80. Pliam MB, Krellenstein DJ, Vassalle M, Brooks C McC. Influence of the sympathetic system on the pacemaker suppression which follows overdrive. Circulation. 1973;48:313-21.
81. Pliam MB, Krellenstein DJ, Vassalle M, Brooks C McC. The influence of norepinephrine, reserpine and propranolol on overdrive suppression. J Electrocardiol. 1975;8:17-24.
82. Qu Y, Karnabi E, Chahine M, Vassalle M, Boutjdir M. Expression of skeletal muscle Na(V)1.4 Na channel isoform in canine cardiac Purkinje myocytes. Biochem Biophys Res Commun. 2007;355:28-33 Epub.
83. Ravens U, Cerbai E. Role of potassium currents in cardiac arrhythmias. Europace. 2008;10:1133-7.
84. Roberts J, Stadter RP. Effect of reserpine on ventricular escape. Science. 1960;132:1836-7
85. Rota M, Vassalle M. Patch-clamp analysis in canine cardiac Purkinje cells of a novel sodium component in the pacemaker range. J Physiol (London). 2003;548:147-65.
86. Satoh H, Hasegawa J, Vassalle M. On the characteristics of the inward tail current induced by calcium overload. J Mol Cell Cardiol. 1989;21: 5-20.
87. Satoh H, Vassalle M. Role of calcium in caffeine-norepinephrine interactions in cardiac Purkinje fibers. Am J Physiol. 1989;257:H226-H37.
88. Shen J-B, Vassalle M. Cesium abolishes the barium-induced pacemaker potential and current in guinea pig ventricular myocytes. J Cardiovasc Electrophysiol. 1994;5:1031-44.
89. Spiegler P, Vassalle M. Role of voltage oscillations in the automaticity of sheep cardiac Purkinje fibers. Can J Physiol Pharmacol. 1995;73:1165-80.
90. Sternlicht JP, Vassalle M. Cesium, Na^+-K^+ pump and pacemaker potential in cardiac Purkinje fibers. J Biomed Sci. 1995;2:366-78.
91. Stuckey JH, Levine MJ, Vassalle M. On the sympathetic control of ventricular automaticity: the effects of a reflex increase of sympathetic discharge. Am J Cardiol. 1969;23:822-9.
92. Szabo B, Sweidan R, Rajagopalan CV, Lazzara R. Role of Na^+:Ca^{2+} exchange current in Cs^+-induced early afterdepolarizations in Purkinje fibers. J Cardiovasc Electrophysiol. 1994;5:933-44.
93. Taal W, van der Dussen DH, van Erven L, van Dijk JG. Neurally-mediated complete heart block. Case Report Lancet Neurol. 2003;2:255-6.
94. Tamargo J, Vassalle M. Mechanisms by which calcium modulates diastolic depolarization in sheep Purkinje fibers. J Electrocardiol. 1991;24:349-61.
95. Trautwein W, Kassebaum DG. On the mechanism of spontaneous impulse generation in the pacemaker of the heart. J Gen Physiol. 1961;45:317-30.
96. Ulbricht W. Effects of veratridine on sodium currents and fluxes. Rev Physiol Biochem Pharmacol. 1998;133:1-54.
97. Valenzuela F, Vassalle M. Interaction between overdrive excitation and overdrive suppression in canine Purkinje fibres. Cardiovasc Res. 1983;17:608-19.
98. Valenzuela F, Vassalle M. Overdrive excitation and cellular calcium load in canine cardiac Purkinje fibers. J Electrocardiol. 1985;18:21-34.
99. Valenzuela F, Vassalle M. On the mechanism of barium induced diastolic depolarization in isolated ventricular myocytes. Cardiovasc Res. 1989;23:390-9.
100. Vassalle M, Lin C-I. Effect of calcium on strophanthidin-induced electrical and mechanical toxicity in cardiac Purkinje fibers. Am J Physiol. 1979;236:H689-H97.
101. Vassalle M, Bocchi L, Du F. Slowly inactivating sodium current (I_{Na2}) in the plateau range in canine cardiac Purkinje single cells. Exper Physiol. 2007;92.1:161-73.
102. Vassalle M, Caress DL, Slovin AJ and Stuckey JH. On the cause of ventricular asystole during vagal stimulation. Circ Res. 1967a;20:228-41.
103. Vassalle M, Catanzaro JN, Nett MP, Rota M. Essential role of diastolic oscillatory potentials in adrenergic control of guinea pig sinoatrial node discharge. J Biomed Sci. 2009;16:101 doi:10.1186/1423-0127-16-101.

104. Vassalle M, Greenspan K, Jomain S, Hoffman BF. Effect of potassium on automaticity and conduction of canine heart. Am J Physiol. 1964;207:334-40.
105. Vassalle M, Greenspan K, Hoffman BF. An analysis of arrhythmias induced by ouabain in intact dogs. Circ Res. 1963;13:132-48.
106. Vassalle M, Greneider JK, Stuckey JH. Role of the sympathetic nervous system in the sinus node resistance to high potassium. Circ Res. 1973;32:348-54.
107. Vassalle M, Karis J, Hoffman BF. Toxic effects of ouabain on Purkinje fibers and ventricular muscle fibers. Am J Physiol. 1962;203:433-9.
108. Vassalle M, Knob RE, Cummins M, Lara GA, Castro C and Stuckey JH. An analysis of fast idioventricular rhythm in the dog. Circ Res. 1977a;41:218-26.
109. Vassalle M, Knob RE, Lara GA, Stuckey JH. The effect of adrenergic enhancement on overdrive excitation. J Electrocardiol. 1976b;9:335-43.
110. Vassalle M, Kotake H, Lin CI. Pacemaker current, membrane resistance, and K^+ in sheep cardiac Purkinje fibres. Cardiovasc Res. 1992;26:383-91.
111. Vassalle M, Krellenstein DJ, Pliam MB, Brooks C, Brooks McC. Potassium-related humoral transmission of overdrive suppression. J Mol Cell Cardiol. 1977b;9:921-31.
112. Vassalle M, Levine MJ, Stuckey JH. On the sympathetic control of ventricular automaticity: the effects of stellate ganglion stimulation. Circ Res. 1968;23:249-58.
113. Vassalle M, Stuckey JH and Levine MJ. Sympathetic control of ventricular automaticity: role of the adrenal medulla. Am J Physiol. 1969;217:930-7.
114. Vassalle M, Vagnini FJ, Gourin A, Stuckey JH. Suppression, initiation of idioventricular automaticity during vagal stimulation. Am J Physiol. 1967b;212:1-7.
115. Vassalle M, Yu H, Cohen IS. The pacemaker current in cardiac Purkinje myocytes. J Gen Physiol. 1995;106:559-78.
116. Vassalle M, Yu H, Cohen IS. Pacemaker channels, cardiac automaticity. In: Cardiac Electrophysiology. From Cell to Bedside. (Eds.DP Zipes and J Jalife), WB Saunders Company, Philadelphia. 1999;94-103.
117. Vassalle M. Cardiac pacemaker potentials at different extra, intracellular K concentrations. Am J Physiol. 1965;208:770-5.
118. Vassalle M. Analysis of cardiac pacemaker potential using a "voltage clamp" technique. Am J Physiol. 1966;210:1335-41.
119. Vassalle M. Electrogenic suppression of automaticity in sheep and dog Purkinje fibers. Circ Res. 1970;27:361-77.
120. Vassalle M. The relationship among cardiac pacemakers: Overdrive suppression. Circ Res. 1977a;41:269-77.
121. Vassalle M. Generation, conduction of impulses in the heart under physiological and pathological conditions. Pharmac Ther B. 1977b;3:1-39.
122. Vassalle M. The role of the electrogenic sodium pump in controlling excitability in nerve, cardiac fibers. In: Electrogenic Ion Pumps (Ed. CL Slayman) Academic Press, New York. 1982;467-83.
123. Vassalle M. Physiological basis of normal, abnormal automaticity. In: Frontiers of Cardiac Electrophysiology (Ed. MB Rosenbaum and MV Elizari), Martinus Nijhoff Publishers Boston. 1983;120-43.
124. Vassalle M. Contribution of the Na^+/K^+-pump to the membrane potential. Experientia. 1987;43:1135-40.
125. Vassalle M. Overdrive suppression, overdrive excitation. In Cardiac Electrophysiology: A textbook (Eds. MR Rosen, MJ Janse and AL Wit), section 2.2 pp. 1-15, Futura Publishing Co., Inc., Mount Kisco, New York. 1990.
126. Vassalle M. Mechanisms underlying cardiac pacemaker activity. J Med Sci. 2003;23:249-64.
127. Vassalle M. The vicissitudes of the pacemaker current I_{Kdd} of cardiac Purkinje fibers. J Biomed Sci 2007;14(6): 699-716. On line 2007, DOI 10.1007/s11373-007-9182-2.

128. Vassalle M and Barnabei O. Norepinephrine, potassium fluxes in cardiac Purkinje fibers. Pflügers Arch. 1971;322:287-303.

129. Vassalle M, Bhattacharyya M. Local anesthetics and the role of sodium in the force development by canine ventricular muscle and Purkinje fibers. Circ Res. 1980;47:666-74.

130. Vassalle M, Bhattacharyya ML. Interactions of norepinephrine and strophanthidin in cardiac Purkinje fibers. Internat J Cardiol. 1981;1:179-94.

131. Vassalle M, Bocchi L. Slow sodium current I_{Na2} and frequency changes in Purkinje cells. FASEB J. 2007;21: Abs. 956.5.

132. Vassalle M, Carpentier R. Hyperpolarizing and depolarizing effects of norepinephrine in cardiac Purkinje fibers. In: Research in Physiology, A Liber Memorialis in Honor of Prof. C. McC. Brooks. (Eds. FF Kao, K Koizumi and M Vassalle) 373-88,Gaggi Publisher, Bologna. 1971.

133. Vassalle M, Carpentier R. Overdrive excitation: the initiation of spontaneous activity in Purkinje fibers following a fast drive in the presence of norepinephrine. Pflügers Arch. 1972;332:198-205.

134. Vassalle M, Di Gennaro M. Caffeine actions on currents induced by calcium overload in Purkinje fibers. Europ J Pharmacol. 1984;106:121-31.

135. Vassalle M, Hoffman BF. The spread of sinus activation during potassium administration. Circ Res. 1965;17:285-95.

136. Vassalle M, Lee, CO. The relationship among intracellular sodium activity, calcium, and strophanthidin inotropy in canine cardiac Purkinje fibers. J Gen Physiol. 1984;83:287-307.

137. Vassalle M, Lin C-I. Calcium overload, cardiac function. J Biomed Sci. 2004;11:542-65.

138. Vassalle M, Mugelli A. An oscillatory current in sheep cardiac Purkinje fibers. Circ Res. 1981;48:618-31.

139. Vassalle M, Musso E. On the mechanisms underlying digitalis toxicity in cardiac Purkinje fibers, in: Recent Advances in Studies on Cardiac Structure and Metabolism. Vol., 9. The Sarcolemma. (Eds P-E Royand and NS Dhalla), 355-76, University Press, Baltimore. 1976.

140. Vick RL. Suppression of latent cardiac pacemaker; relation to slow diastolic depolarization. Am J Physiol. 1969;271:451-7.

141. Wang Q, Shen J, Splawski I, Atkinson D, Li Z, Robinson JL, Moss AJ, Towbin JA and Keating MT. SCN5A mutations associated with an inherited cardiac arrhythmia, long QT syndrome Cell. 1995;80:805-11.

142. Weidmann S. Elektrophysiologie der Herzmuskelfaser. Bern: Medizinischer Verlag Hans Huber. 1956.

143. Yu H, Chang F and Cohen IS. Pacemaker current exists in ventricular myocytes. Circ Res. 1993;72:232-6.

144. Zhang H, Vassalle M. Role of dual pacemaker mechanisms in sinoatrial node discharge. J Biomed Sci. 2000;7:100-13.

Chapter

4

Sympathetic Innervations in Human Heart

Marcellino Monda, Giovanni Messina, Andrea Viggiano, Gennaro Izzo, Domenico Tafuri, Vincenzo De Luca

Abstract. This chapter reports the role played by the sympathetic innervation on physilogical and pathophysiological mechanisms of heart functions. The sympathetic activity increases the cardiac variables: Frequency of beats, velocity of conduction, excitability and inotropic properties. Aspects of anatomical development of the cardiac sympathetic nerves are reported to underline the influence of nerve sprouting on heart diseases. The importance of heart rate variability as a tool of sympathetic activity measurement is discussed.

Keywords. Cardiac properties, heart diseases, heart rate variability, vegetative regulation.

INTRODUCTION

The heart is extensively innervated by autonomic nervous system. The sympathetic nerves release norepinephrine that increases the heart rate, velocity of conduction, as well as myocardial contraction and relaxation. Density of sympathetic innervations, which is high in the subepicardium and the central conduction and it is stringently controlled in the heart (Ieda et al 2007). Regional differences in sympathetic innervation correspond to different areas of influence over cardiac function to effectively control heart rate and myocardial contraction and relaxation.

Autonomic control of pacemaker activity *in vivo* is based on concomitant input from sympathetic and parasympathetic limbs. However, the ratio between vagal and sympathetic input varies in a species-dependent way. The impact of sympathovagal balance on the heart rate can be appreciated by comparing basal rates in different mammalian species in the presence and in the absence of autonomic input. In mammals, basal heart rates are inversely correlated with the body weight. Smaller mammals such as mice and bats have fast heart rate, ranging from ~500 beats/min in mice during daytime to 800–1,000 beats/min in flying bats. In contrast, the heart rate in medium-sized and larger mammals can vary between 60 and 70 beats/min in humans and ~20 beats/min in whales (Opthof 2000). Isolated hearts and sinoatrial node (SAN) pacemaker cells also show a wide range of basal rates and maintain the same rate-to-animal weight ratio as in the presence of an autonomic input. The intrinsic properties of pacemaker cells in different species are one of the bases of the variability of heart rate in mammals. However, the species-dependent balance between sympathetic and parasympathetic input also contributes to this wide range of pacemaking frequencies. The two branches of the autonomic nervous system interact to generate an adaptable equilibrium so that SAN automaticity can be under dominance of the sympathetic or parasympathetic limb. Sympathovagal dominance is generally assessed *in vivo* by pharmacological inhibition of the autonomic input by combined injection of atropine and propranolol. Even if propranolol does not block α-adrenergic receptors, the heart rate measured under these conditions constitutes a reliable estimate of the intrinsic pacing rate of a "denervated" heart (Beau et al 1995).

In animals, the beating frequency of the isolated SAN is also an index of the intrinsic heart rate. In the mouse, the intrinsic SAN rate is significantly lower than the *in vivo* heart rate, indicating the existence of a significant sympathetic tone in this species (Gehrmann et al 2000). In contrast, it can be shown that dogs and humans are under prominent vagal tone, since pharmacological block of the autonomic input significantly accelerates the basal heart rate (Opthof 2000). However, adrenergic dominance does not demonstrate the absence of a vagal tone. For example, the presence of vagal tone in small rodents can be easily demonstrated by injection of atropine in freely moving mice.

SYMPATHETIC REGULATION OF PACEMAKER ACTIVITY

Activation of the β-adrenergic receptor underlies the positive chronotropic effect induced by catecholamines on automaticity. Catecholamines enhance the activity of ion channels as well as intracellular Ca^{2+} release. The relative importance of sarcolemmal ion channels in the β-adrenergic regulation of pacemaker activity is still debated.

I_f and $I_{Ca,L}$ have been proposed to constitute important mechanisms in heart rate acceleration by catecholamines (Brown et al 1979, Bucchi et al 2003, DiFrancesco 1993). The open probability of f-channels increases even for a small augmentation of intracellular cAMP. A rise in cAMP positively shifts the I_f activation curve, thereby supplying more inward current during the linear part of diastolic depolarization. DiFrancesco has proposed that I_f is the predominant mechanism for increasing the slope of the diastolic depolarization at low adrenergic tone. This is based on the observation that low doses of the β-adrenergic agonist isoproterenol (which is supposed to mimic weak adrenergic activity) increase the slope of the diastolic depolarization without affecting the action potential waveform (DiFrancesco 1993). Remarkably, specific regulation of the diastolic depolarization slope is a common property of low doses of autonomic agonists and selective I_f blockers (Baruscotti et al 2005).

The functional role of $I_{Ca,L}$ in adrenergic regulation of heart rate is still unresolved. Three lines of indirect evidence are suggestive of a role of $I_{Ca,L}$ in the sympathetic regulation of heart rate. First, catecholamines robustly enhance $I_{Ca,L}$ in the same concentration range as pacemaker activity. I_f and $I_{Ca,L}$ have similar sensitivity to isoproterenol in rabbit SAN cells. Second, it has been reported that DHPs reduce the positive chronotropic response of mouse atria to stimulation of the stellate ganglion. Third, the contribution of $Ca_v1.3$ channels in the generation of the diastolic depolarization in mouse SAN cells suggests that $I_{Ca,L}$ can constitute an important mechanism for accelerating the diastolic depolarization slope upon activation of β-adrenergic receptors. Consistent with this hypothesis, the positive chronotropic response to isoproterenol of isolated $Ca_v1.3^{-/-}$ hearts is moderately reduced. However, the *in vivo* heart rate of mice lacking $Ca_v1.3$ channels is comparable to that of wild-type mice. The maximal heart rates of wild-type and $Ca_v1.3^{-/-}$ mice are significantly reduced by selective I_f block by ivabradine. Taken together, these observations are suggestive of a distinct role of f-channels and $Ca_v1.3$ channels in the autonomic regulation of heart rate (Herrmann et al 2007).

SYMPATHETIC NERVES AND HEART DISEASES

Sympathetic nerve fibers are located subepicardially and travel along the routes of the major coronary arteries. In contrast, the vagus nerve is subendocardial in its location after it crosses the atrioventricular groove. A lesion of the heart produced by infarct or fibrosis can result in denervation of otherwise normal myocardium by interruption of neural axons traveling through the lesion. A defect in sympathetic function following myocardial infarction (MI) has been demonstrated in both animals and humans as measured by iodine-123-metaiodobenzylguanidine (MIBG) and C-11 hydroxyephedrine (Stanton et al 1989).

Reduced uptake of MIBG in the inferior wall has recently been observed in patients with idiopathic ventricular fibrillation as compared with controls. Although no difference in survival could be detected between the two groups, patients with reduced uptake of MIBG had an increased incidence of ventricular tachyarrhythmias compared with those who did not have such a defect (Paul et al 2006).

Similar observations of sympathetic dysfunction have been made in a variety of animal models and humans with heart failure, coronary disease, and ventricular tachycardia in the absence of structural heart disease. In such instances, the speculation is that sympathetic heterogeneity may produce electrical heterogeneity and spur the development of ventricular arrhythmias. The arrhythmic mechanism is probably more complex than this description, however, because the response to sympathetic inhibition using β-blockers is not uniform.

Since the cardiac sympathetic discharge plays a significant role in clinical aspects of heart diseases, it is important to know the developmental and regulatory mechanisms underlying cardiac sympathetic innervation patterning. The density of cardiac innervation is altered in diseased hearts, as in cases of congestive heart failure and myocardial infarction. Following myocardial injury, cardiac nerves undergo Wallerian degeneration, which may be followed by neurilemmal cell proliferation and axonal regeneration, resulting in heterogeneous innervation.

Unbalanced sympathetic innervation may trigger lethal arrhythmia through ion channel modulation in cardiomyocytes (Chen et al 2007). Also of clinical concern is the development of cardiac sensory denervation in diabetic patients. As the sensory nervous system is responsible for pain perception, cardiac sensory denervation can lead to diabetic sensory neuropathy and silent myocardial ischemia. This condition is characterized by loss of pain perception during myocardial ischemia and frequently leads to sudden cardiac death (SCD) in diabetic patients.

DEVELOPMENT OF CARDIAC INNERVATION

Neural crest cells migrate and form sympathetic ganglia by mid-gestation and subsequently proliferate and differentiate into mature neurons (Loring and Erickson 1987). The cardiac sympathetic nerves extend from the sympathetic neurons in stellate ganglia, which are located bilateral to the vertebra. Sympathetic nerve fibers project from the base of the heart into the myocardium and are located predominantly in the subepicardium of the ventricle. The central conduction system, which includes the sinoatrial node, atrioventricular node, and His bundle, is abundantly innervated compared with the working myocardium. This regional difference in cardiac sympathetic innervation (innervation patterning) is highly conserved among mammals.

The cardiac nervous system also involves afferent nerves. The sensory signals generated in the heart are conducted through cardiac afferent nerves, primarily thinly myelinated Aδ-fibers and nonmyelinated C-fibers. The sensory nerve fibers project to the upper thoracic dorsal horn via dorsal root ganglia neurons, which are also derived from neural crest cells. A major challenge to analysis of cardiac innervation of the heart has been the lack of suitable molecular markers. Recent advances in immunohistochemical technology now allow autonomic nerves to be stained using antibodies against nerve-specific markers, such as tyrosine hydroxylase (TH), a sympathetic marker; calcitonin gene-related peptide (CGRP), a sensory marker; protein gene product 9.5, a general peripheral nerve marker; and growth-associated protein 43, a nerve sprouting marker.

These specific neural markers to demonstrate that the organization of cardiac innervation is strictly controlled in the heart during development, whereas in diseased hearts, innervation density and organization are dramatically altered. Cardiac nerves are highly plastic, and innervation patterning is strictly controlled by the balance between NGF and Sema3a synthesized in the heart.

NERVE SPROUTING AND SCD

Sympathetic stimulation is important in the generation of SCD in diseased hearts. There is circadian variation in the frequency of SCD that parallels sympathetic nerve activity. β-blocker therapy prevents SCD secondary to ventricular tachyarrhythmia in ischemic heart disease or congestive heart failure. Immunohistochemical analysis of cardiac nerves in explanted hearts of transplant recipients reveals a positive correlation between nerve density and clinical history of ventricular tachyarrhythmia (Cao et al 2000b).

ROLE OF NERVE GROWTH FACTOR (NGF)

Sympathetic hypersensitivity has been shown in areas of denervation, which may be related in part to nerve sprouting. Other sympathetic and electrical phenomena following myocardial injury include an upregulation of NGF, a heterogeneous distribution of sympathetic innervation, and electrical heterogeneity with areas of denervation, hyperinnervation, and normal nerve density. NGF which is critical for sympathetic nerve sprouting, is upregulated after myocardial infarction (MI) in animal models, resulting in the regeneration of cardiac sympathetic nerves and heterogeneous innervation (Zhou et al 2004). Augmented myocardial nerve sprouting through NGF infusion after MI results in a dramatic increase in SCD and a high incidence of ventricular tachyarrhythmia, compared with animals not receiving NGF infusion (Cao et al 2000a). These results demonstrate that NGF upregulation and nerve sprouting in diseased hearts may cause lethal arrhythmia and SCD. However, the molecular mechanisms that regulate NGF expression and sympathetic innervation in the heart are poorly understood. The endothelin-1 (ET-1) / NGF pathway is critical for cardiac sympathetic innervation. In general, the growth-cone behavior of nerves is modulated by coincident signaling modulated by neural chemoattractants and chemorepellents synthesized in the innervated tissue. NGF, a potent neural chemoattractant, is a prototypic member of the neurotrophin family that plays critical roles in the differentiation, survival, and synaptic activity of the peripheral sympathetic and sensory nervous systems (Snider 1994). The level of NGF expression within innervated tissue corresponds approximately to innervation density. NGF expression increases during development and is altered in diseased hearts. ET-1 is a critical factor in the pathogenesis of cardiac hypertrophy, hypertension, and atherosclerosis. Gene targeting of ET-1 and its receptor ETA results in unexpected craniofacial and cardiovascular abnormalities not observed in other hypertrophic factor–deficient mice (Kurihara et al 1995). Although these phenotypes are consistent with interference of neural crest differentiation, the role of ET-1 in neural crest development remains undetermined.

ET-1 affects the induction of neurotrophic factors and that the disruption of ET-1 contributes to the immature development of neural crest–derived cells. ET-1, but not angiotensin II, phenylephrine, leukemia inhibitory factor, or IGF-1, upregulates NGF expression in primary cultured cardiomyocytes (Ieda et al 2004). ET-1–induced NGF augmentation is not observed in cardiac fibroblasts and is specific to cardiomyocytes. ET-1–induced NGF augmentation is mediated via the ETA receptor, Giβγ, PKC, the Src family, EGFR, extracellular signal-regulated kinase, p38MAPK, activator protein-1, and the CCAAT/enhancer-binding protein δ element. To study the role of the ET-1/NGF pathway in the development of the cardiac sympathetic nervous system, various mouse models of modified genes have been analyzed. NGF expression, cardiac sympathetic innervation, and norepinephrine concentration are reduced in ET-1–deficient mouse (Edn1–/–) hearts, but not in the hearts of angiotensinogen-deficient mice (Atg–/–). In Edn1–/– mice, the sympathetic stellate ganglia exhibited excessive apoptosis and display loss of neurons at the late embryonic stage. Moreover, we demonstrate that cardiac-specific overexpression of NGF in Edn1–/– mice rescues the heart from sympathetic nerve retardation.

These findings indicate that ET-1 is a key regulator of NGF expression in cardiomyocytes and that the ET-1 /NGF pathway is critical for sympathetic innervation in the heart. Given that ET-1 is strongly induced in pathological conditions, the ET-1/NGF pathway may also be involved in NGF upregulation and nerve regeneration after myocardial infarction.

Infusion of nerve growth factor into the stellate ganglion prolongs the QT interval and prolongs ventricular arrhythmias (Cao et al 2000a). A relationship has been established between the hyperinnervation that occurs following myocardial injury and ventricular arrhythmias. Using immunocytochemical staining in explanted native hearts of transplant recipients, Chen and colleagues demonstrated colocalization of Schwann cells, sympathetic nerves, and nerve axons, as well as regional cardiac hyperinnervation, with the most abundant nerve sprouting in the areas bordering myocardial injury and normal myocardium. In addition, they demonstrated positive tyrosine hydroxylase staining of cardiac nerves in areas around coronary arteries in patients with coronary disease and idiopathic dilated nonischemic cardiomyopathy. At the origin of ventricular tachycardia (prior to transplant), nerve sprouting was shown by staining for S100 protein and tyrosine hydroxylase. The authors hypothesized that nerve sprouting may give rise to ventricular arrhythmia and sudden cardiac death, in which MI results in nerve injury, followed by sympathetic nerve sprouting and regional myocardial hyperinnervation (Cao et al 2000a).

ROLE OF THE CLASS 3 SECRETED SEMAPHORIN (SEMA3A)

Sema3a is critical for cardiac sympathetic innervation patterning, NGF plays critical roles in cardiac nerve development. In contrast, the neural chemorepellent that induces growth-cone collapse and repels nerve axons has not been identified in the heart. Sema3a, has been cloned and identified as a potent neural chemorepellent and a directional guidance molecule for nerve fibers (Puschel et al 1995, Kawasaki et al 2002, Taniguchi et al 1997).

However, it is not known whether cardiomyocytes produce Sema3a, and if so, whether this protein affects sympathetic neural patterning and cardiac performance. TH-immunopositive sympathetic nerve endings appear on the epicardial surface at embryonic day (E)15 and gradually increase in number in the myocardium after postnatal day (P)7 and P42. In the ventricular myocardium, sympathetic nerves are more abundant in the subepicardium than in the subendocardium, suggesting an epicardial-to-endocardial gradient. Various studies analyzed heterozygous Sema3a knocked-in lacZ mice (Sema3alacZ/+) to identify the Sema3a expression pattern and its relationship to innervation patterning in the heart.

At E12, lacZ expression was detected strongly in the heart, especially in the trabecular components of the ventricles. In E15 hearts, lacZ expression was observed in the subendocardium but not in the subepicardium of the atria and ventricles. At P1 and P42, lacZ expression was reduced in certain regions and highlighted the Purkinje fiber network along the ventricular free wall. Quantitative RT-PCR of Sema3a in developing hearts confirmed the presence of Sema3a from E12 and the subsequent linear decrease in expression. The spatial and temporal expression pattern of Sema3a contrasts directly with the patterning of sympathetic innervation in developing hearts. These results indicate that Sema3a is a negative regulator of cardiac innervation.

Studies have analyzed Sema3a-deficient mice (Sema3a−/−) to investigate whether Sema3a is critical for cardiac sympathetic nerve development. The WT hearts show a clear epicardial-to-endocardial gradient of sympathetic innervation. In contrast, the sympathetic nerve density is lower in the subepicardium and higher in the subendocardium of Sema3a−/− mice, resulting in disruption of the innervation gradient in Sema3a−/− ventricles. The Sema3a−/− mice also exhibit malformation of the stellate ganglia that extend sympathetic nerves to the heart. To investigate whether the abnormal sympathetic innervation patterning in Sema3a−/− hearts is a secondary effect of stellate ganglia malformation, transgenic mice overexpressing Sema3a specifically in the heart (SemaTG) have been generated. SemaTG mice are associated with reduced sympathetic innervation and attenuation of the epicardialto-endocardial innervation gradient. These results indicate that cardiomyocyte-derived Sema3a plays critical roles in cardiac sympathetic innervation by inhibiting neural growth. Since cardiomyocyte-derived NGF acts as a chemoattractant, it is possible that the balance between NGF and Sema3a synthesized in the heart determines cardiac sympathetic innervation patterning. The growth-cone behavior of somatic sensory axons is also modulated by the coincident signaling of NGF and Sema3a (Kitsukawa et al 1997, Wright et al 1995). During development, NGF and Sema3a are expressed within the spinal cord and influence the guidance pathway of sensory axons.

Sema3a is specifically expressed in the ventral half of the spinal cord and mediates the termination of NGFresponsive sensory axons at the dorsal part of the spinal cord. The targeted inactivation of Sema3a disrupts neural patterning and projections in the spinal cord, thereby highlighting the critical role of Sema3a signaling in the directional guidance of nerve fibers (Behar et al 1996).

Most Sema3a−/− mice die within the first postnatal week, with only 20% surviving until weaning. Telemetric electrocardiography and heart rate variability analysis has been performed to identify the cause of death and the effects of abnormal sympathetic neural distribution in Sema3a−/− hearts (Ieda et al 2007). In addition to multiple premature ventricular contractions, Sema3a−/− mice develop sinus bradycardia and abrupt sinus arrest due to sympathetic neural dysfunction. By comparison, the SemaTG mice die suddenly at 10 months of age without symptoms. Sustained ventricular tachyarrhythmia is induced in SemaTG mice, but not in WT mice, after epinephrine administration, and programmed electrical stimulation reveals that SemaTG mice are highly susceptible to ventricular tachyarrhythmia.

The β1-adrenergic receptor density is upregulated and the cAMP response after catecholamine injection is exaggerated in SemaTG ventricles. Action potential duration is significantly prolonged in hypoinnervated SemaTG ventricles, presumably via ion channel modulation. These results suggest that the higher susceptibility of SemaTG mice to ventricular arrhythmia is due, at least in part, to catecholamine supersensitivity and prolonged action potential duration, both of which can augment triggered activity in cardiomyocytes. Thus, Sema3a mediated sympathetic innervation patterning is critical for the maintenance of arrhythmia-free hearts. Sympathetic nerves modulate the function of ion channels and trigger various arrhythmias in diseased hearts (Dae et al 1997, Qu and Robinson 2004). Various studies highlight the importance of regulatory factors in sympathetic innervation patterning. For example, Sema3a–/– mice exhibit sinus bradycardia, abrupt sinus slowing, and stellate ganglia defects. Right stellectomy induces sinus bradycardia and sudden, asystolic death in dogs (Sosunov et al 2001). In addition, Stramba-Badiale et al. report that developmental abnormalities in cardiac innervation may play a role in the genesis of some cases of sudden infant death syndrome (Stramba-Badiale et al 1992). The SemaTG hearts are also highly susceptible to ventricular arrhythmias, albeit without contractile dysfunction or structural defects. Given that catecholamine augments systolic function, it is surprising that SemaTG mice show normal cardiac function. Patients with denervated hearts who undergo heart transplantation do not develop heart failure but approximately 10% of the patients develop SCD (Chantranuwat et al 2004). Together, these studies highlight the significance of cardiac nerve regulation as a new paradigm for the management of SCD.

How sympathetic hyperinnervation promotes cardiac arrhythmias is speculative, but increased density of sympathetic nerve endings could promote the release of sympathetic neurotransmitters during sympathetic excitation. The autonomic remodeling is associated with heterogeneous electrical remodeling of cardiomyocytes, resulting in prolongation of action potentials in hyperinnervated regions. Further, acute release of sympathetic neurotransmitters probably accentuates the heterogeneity of excitability and refractoriness, likely contributing to arrhythmia susceptibility.

PHARMACOLOGIC SYMPATHETIC BLOCKADE

Inhibiting sympathetic activity pharmacologically reduces the incidence of sudden cardiac death in patients with heart failure. In the Eplerenone Postacute Myocardial Infarction Heart Failure Efficacy and Survival Study (EPHESUS), the aldosterone inhibitor eplerenone was associated with a clear reduction in sudden cardiac arrest in patients with acute MI complicated by left ventricular dysfunction (Pitt et al 2006). β-blockers and angiotensin-converting enzyme inhibitors have had the same effect. These findings indicate that adverse electrophysiologic consequences from sympathetic stimulation may contribute to the development of a proarrhythmic substrate, and that antagonizing sympathetic activation can reduce the extent of adverse electrical remodeling to reduce the risk of sudden cardiac death.

HEART RATE VARIABILITY

Heart rate variability is a tool to investigate the activity of the autonomic nervous system. The neural regulation of circulatory function is mainly effected through the interplay of the sympathetic and vagal outflows. This interaction can be explored by assessing cardiovascular rhythmicity with appropriate spectral methodologies. Spectral analysis of cardiovascular signal variability, and in particular of RR period (heart rate variability, HRV), is a widely used procedure to investigate autonomic cardiovascular control and/or target function impairment. The oscillatory pattern which characterizes the spectral profile of heart rate and arterial pressure short-term variability consists of two major components, at low (LF, 0.04-0.15Hz) and high (HF, synchronous with respiratory rate) frequency, respectively, related to vasomotor and respiratory activity. With this procedure the state of sympathovagal balance modulating sinus node pacemaker activity can be quantified in a variety of physiological and pathophysiological conditions. Changes in sympathovagal balance can be often detected in basal conditions, however a reduced responsiveness to an excitatory stimulus is the most common feature that characterizes numerous pathophysiological states. Moreover the attenuation of an oscillatory pattern or its impaired responsiveness to a given stimulus can also reflect an altered target function and thus can furnish interesting prognostic markers. The dynamic assessment of these autonomic changes may provide crucial diagnostic, therapeutic and prognostic information, not only in relation to cardiovascular, but also noncardiovascular disease. As linear methodologies fail to provide significant information in conditions of extremely reduced variability, (e.g. strenuous exercise, heart failure) and in presence of rapid and transients changes or coactivation of the two branches of autonomic nervous system, the development of new nonlinear approaches seems to provide a new perspective in investigating neural control of cardiovascular system.

CONCLUSION

The cardiac sympathetic nerves play an important role in the control of cardiac functions and they exert relevant influences on pathophysiological mechanisms of various heart diseases.

BIBLIOGRAPHY

1. Baruscotti M, Bucchi A, Difrancesco D. Physiology, pharmacology of the cardiac pacemaker ("funny") current. Pharmacol Ther. 2005;107:59-79.
2. Beau SL, Hand DE, Schuessler RB, Bromberg BI, Kwon B, Boineau JP, et al. Relative densities of muscarinic cholinergic, beta-adrenergic receptors in the canine sinoatrial node and their relation to sites of pacemaker activity. Circ Res. 1995;77:957-63.
3. Behar O, Golden JA, Mashimo H, Schoen FJ, Fishman MC. Semaphorin III is needed for normal patterning, growth of nerves, bones, heart. Nature. 1996;383:525-8.
4. Brown HF, DiFrancesco D, Noble SJ. How does adrenaline accelerate the heart? Nature. 1979;280:235-6.
5. Bucchi A, Baruscotti M, Robinson RB, DiFrancesco D. I_f-dependent modulation of pacemaker rate mediated by cAMP in the presence of ryanodine in rabbit sino-atrial node cells. J Mol Cell Cardiol. 2003;35:905-13
6. Cao JM, Chen LS, KenKnight BH, Ohara T, Lee MH, Tsai J. Nerve sprouting and sudden cardiac death. Circ Res. 2000a;86:816-21.
7. Cao JM, Fishbein MC, Han JB, Lai WW, Lai AC, Wu TJ. Relationship between regional cardiac hyperinnervation, ventricular arrhythmia. Circulation. 2000b;101:1960-9.
8. Chantranuwat C, Blakey JD, Kobashigawa JA, Moriguchi JD, Laks H, Vassilakis ME. Sudden, unexpected death in cardiac transplant recipients: An autopsy study. J Heart Lung Transplant. 2004;23:683-9.

9. Chen LS, Zhou S, Fishbein MC, Chen PS. New perspectives on the role of autonomic nervous system in the genesis of arrhythmias. J Cardiovasc Electrophysiol. 2007;18:123-7.
10. Dae MW, Lee RJ, Ursell PC, Chin MC, Stillson CA, Moise NS. Heterogeneous sympathetic innervation in German shepherd dogs with inherited ventricular arrhythmia and sudden cardiac death. Circulation. 1997;96:1337-42.
11. DiFrancesco D. Pacemaker mechanisms in cardiac tissue. Annu Rev Physiol. 1993;55:455-72.
12. Gehrmann J, Hammer PE, Maguire CT, Wakimoto H, Triedman JK, Berul CI. Phenotypic screening for heart rate variability in the mouse. Am J Physiol Heart Circ Physiol. 2000;279:H733-H40.
13. Herrmann S, Stieber J, Stockl G, Hofmann F, Ludwig A. HCN4 provides a "depolarization reserve", is not required for heart rate acceleration in mice. EMBO J. 2007;26:4423-32.
14. Ieda M, Fukuda K, Hisaka Y, Kimura K, Kawaguchi H, Fujita J. Endothelin-1 regulates cardiac sympathetic innervation in the rodent heart by controlling nerve growth factor expression. J Clin Invest. 2004;113:876-84.
15. Ieda M, Kanazawa H, Kimura K, Hattori F, Ieda Y, Taniguchi M. Sema3a maintains normal heart rhythm through sympathetic innervation patterning. Nat Med. 2007;13:604-12.
16. Kawasaki T, Bekku Y, Suto F, Kitsukawa T, Taniguchi M, Nagatsu I. Requirement of neuropilin 1-mediated Sema3A signals in patterning of the sympathetic nervous system. Development. 2002;129:671-80.
17. Kitsukawa T, Shimizu M, Sanbo M, Hirata T, Taniguchi M, Bekku Y. Neuropilin-semaphorin III /D-mediated chemorepulsive signals play a crucial role in peripheral nerve projection in mice. Neuron. 1997;19:995-1005.
18. Kurihara Y, Kurihara H, Oda H, Maemura K, Nagai R, Ishikawa T. Aortic arch malformations, ventricular septal defect in mice deficient in endothelin-1. J Clin Invest. 1995;96:293-300.
19. Loring JF, Erickson CA. Neural crest cell migratory pathways in the trunk of the chick embryo. Dev Biol. 1987;121:220-36.
20. Opthof T. The normal range and determinants of the intrinsic heart rate in man. Cardiovasc Res. 2000;45:177-84
21. Paul M, Schäfers M, Kies P. Impact of sympathetic innervation on recurrent life-threatening arrhythmias in the follow-up of patients with idiopathic ventricular fibrillation. Eur J Nucl Med Mol Imaging. 2006;33:862-5.
22. Pitt B, Gheorghiade M, Zannad F. Evaluation of eplerenone in the subgroup of EPHESUS patients with baseline left ventricular ejection fraction -30%. Eur. J Heart Fail. 2006;8:295-301.
23. Puschel AW, Adams RH, Betz H. Murine semaphorin D/collapsin is a member of a diverse gene family, creates domains inhibitory for axonal extension. Neuron. 1995;14:941-8.
24. Qu J, Robinson RB. Cardiac ion channel expression and regulation: the role of innervation. J Mol Cell Cardiol. 2004;37:439-48.
25. Snider WD. Functions of the neurotrophins during nervous system development: What the knockouts are teaching us. Cell. 1994;77:627-38.
26. Sosunov EA, Anyukhovsky EP, Gainullin RZ, Plotnikov A, Danilo P Jr, Rosen MR. Long-term electrophysiological effects of regional cardiac sympathetic denervation of the neonatal dog. Cardiovasc Res. 2001;51:659-69.
27. Stanton MS, Tuli MM, Radtke NL. Regional sympathetic denervation after myocardial infarction in humans detected noninvasively using I-123-metaiodobenzylguanidine. J Am Coll Cardiol. 1989;14:1519-26.
28. Stramba-Badiale M, Lazzarotti M, Schwartz PJ. Development of cardiac innervation, ventricular fibrillation, and sudden infant death syndrome. Am J Physiol. 1992;263:H1514-22.
29. Taniguchi M, Yuasa S, Fujisawa H, Naruse I, Saga S, Mishina M. Disruption of semaphorin III /D gene causes severe abnormality in peripheral nerve projection. Neuron. 1997;19:519-30.
30. Wright DE, White FA, Gerfen RW, Silos-Santiago I, Snider WD. The guidance molecule semaphorin III is expressed in regions of spinal cord and periphery avoided by growing sensory axons. J Comp Neurol. 1995;361:321-33.
31. Zhou S, Chen LS, Miyauchi Y, Miyauchi M, Kar S, Kangavari S. Mechanisms of cardiac nerve sprouting after myocardial infarction in dogs. Circ Res. 2004;95:76-83.

Chapter

5

Stepwise Approach for Ablation of Persistent Atrial Fibrillation

Matthew Wright, Sebastien Knecht

Abstract. Mechanisms of Chronic AF, Ablation for Persistent AF. The overall prevalence of AF in the Framingham Heart Study was 6% and in people over 40 there was a 16% lifetime chance of developing AF without a history or precedent heart failure or myocardial infarction. Although catheter ablation of persistent AF is a difficult procedure, advances in catheter design and identification of areas that actively participate in the AF process should increase the number of patients that can receive treatment.

Keywords. Atrial fibrillation, catheter ablation, pulmonary vein isolation, electrophysiological mechanisms.

INTRODUCTION

Atrial fibrillation (AF) is the most common cardiac arrhythmia responsible for approximately a third of all hospital admissions with a cardiac rhythm disturbance (Fuster et al 2006). The incidence and prevalence of AF in the general population are rising (Stewart et al 2001), and it is estimated that 15.9 million people will have AF by 2050 in the USA alone (Miyasaka et al 2006) if the incidence continues to rise at it has in the past 2 decades. The overall prevalence of AF in the Framingham Heart Study was 6% and in people over 40 there was a 16% lifetime chance of developing AF without a history or precedent heart failure or myocardial infarction. In those over 75 years of age the prevalence is estimated at 10% (Hobbs et al 2005). AF is associated with an increased risk of all cause mortality, heart failure and stroke (Stewart et al 2001, Benjamin et al 1998, Stewart et al 2002) and it is also responsible for about one third of all hospitalisations with cardiac rhythm disturbance. It is responsible for an increased risk of stroke, heart failure and all-cause mortality (Stewart et al 2002, Krahn et al 1995). The vast improvement in results of catheter ablation compared to pharmacological treatment. Over the last decade means that catheter ablation can be considered early in the management of patients. Yet there is room for improvement before this can be the initial treatment of choice, particularly in the case of chronic AF. As a consequence, AF constitutes a major socioeconomic and healthcare problem. It has been calculated that for the ageing UK's population over 0.9% of the entire NHS budget is already spent on managing AF and its consequences, principally that of stroke (Stewart et al 2004) and in the USA an estimated $6-7 billion dollars is spent on AF management per year (Kozak et al 2003).

Although no difference in mortality has been proven using antiarrhythmic medication (Wyse et al 2002), a rhythm or a rate control strategy has to be considered in symptomatic patients (Van Gelder et al 2002). If a rhythm control strategy is preferred, the first step still consists of trying at least one antiarrhythmic drug. In patients with symptomatic persistent AF maintenance of sinus rhythm at 1 year varies between 41% and 62% for sotalol and amodarone respectively (Singh et al 2005). In the combined results from EURIDIS and ADONIS which enrolled a combination of patients with typical atrial flutter, paroxysmal and persistent AF, only 38% had remained in sinus rhythm at 1 year with dronedarone (Singh et al 2007).

In comparison catheter ablation for paroxysmal AF has a one year success rate of between 69 and 87% (Oral et al 2002, 2004, Jais et al 2004, Hocini et al 2005, Gerstenfeld et al 2006, Mainigi et al 2007), and many groups report success rates over 70% for persistent AF (O'Neill et al 2009, Della Bella et al 2009, Estner et al 2008, Chen et al 2008, Fiala et al 2008, Verma et al 2007, Seow et al 2007, Sanders et al 2007, Calo et al 2006, Willems et al 2006, Fassini et al 2005, Haissaguerre et al 2005, Haissaguerre et al 2005, Oral et al 2005), including patients with long-standing persistent AF, off antiarrhythmic drugs.

From this data, it seems clear that catheter ablation is superior to anti-arrhythmic drugs in restoring and maintaining sinus rhythm over the long-term in patients with both paroxysmal and persistent AF. However, it has to be emphasized that the endpoints were not all the same in the different studies, as in ablation studies, success is defined as the absence of arrhythmia recurrences (AF and atrial tachycardia(AT)) whereas in several pharmacological studies the presence of sinus rhythm at the final follow-up has been considered a success regardless of any intervening periods of AF. For example, in AF-CHF, 73% of patients in the antiarrhythmic group were in sinus rhythm at last follow-up, however 58% of patients in this same group had experienced at least 1 episode of AF during the study period (Roy et al 2008). Additionally, patients in ablation studies are for the most part attempting second-line therapy as opposed to antiarrhythmic drug trials, where a significant proportion of patients were enrolled after a first episode, and may represent a lower risk and easier to treat population.

Great efforts are being made in order to improve the success rates of catheter ablation for AF, which, correctly, are not deemed good enough when compared to ablation of other cardiac arrhythmias. However, the success rates of antiarrhythmic drugs in preventing AF are poor when judged by similar standards. The current HRS/EHRA/ECAS guidelines on catheter ablation of AF support catheter ablation for symptomatic patients in whom at least one antiarrhythmic drug has failed or has not been tolerated (Calkins et al 2007).

MECHANISMS OF CHRONIC AF

Catheter ablation of AF has been successful without a complete understanding of the mechanisms underlying the fibrillatory process. The multiple wavelet hypothesis, proposed by Moe (Moe and Abildskov 1959), with supportive/contributory experimental work by Alessie (Allessie et al 1985) was the predominant hypothesis prior to the late 1990s, and was the premise on which Cox's Maze procedure was developed. The developments of the Maze procedure, culminated in the Maze III (Cox et al 1991), which incorporates 4 lesions sets; (i) Encirclement of the pulmonary veins; (ii) A lesion joining the circumferential PV lesion to the mitral annulus; (iii) A circumferential lesion in the coronary sinus; (iv) Cryoablation of the cavotricuspid isthmus. Although catheter ablation approaches based on the early surgical approaches were tried by a number of groups, the success rate was disappointing, with an unacceptable high complication rate (Schwartz et al 1993, Haissaguerre 1996).

In the late 1990s, the pivotal role of the pulmonary veins (PV) in triggering paroxysmal AF was recognised (Haissaguerre et al 1998). This led to attempts at treating focal sources that triggered AF rather than compartmentalising the atria (Haissaguerre et al 2000). By mapping the atria it was observed that paroxysmal AF was triggered by ectopic beats originating from within the PV's, and that by electrically isolating the PV's, AF was eliminated (Haissaguerre et al 2000). Other reports also demonstrated the importance of PV's for AF perpetuation through automatic or reentrant mechanisms (Hocini et al 2002, Jais et al 2002). A "venous wave hypothesis" has therefore been proposed as the main electrophysiological mechanisms of paroxysmal AF, implicating PV's as the exclusive sources of "venous waves/drivers" maintaining the atria in fibrillation (Haissaguerre et al 2004). For both paroxysmal and persistent AF, isolated sources maintaining AF within the left atrium and coronary sinus have been observed (Mainigi et al 2007, Rostock et al 2006, Haissaguerre et al 2006, Knecht et al 2007).

ABLATION FOR PERSISTENT AF

Although pulmonary vein isolation (PVI) without additional ablation has been attempted for patients with persistent AF, the success rates with this approach are disappointing. Pulmonary vein isolation without additional ablation has been reported to be successful in between 20% to 61% of cases, and ablation at sites of complex fractionated atrial electrograms (CFAE) alone has been reported to be successful in between 9% and 85% of cases (Estner et al 2008, Willems et al 2006, Fassini et al 2005, Yoshida et al 2008, Neumann et al 2008, Elayi et al 2008, Nademanee et al 2008, Oral et al 2007, Arentz et al 2007, Lim et al 2006, Nademanee et al 2004, Arentz et al 2003, Estner et al 2008), although some investigators have reported success rates of up to 95% with PVI alone (Ouyang et al 2005, Chen et al 2004). For the majority of patients with persistent AF however, PVI alone is insufficient (Oral et al 2002). Strategies that have combined two techniques such as PVI and complex and fractionated atrial electrogram ablation, or PVI and linear ablation, or PVI, ablation of complex and fractionated electrograms and linear lesions have achieved success rates of between 42% to 95% without antiarrhythmic drugs, with most centers reporting success rates of over 70% in the short to medium term (O'Neill et al 2009, Della Bella et al 2009, Estner et al 2008, Chen et al 2008, Fiala et al 2008, Verma et al 2007, Seow et al 2007, Sanders et al 2007, Calo et al 2006, Willems et al 2006, Fassini et al 2005, Haissaguerre et al 2005, Haissaguerre et al 2005, Oral et al 2005) Importantly, two or more procedures are often necessary in order to cure persistent AF or secondary atrial tachycardia, and patients considering ablative treatment should be aware that approximately half require more than one procedure (O'Neill et al 2009).

CATHETER ABLATION OF PERSISTENT AF: THE STEPWISE APPROACH

During persistent AF, catheter ablation progressively targets all structures potentially contributing to initiation and maintenance of AF: PV's, left atrial (LA) tissue, linear ablation of the LA roof and mitral isthmus, and right atrial (RA) targets. Each region is ablated following a sequential approach until AF termination, and the impact of ablation is assessed by measurement of AF cycle length in both appendages. Each step is accompanied by an increase in AF cycle length until conversion of AF directly to sinus rhythm or more often to multiple ATs that are then systematically ablated (O'Neill et al 2009, Haissaguerre et al 2005, Haissaguerre et al 2005).

This sequential approach has resulted in unprecedented success in maintaining sinus rhythm in the medium term with recovery of atrial mechanical function in patients with longstanding persistent AF (Takahashi et al 2007). Termination of AF occurs in 82 to 87% (O'Neill et al 2009, Knecht et al 2008),with 95% of the patients in sinus rhythm at 1 year and 90% after more than 2 years (O'Neill et al 2009); however with a second procedure needed in about 50% of the patients, mainly for AT (O'Neill et al 2009, Knecht et al 2008).

ATRIAL FIBRILLATION CYCLE LENGTH: A REAL-TIME GUIDE TO ABLATION

The AF cycle length can be reliably monitored during the procedure by averaging 30 consecutive cycles at the left and right atrial appendages, which display unambiguous high voltage and reproducible electrograms (Haissaguerre et al 2007). Various early studies have shown that AF cycle length correlates with the local refractory period, that it shortens in parallel with the duration of AF and that drugs may affect it (Kim et al 1996). However, AF cycle length prolongation during ablation at remote sites is evidence that the AFCL is not just a representation of the local refractory period (Haissaguerre et al 2004). A study using an advanced computer simulation demonstrated that the AF cycle length, as measured in the LA appendage, represents the sum of all fibrillatory activities converging to this area (Haissaguerre et al 2007). The higher the number of elements participating in the

AF process, the shorter the AF cycle length and the more complex the ablation. Of note the surface AF cycle length is also a marker for resistance to AAD and DC cardioversion (Biffi et al 2002, Fujiki et al 2004).

Both the impact of ablation at each region, and the amount of work remaining can be followed and estimated by monitoring the AF cycle length respectively. After each step of ablation, a gradual prolongation of AF cycle length is observed (Haissaguerre et al 2005). Conversion to sinus rhythm or AT usually occurs when AF cycle length reaches 180 and 200 ms in patients off drugs (Haissaguerre et al 2005). If AF persists during ablation of the LA despite a prolonged LA appendage cycle length, a lesser prolongation of the right atrial appendage cycle length would suggest that the right atrium may contain independent elements that participate to the AF process (Haissaguerre et al 2007).

Importantly, the surface ECG AF cycle length (manually measured by taking the mean cycle length from 10 unambiguous fibrillatory waves on lead VI) has also been shown to be a clinically useful preablation tool (Matsuo et al 2009). Indeed, among 90 patients ablated for persistent AF, the surface ECG AF cycle length was the only independent predictor of AF termination ($p<0.01$) and predicted clinical success of persistent AF ablation (Matsuo et al 2009).

PULMONARY VEIN ISOLATION

Pulmonary vein isolation (either antral, ostial or circumferential) invariably results in a better clinical prognosis in patients with paroxysmal as compared to persistent AF (Haissaguerre et al 2005, Pappone et al 2008, Ouyang et al 2004, Marrouche et al 2003, Kanagaratnam et al 2001). Despite these poor results when used as a stand alone strategy, PVI is still performed as the initial ablation step in all patients with persistent AF, because spared PVs can lead to arrhythmia recurrence due to triggering foci (Gerstenfeld et al 2004). A circumferential catheter is used to map and guide ablation of PV's, which can be isolated individually or as ipsilateral pairs depending on venous anatomy, catheter stability and the operator's preference. In all cases, ablation is performed at least 0.5 to one centimetre way from PV ostia to avoid the risk of PV stenosis when possible. However, it is sometimes necessary to go more distally to achieve PVI, for example at the anterior part of the left superior PV catheter stability is sometimes extremely difficult, necessitating ablation at the ostium and even just inside the vein. For all veins, isolation is assessed by either electrical elimination or dissociation of the PV potentials (Haissaguerre et al 2000).

COMPLEX FRACTIONATED ATRIAL ELECTROGRAMS

Electrophysiological Mechanisms

Complex fractionated atrial electrograms are defined as electrograms displaying more than two deflections that are fractionated or have a short cycle length (≤120ms), in its maximal form giving continuous electrical activity. The mechanisms underlying such fractionated potentials are still disputed. Important progress has been made since the first report from Cosio describing fragmentation in zones of slow interatrial conduction produced by extrastimulation in patients with AF (Cosio et al 1983). Jaïs et al proposed that CFAE represents the ultimate degree of temporal asynchrony and demonstrated a heterogeneous distribution during paroxysmal AF, mostly in the posterior LA and septum (Jais et al 1996). Spach et al. and then Konings et al. showed that fractionation may be caused by asynchronous activation of local muscles bundles, due to tissue anisotropy and the presence of insulating collagenous septa between atrial muscle bundles (Spach et al 1982, Konings et al 1997). From these studies, fractionation may represent zones of colliding wavefronts or pivoting points between different wavelets participating in the AF process. These areas of slow conduction could shorten the wavelength of the wandering wavelets, thereby increasing the number that can coexist in the atria and the complexity of AF. Rostock et al. reported that occurrence of CFAE was associated with prior acceleration of the AF cycle length and that duration of CFAE was inversely correlated with the preceding AF cycle length (Rostock et al 2006). Consequently, a given region may harbour apparently normal potentials during slow AFCL episodes, while fractionation may be observed after acceleration of the AFCL. Kalifa et al analyzed the relationship between local frequency, AF wave propagation and electrogram fractionation in the posterior LA of the isolated sheep heart the relation during sustained AF (Kalifa et al 2006). They demonstrated that the sites where the most fractionation occurs are located at the margin of rapidly activating areas. Fractionation, therefore, arises from slow conduction at the outer limit of a region displaying higher frequency activity.

All the above studies reinforce the concept that fractionation is a manifestation of either active reentrant mechanisms, or passive slow conduction with a tight functional relationship with local cycle length. Therefore, location of CFAE may sometimes not represent a critical region of AF perpetuation but a consequence of nearby rapid activity.

Alternatively, the autonomic nervous system is also thought to be implicated in the genesis of fractionated atrial electrograms. Acetylcholine administration has been shown to be capable of inducing AF and a spatial correlation between ganglionated plexi and CFAE localization has been observed (Scherlag et al 2005, Sharifov et al 2000). The release of acetylcholine from ganglionated plexi on the surface of the heart causes a shortening of the action potential and effective refractory period (Scherlag et al 2005, Lemery et al 2006, Schauerte et al 2000), which could promote fibrillatory conduction.

We have evaluated the impact of pharmacological autonomic blockade on CFAE (unpublished data). Autonomic blockade was achieved with intravenous injection of propanolol and atropine sulphate in 29 consecutive patients during AF. Three dimensional maps of the fractionation degree were made before and after autonomic blockade using the Ensite Navx® system. We observed that CFAE as a proportion of all atrial electrogram samples were indeed significantly reduced after autonomic blockade, but only for paroxysmal AF (and not persistent AF.) Furthermore, fractionation decreased only in patients with a significant prolongation of the AF cycle length, suggesting that the effect on CFAE is mediated by a prolongation of the AF cycle length [Knecht et al 2010 (in press)].

Clinical Results

Nademanee was the first to target exclusively CFAE in both atria in patients with paroxysmal and persistent AF. He reported maintenance of sinus rhythm of 91% at 1 year, with an average of 1.2 procedures per patient, most patients being treated by antiarrhythmic drugs. However, another group reported only modest short-term efficacy (57% persistent AF patients) with ablation of persistent AF only guided by CFAE (Oral et al 2007). In this latter study, a significant amount of the patients developed AT finally necessitating PV isolation or LA linear lesions to be controlled. Results from other groups (Verma et al 2008) also confirmed that the addition of CFAE ablation to PV isolation provides an increased clinical success rate, but at the cost of numerous subsequent iatrogenic AT (Haissaguerre et al 2005a, Haissaguerre et al 2005b, Knecht et al 2008).

Linear Lesions

The most common LA linear lesions consist of the roof line which connects the two superior PVs (Hocini et al 2005) and the mitral line which joins the mitral annulus to the PV either anteriorly or laterally (Jais et al 2004, Hocini et al 2005, Sanders et al 2004). The observed therapeutic efficacy of these linear lesions drawn during AF may be related to interruption of wavelet and macroreentrant tachycardias, alteration of autonomic innervation, atrial debulking or an effect on local complex electrograms.

A recent study highlights that although PV isolation and electrogram based ablation without linear lesions may be effective for terminating persistent AF in a significant number of patients, macro reentrant AT requiring LA linear ablation is very likely to occur during the overall follow-up period (Knecht et al 2008). In this study, 96% of the patients ultimately required a roofline and 86% a mitral line after a mean follow-up of 2 years, despite attempts to avoid LA linear lesions. These data suggest that at least the roofline (which is easier and simpler to perform as compared to the mitral isthmus line) could be used in the case of AF persistence after PV isolation and CFAE ablation. This study also confirmed the high risk of AT recurrence in cases of incomplete conduction block at LA lines.

Autonomic Targets

Macroreentrant tachycardias that occur at follow up are frequently associated with gaps in linear lesions, either due to lesion recovery or an initial incomplete line (Fassini et al 2005, Haissaguerre P et al 2005a). That linear lesions are useful in persistent AF, despite the potential proarrhythmic effect suggests that their benefit is not solely related to disrupting macroreentry. Both the left atrial roof line and the mitral isthmus line inadvertently incorporate the locations of known vagal ganglia, with the highest density of cardiac autonomic nerves occurring within 5 mm of the LA-PV junction (Tan et al 2006). Although it is feasible to map and locate individual vagal ganglia (Lemery et al 2006) with high frequency stimulation, this is not routinely performed in clinical practice, nor may it be necessary, given the overlap between the PV ostia and the vagal ganglia.

The autonomic nervous system is known to play a role in the generation of AF, with increased sympathetic and parasympathetic activity preceding pulmonary vein firing, and shortening the atrial refractory period (Takahashi et al 2006). In patients with drug refractory paroxysmal AF, the abolition of evoked vagal responses seen during circumferential PV ablation rendered 99% of patients free of AF at 12 months compared with 85% in those in whom vagal responses could not be evoked (Pappone et al 2004).

Right Atrium

Early work by several groups investigated the utility of right atrial linear lesions, with or without additional left atrial linear lesions with only modest success in patients with either paroxysmal and persistent AF (Haissaguerre et al 1996, Jais et al 1998). This does not mean, however, that the right atrium does not contribute to AF. There is accumulating evidence that in a subset of patients, possibly up to 20% of patients with long lasting persistent AF, the right atrium plays an active role in the perpetuation of AF (Wright et al 2008).

Atrial Tachycardia: Mapping Approach

In the stepwise approach the endpoint of ablation is restoration of sinus rhythm with confirmation of pulmonary vein isolation and electrically confirmed block of any linear lesion performed; however sinus rhythm is rarely restored directly and in more than 70% of patients, AF terminates by conversion to AT (Haissaguerre et al 2005b). Those may also appear late after the healing process of ablation (Haissaguerre et al 2005a, Knecht et al 2008). They are multiple in numbers and mechanisms and add significantly to the complexity of ablation. They are considered as the last step of persistent and long standing AF ablation (during the initial procedure or during follow-up), and results of their mapping and ablation will achieve either subsequent success or failure of the procedure for patients. Mechanisms of AT after an AF ablation varies with the ablation approach. While focal origins from reconnected PVs are more usual using a segmental PV isolation (Gerstenfeld et al 2004, Ouyang et al 2005), macro reentrant mechanisms are more frequent after an anatomical approach (Calkins et al 2007, Knecht et al 2008, Gerstenfeld et al 2004, Ouyang et al 2005, Mesas et al 2004, Pappone et al 2004), and "small circuits" (corresponding to localized reentries) are common after a stepwise approach (Deisenhofer et al 2006).

Although 3D electro anatomical mapping systems may assist in mapping AT, using these technologies is often impractical because of AT instability or multiple AT which each require mapping. For this reason, a deductive diagnostic electrophysiological approach has recently been validated (Jais et al 2009), based upon the common mechanisms of atrial tachycardias that are encountered. Macroreentrant circuits (either around the ipsilateral veins, and thus being roof dependent or around the mitral or tricuspid valve annulus) are easily diagnosed by activation mapping and confirmed with entrainment at two opposite parts of the circuit. Macroreentry accounts for approximately 50% of all ATs post AF ablation, the other 50% are 'focal", which again can be mapped using a combination of activation and entrainment mapping. This prospective study also highlighted the dominant role of localized reentry as a novel mechanism of 'focal' AT.

The Procedural Endpoint for Persistent AF Ablation

Although there are a number of different strategies to ablation of persistent AF, there are more similarities than differences in the targets that are approached. However there is wide variation in the procedural endpoint of ablation of persistent AF. Besides, it is important to emphasize that while for CFAE ablation there is no clear technical endpoint during ablation, electrical isolation of PV's as well as bidirectional electrical conduction block at linear lesions are essential for the global success of the procedure (Stewart et al 2004, Sanders et al 2007, Allessie et al 1985, Arentz et al 2007).

Concerning the procedural endpoint of the ablation procedure itself, some authors prefer to perform a standardized lesion set; however it appears that AF termination by catheter ablation is associated with the best clinical outcome (O'Neill et al 2009).

PREDICTORS OF SUCCESS

During the procedure, when AF can be terminated by catheter ablation (without drug or external cardioversion), only 5% of these patients will recur AF (O'Neill et al 2009, Rostock et al 2008); however almost 50% will have AT recurrence, which may be more symptomatic than AF (O'Neill et al 2009, Haissaguerre et al 2005a). Thankfully, in experienced centers, catheter ablation of subsequent AT's is associated with high success rate (Jais et al 2009). Other important predictors of success have been reported by investigators: Preexisting LA scarring (Verma et al 2005), voltage abatement (Pappone et al 2001), the percentage of left atrium ablated or vagal denervation, electrical block at linear lesions (O'Neill et al 2009, Knecht et al 2008, Matsuo et al 2007).

More practically, the main predictors of success before the ablation procedure are the following: AF cycle length, duration of continuous AF (with a very low success rate for AF of continuous duration of more than 5 years (O'Neill et al 2009, Knecht et al 2008, Matsuo et al 2007), history of hypertension and LA dimensions (Berruezo et al 2007).

We have evaluated the clinical predictors of success in 90 consecutive patients with persistent AF followed during 2 years (Matsuo et al 2009). The duration of AF, LA dimensions, presence of structural heart disease and the surface ECG AF cycle length were assessed prior to ablation and analyzed with respect to long-term clinical outcome. The surface ECG AF cycle length was manually measured from 10 unambiguous fibrillatory waves on lead VI (minimal voltage> 0.01mV) that were not fused with QRST segments at a paper speed of 50 mm/s and a gain setting of 20, 40 or 80 mm/mV. Long-term maintenance of sinus rhythm was associated with a shorter duration of continuous AF ($p<0.0001$), a longer surface ECG AF cycle length ($p<0.001$) and a smaller LA ($p<0.05$) compared to those with recurrent arrhythmia. In multivariate analysis the surface ECG AF cycle length and the AF duration predicted clinical success of persistent AF ablation ($p<0.01$ and $p<0.05$, respectively). Furthermore, using a ROC curve, the optimal cut-off for the AF cycle length as a predictor of AF termination was 142 msec with specificity and sensitivity of 92.9 % and 69.7 %, respectively. On the other hand, the optimal cut-off point for the duration of continuous AF was 21 months for AF termination (specificity 92.9 % and sensitivity 61.8 %). The combined cut-off using a surface ECG AFCL>142 msec and a duration of continuous AF<21 months had 100.0 % specificity in predicting procedural termination of AF (sensitivity: 39.5 %, positive predict value; 100.0%, negative predictive value; 23.3%).

RELATED COMPLICATIONS AND POTENTIAL BENEFITS

The most frequent complications related to catheter ablation of persistent AF occur in 1 to 2% of the patients and mainly include stroke, which is fortunately rare, and pericardial tamponade (Cappato et al 2005). Stroke or transient ischemic attacks are mainly the consequences of thrombi adherent to catheters and sheaths, endocardial disruption from the ablation lesions and air passing through trans septal sheaths. For this reason it is important to have ready access to vascular imaging of the brain, and protocols for acute thrombolysis for stroke. Anticoagulation is used to prevent thrombi forming, but this increases the risk of pericardial tamponade, due to ooze from the ablated tissue. Other possible complications are PV stenosis, which has dramatically reduced with a more proximal ablation strategy compared to the initial reports of isolation within the vein (Packer et al 2005), atrioesophageal fistula (exceedingly rare but almost always fatal) (Pappone et al 2004) and phrenic nerve paralysis, which almost always recovers (Sacher et al 2006).

On the other hand, catheter ablation of persistent AF has shown promising results concerning improved morbidity (Pappone et al 2003, Hsu et al 2004) and quality of life (Purerfellner et al 2004, Weerasooriya et al 2005) (especially in patients with preexisting heart failure (Hsu et al 2004, Khan et al 2008), but also potential benefits in term of mortality (Nademanee et al 2008, Pappone et al 2003). A nonrandomized study comparing catheter ablation versus medical therapy patients showed that patients treated with catheter ablation were approximately half as likely to die during the follow-up period and half as likely to have a stroke or other major adverse cardiovascular event as those treated medically (Pappone et al 2003). Another study showed that, after catheter ablation of symptomatic persistent AF in high-risk patients, patients remaining in sinus rhythm had a significant benefit in term of mortality as compared with patients recurring AF (Nademanee et al 2008).

INDICATIONS FOR PERSISTENT AF ABLATION

The latest guidelines published by the ACC/ AHA/ESC societies have recommended not differentiating between patients on the basis of the duration of AF (Calkins et al 2007). Briefly, patients are considered for ablation in case of symptomatic recurrent AF despite after failure of at least one antiarrhythmic drug, electrical cardioversion, or both. Importantly, as mentioned earlier, one has to consider that catheter ablation for patients with very long duration persistent AF (especially more than 5 years), very short cycle length on a 12 lead ECG, and extremely dilated LA have very poor chance of clinical success.

Of note, data has suggested that patients with heart failure (NYHA II or more) or evidence of left ventricular dysfunction without an alternative explanation have the most to gain from catheter ablation (Hsu et al 2004), even if the success rate is lower compared to patients with normal left ventricular function. It has been suggested that asymptomatic patients with AF related thromboembolism should be treated by catheter ablation (Oral et al 2006), even though there have been no trials that have reported a reduction in events postablation, due to the large number of patients that would need to be recruited. Therefore the ACC/AHA/ESC recommendations for anticoagulation remain the same following catheter ablation (Calkins et al 2007).

FUTURE PERSPECTIVES

In order to make progress in our understanding of the mechanisms underlying persistent AF improved mapping tools are required to allow identification of the precise electrophysiological substrate. Indeed, although some CFAE may indicate focal sources or localised reentrant circuits, there is currently no accurate mapping technology that has been shown to be clinically effective in differentiating active from passive areas of activation. Although dominant frequency mapping has been used to try and determine the areas with the highest frequency of activation, it has so far been disappointing in the treatment of persistent AF (Sanders et al 2005).

There is room for improvement in ablation technology. There are a number of "single shot" catheters that have been developed using a variety of energy sources: For example, radiofrequency (Meissner et al 2009), high intensity focused ultrasound (Nakagawa et al 2007) and cryothermal balloons (Sarabanda et al 2005). Currently, only limited data are available on the efficacy and safety profile of such catheters. One major limitation of such technology is the variation in pulmonary venous anatomy. Furthermore these catheters are very specific to pulmonary vein isolation; and although this could be appropriate for most patients with paroxysmal AF, patients with persistent AF require ablation of more than just the pulmonary veins, thereby increasing the cost and limiting their applicability.

CONCLUSION

Since the initial report that AF was triggered from ectopic beats within the pulmonary veins, we have learnt a tremendous amount about the underlying physiopathology of AF. Catheter ablation of persistent AF is undergoing a massive expansion because of very promising results, and persistent AF patients can now look forward to a cure for their arrhythmia and the morbidity and mortality risk that this brings. Although catheter ablation of persistent AF is a difficult procedure, advances in catheter design and identification of areas that actively participate in the AF process should increase the number of patients that can receive treatment.

ACKNOWLEDGEMENTS

Matthew Wright receives financial support from the Department of Health via the National Institute for Health Research (NIHR) comprehensive Biomedical Research Centre award to Guy's and St Thomas' NHS Foundation Trust in partnership with King's College London and King's College Hospital NHS Foundation Trust.

BIBLIOGRAPHY

1. Allessie MA, Lammers WJEP, Bonke FIM, et al. Experimental evaluation of Moe's multiple wavelet hypothesis of atrial fibrillation. In: Zipes DP, Jalife J, eds. Cardiac Electrophysiology and Arrhythmias. NY Grune and Stratton. 1985;265-75.
2. Arentz T, von Rosenthal J, Blum T, et al. Feasibility and safety of pulmonary vein isolation using a new mapping and navigation system in patients with refractory atrial fibrillation. Circulation. 2003;108:2484-90.
3. Arentz T, Weber R, Burkle G, et al. Small or large isolation areas around the pulmonary veins for the treatment of atrial fibrillation? Results from a prospective randomized study. Circulation. 2007;115:3057-63.
4. Benjamin EJ, Wolf PA, D'Agostino RB, et al. Impact of atrial fibrillation on the risk of death: the Framingham Heart Study. Circulation. 1998;98:946-52.
5. Berruezo A, Tamborero D, Mont L, et al. Pre-procedural predictors of atrial fibrillation recurrence after circumferential pulmonary vein ablation. Eur Heart J. 2007;28:836-41.
6. Biffi M, Boriani G, Bartolotti M, et al. Atrial fibrillation recurrence after internal cardioversion: prognostic importance of electrophysiological parameters. Heart. 2002;87:443-8.
7. Calkins H, Brugada J, Packer DL, et al. HRS/EHRA/ECAS expert Consensus Statement on catheter and surgical ablation of atrial fibrillation: recommendations for personnel, policy, procedures and follow-up. A report of the Heart Rhythm Society (HRS) Task Force on catheter and surgical ablation of atrial fibrillation. Heart Rhythm. 2007;4:816-61.
8. Calo L, Lamberti F, Loricchio ML, et al. Left atrial ablation versus biatrial ablation for persistent and permanent atrial fibrillation: A prospective and randomized study. J Am Coll Cardiol. 2006;47:2504-12.
9. Cappato R, Calkins H, Chen SA, et al. Worldwide survey on the methods, efficacy, and safety of catheter ablation for human atrial fibrillation. Circulation. 2005;111:1100-5.
10. Chen J, Off MK, Solheim E, et al. Treatment of atrial fibrillation by silencing electrical activity in the posterior inter-pulmonary-vein atrium. Europace. 2008;10:265-72.
11. Chen MS, Marrouche NF, Khaykin Y, et al. Pulmonary vein isolation for the treatment of atrial fibrillation in patients with impaired systolic function. J Am Coll Cardiol. 2004;43:1004-9.
12. Cosio FG, Palacios J, Vidal JM, et al. Electrophysiologic studies in atrial fibrillation. Slow conduction of premature impulses: A possible manifestation of the background for reentry. Am J Cardiol. 1983;51:122-30.
13. Cox JL, Schuessler RB, D'Agostino HJJ, et, al. The surgical treatment of atrial fibrillation. III. Development of a definitive surgical procedure. J Thorac Cardiovasc Surg. 1991;101:569-83.
14. Deisenhofer I, Estner H, Zrenner B, et al. Left atrial tachycardia after circumferential pulmonary vein ablation for atrial fibrillation: Incidence, electrophysiological characteristics, and results of radiofrequency ablation. Europace. 2006;8:573-82.
15. Della Bella P, Fassini G, Cireddu M, et al. Image integration-guided catheter ablation of atrial fibrillation: A prospective randomized study. J Cardiovasc Electrophysiol. 2009;20:258-65.

16. Elayi CS, Verma A, Di Biase L, et al. Ablation for longstanding permanent atrial fibrillation: Results from a randomized study comparing three different strategies. Heart Rhythm. 2008;5:1658-64.
17. Estner HL, Hessling G, Ndrepepa G, et al. Electrogram-guided substrate ablation with or without pulmonary vein isolation in patients with persistent atrial fibrillation. Europace. 2008a;10:1281-7.
18. Estner HL, Hessling G, Ndrepepa G, et al. Acute effects and long-term outcome of pulmonary vein isolation in combination with electrogram-guided substrate ablation for persistent atrial fibrillation. Am J Cardiol. 2008b;101:332-7.
19. Fassini G, Riva S, Chiodelli R, et al. Left mitral isthmus ablation associated with PV Isolation: Long-term results of a prospective randomized study. J Cardiovasc Electrophysiol. 2005;16:1150-6.
20. Fiala M, Chovancik J, Wojnarova D, et al. Results of complex left atrial ablation of long-lasting persistent atrial fibrillation. J Interv Card Electrophysiol. 2008;23:189-98.
21. Fujiki A, Tsuneda T, Sakabe M, et al. Maintenance of sinus rhythm and recovery of atrial mechanical function after cardioversion with bepridil or in combination with aprindine in long-lasting persistent atrial fibrillation. Circ J. 2004;68:834-9.
22. Fuster V, Ryden LE, Cannom DS, et al. ACC/AHA/ESC 2006 Guidelines for the Management of Patients with Atrial Fibrillation: a report of the American College of Cardiology/American Heart Association Task Force on Practice Guidelines and the European Society of Cardiology Committee for Practice Guidelines (Writing Committee to Revise the 2001 Guidelines for the Management of Patients With Atrial Fibrillation): Developed in collaboration with the European Heart Rhythm Association and the Heart Rhythm Society. Circulation. 2006;114:e257-354
23. Gerstenfeld EP, Callans DJ, Dixit S, et al. Mechanisms of organized left atrial tachycardias occurring after pulmonary vein isolation. Circulation. 2004;110:1351-7.
24. Gerstenfeld EP, Sauer W, Callans DJ, et al. Predictors of success after selective pulmonary vein isolation of arrhythmogenic pulmonary veins for treatment of atrial fibrillation. Heart Rhythm. 2006;3:165-70
25. Haissaguerre M, Hocini M, Sanders P, et al. Catheter ablation of long-lasting persistent atrial fibrillation: Clinical outcome and mechanisms of subsequent arrhythmias. J Cardiovasc Electrophysiol. 2005b;16:1138-47.
26. Haissaguerre M, Hocini M, Sanders P, et al. Localized sources maintaining atrial fibrillation organized by prior ablation. Circulation. 2006;113:616-25.
27. Haissaguerre M, Jais P, Shah DC, et al. Right and left atrial radiofrequency catheter therapy of paroxysmal atrial fibrillation. J Cardiovasc Electrophysiol. 1996;7:1132-44.
28. Haissaguerre M, Jais P, Shah DC, et al. Spontaneous initiation of atrial fibrillation by ectopic beats originating in the pulmonary veins. N Engl J Med. 1998;339:659-66.
29. Haissaguerre M, Jais P, Shah DC, et al. Catheter ablation of chronic atrial fibrillation targeting the reinitiating triggers. J Cardiovasc Electrophysiol. 2000a;11:2-10.
30. Haissaguerre M, Jais P, Shah DC, et al. Electrophysiological end point for catheter ablation of atrial fibrillation initiated from multiple pulmonary venous foci. Circulation. 2000b;101:1409-17.
31. Haissaguerre M, Lim KT, Jacquemet V, et al. Atrial fibrillatory cycle length: computer simulation and potential clinical importance. Europace 2007;9 Suppl 6:vi64-vi70.
32. Haissaguerre M, Sanders P, Hocini M, et al. Changes in atrial fibrillation cycle length and inducibility during catheter ablation and their relation to outcome. Circulation. 2004a;109:3007-13.
33. Haissaguerre M, Sanders P, Hocini M, et al. Pulmonary veins in the substrate for atrial fibrillation: The "venous wave" hypothesis. J Am Coll Cardiol. 2004b;43:2290-2.

34. Haissaguerre M, Sanders P, Hocini M, et al. Catheter ablation of long-lasting persistent atrial fibrillation: Critical structures for termination. J Cardiovasc Electrophysiol. 2005a;16:1125-37.
35. Haissaguerre M, Shah DC, Jais P, et al. Electrophysiological breakthroughs from the left atrium to the pulmonary veins. Circulation. 2000c;102:2463-5.
36. Hobbs FD, Fitzmaurice DA, Mant J, et al. A randomised controlled trial and cost-effectiveness study of systematic screening (targeted and total population screening) versus routine practice for the detection of atrial fibrillation in people aged 65 and over. The SAFE study. Health Technol Assess. 2005;9(40):iii-iv, ix-x, 1-74.
37. Hocini M, Ho SY, Kawara T, et al. Electrical conduction in canine pulmonary veins: electrophysiological and anatomic correlation. Circulation. 2002;105:2442-8.
38. Hocini M, Jais P, Sanders P, et al. Techniques, evaluation, and consequences of linear block at the left atrial roof in paroxysmal atrial fibrillation: A prospective randomized study. Circulation. 2005;112:3688-96.
39. Hsu LF, Jais P, Sanders P, et al. Catheter ablation for atrial fibrillation in congestive heart failure. N Engl J Med. 2004;351:2373-83.
40. Jais P, Haissaguerre M, Shah DC, et al. Regional disparities of endocardial atrial activation in paroxysmal atrial fibrillation. Pacing Clin Electrophysiol. 1996;19:1998-2003.
41. Jais P, Hocini M, Hsu LF, et al. Technique and results of linear ablation at the mitral isthmus. Circulation. 2004;110:2996-3002.
42. Jais P, Hocini M, Macle L, et al. Distinctive electrophysiological properties of pulmonary veins in patients with atrial fibrillation. Circulation. 2002;106:2479-85.
43. Jais P, Matsuo S, Knecht S, et al. A deductive mapping strategy for atrial tachycardia following atrial fibrillation ablation: importance of localized reentry. J Cardiovasc Electrophysiol. 2009;20:480-91.
44. Jais P, Shah DC, Takahashi A, et al. Long-term follow-up after right atrial radiofrequency catheter treatment of paroxysmal atrial fibrillation. Pacing Clin Electrophysiol. 1998;21:2533-8.
45. Kalifa J, Tanaka K, Zaitsev AV, et al. Mechanisms of wave fractionation at boundaries of high-frequency excitation in the posterior left atrium of the isolated sheep heart during atrial fibrillation. Circulation. 2006;113:626-33.
46. Kanagaratnam L, Tomassoni G, Schweikert R, et al. Empirical pulmonary vein isolation in patients with chronic atrial fibrillation using a three-dimensional nonfluoroscopic mapping system: Long-term follow-up. Pacing Clin Electrophysiol. 2001;24:1774-9.
47. Khan MN, Jais P, Cummings J, et al. Pulmonary-vein isolation for atrial fibrillation in patients with heart failure. N Engl J Med. 2008;359:1778-85.
48. Kim KB, Rodefeld MD, Schuessler RB, et al. Relationship between local atrial fibrillation interval and refractory period in the isolated canine atrium. Circulation. 1996;94:2961-7.
49. Knecht S, Hocini M, Wright M, et al. Left atrial linear lesions are required for successful treatment of persistent atrial fibrillation. Eur Heart J. 2008;29(19):2359-66.
50. Knecht S, O'Neill MD, Matsuo S, et al. Focal arrhythmia confined within the coronary sinus and maintaining atrial fibrillation. J Cardiovasc Electrophysiol. 2007;18:1140-6.
51. Knecht S, Wright M, Matsuo S, et al. Impact of pharmacological autonomic blockade on complex fractionated atrial electrograms. J Cardiovasc Electrophysiol. 2010. (In Press)
52. Konings KT, Smeets JL, Penn OC, et al. Configuration of unipolar atrial electrograms during electrically induced atrial fibrillation in humans. Circulation. 1997;95:1231-41.
53. Kozak LJ, Lees KA, DeFrances CJ. National Hospital Discharge Survey: 2003 annual summary with detailed diagnosis and procedure data. Vital Health Stat. 2006;13:1-206.
54. Krahn AD, Manfreda J, Tate RB, et al. The natural history of atrial fibrillation: incidence, risk factors, and prognosis in the Manitoba Follow-Up Study. Am J Med. 1995;98:476-84.
55. Lemery R, Birnie D, Tang AS, et al. Feasibility study of endocardial mapping of ganglionated plexuses during catheter ablation of atrial fibrillation. Heart Rhythm. 2006;3:387-96.

56. Lim TW, Jassal IS, Ross DL, et al. Medium-term efficacy of segmental ostial pulmonary vein isolation for the treatment of permanent and persistent atrial fibrillation. Pacing Clin Electrophysiol. 2006;29:374-9.
57. Mainigi SK, Sauer WH, Cooper JM, et al. Incidence and predictors of very late recurrence of atrial fibrillation after ablation. J Cardiovasc Electrophysiol. 2007;18:69-74.
58. Marrouche NF, Martin DO, Wazni O, et al. Phased-array intracardiac echocardiography monitoring during pulmonary vein isolation in patients with atrial fibrillation: Impact on outcome and complications. Circulation. 2003;107:2710-6.
59. Matsuo S, Lellouche N, Wright M, et al. Clinical Predictors of Termination and Clinical Outcome of Catheter Ablation for Persistent Atrial Fibrillation. J Am Coll Cardiol. 2009;25;54(9):788-95.
60. Matsuo S, Lim KT, Haissaguerre M. Ablation of chronic atrial fibrillation. Heart Rhythm. 2007;4:1461-3.
61. Meissner A, Plehn G, Van Bracht M, et al. First experiences for pulmonary vein isolation with the high-density mesh ablator (HDMA): A novel mesh electrode catheter for both mapping and radiofrequency delivery in a single unit. J Cardiovasc Electrophysiol. 2009;20:359-66.
62. Mesas CE, Pappone C, Lang CC, et al. Left atrial tachycardia after circumferential pulmonary vein ablation for atrial fibrillation: electroanatomic characterization and treatment. J Am Coll Cardiol. 2004;44:1071-9.
63. Miyasaka Y, Barnes ME, Gersh BJ, et al. Secular trends in incidence of atrial fibrillation in Olmsted County, Minnesota, 1980 to 2000, and implications on the projections for future prevalence. Circulation. 2006;114:119-25.
64. Moe GK, Abildskov JA. Atrial fibrillation as a self-sustaining arrhythmia independent of focal discharge. Am Heart J. 1959;58:59-70.
65. Nademanee K, McKenzie J, Kosar E, et al. A new approach for catheter ablation of atrial fibrillation: Mapping of the electrophysiologic substrate. J Am Coll Cardiol. 2004;43:2044-53.
66. Nademanee K, Schwab M, Kosar EM, et al. Clinical outcomes of catheter substrate ablation for high-risk patients with atrial fibrillation. J Am Coll Cardiol. 2008;51:843-9.
67. Nakagawa H, Antz M, Wong T, et al. Initial experience using a forward directed, high-intensity focused ultrasound balloon catheter for pulmonary vein antrum isolation in patients with atrial fibrillation. J Cardiovasc Electrophysiol. 2007;18:136-44.
68. Neumann T, Vogt J, Schumacher B, et al. Circumferential pulmonary vein isolation with the cryoballoon technique results from a prospective 3-center study. J Am Coll Cardiol. 2008;52:273-8.
69. Oral H, Chugh A, Good E, et al. Randomized comparison of encircling and nonencircling left atrial ablation for chronic atrial fibrillation. Heart Rhythm. 2005;2:1165-72.
70. Oral H, Chugh A, Good E, et al. Radiofrequency catheter ablation of chronic atrial fibrillation guided by complex electrograms. Circulation. 2007;115:2606-12.
71. Oral H, Chugh A, Ozaydin M, et al. Risk of thromboembolic events after percutaneous left atrial radiofrequency ablation of atrial fibrillation. Circulation. 2006;114:759-65.
72. Oral H, Knight BP, Ozaydin M, et al. Clinical significance of early recurrences of atrial fibrillation after pulmonary vein isolation. J Am Coll Cardiol. 2002;40:100-4.
73. Oral H, Knight BP, Tada H, et al. Pulmonary vein isolation for paroxysmal and persistent atrial fibrillation. Circulation. 2002;105:1077-81.
74. Oral H, Veerareddy S, Good E, et al. Prevalence of asymptomatic recurrences of atrial fibrillation after successful radiofrequency catheter ablation. J Cardiovasc Electrophysiol. 2004;15:920-4.
75. Ouyang F, Antz M, Ernst S, et al. Recovered pulmonary vein conduction as a dominant factor for recurrent atrial tachyarrhythmias after complete circular isolation of the pulmonary veins: Lessons from double Lasso technique. Circulation. 2005a;111:127-35.

76. Ouyang F, Bansch D, Ernst S, et al. Complete isolation of left atrium surrounding the pulmonary veins: New insights from the double-Lasso technique in paroxysmal atrial fibrillation. Circulation. 2004;110:2090-6.
77. Ouyang F, Ernst S, Chun J, et al. Electrophysiological findings during ablation of persistent atrial fibrillation with electroanatomic mapping and double Lasso catheter technique. Circulation. 2005b;112:3038-48.
78. O'Neill MD, Wright M, Knecht S, et al. Long-term follow-up of persistent atrial fibrillation ablation using termination as a procedural endpoint. Eur Heart J. 2009;30:1105-12.
79. Packer DL, Keelan P, Munger TM, et al. Clinical presentation, investigation, and management of pulmonary vein stenosis complicating ablation for atrial fibrillation. Circulation. 2005;111:546-54.
80. Pappone C, Manguso F, Vicedomini G, et al. Prevention of iatrogenic atrial tachycardia after ablation of atrial fibrillation: A prospective randomized study comparing circumferential pulmonary vein ablation with a modified approach. Circulation. 2004c;110:3036-42.
81. Pappone C, Oral H, Santinelli V, et al. Atrio-esophageal fistula as a complication of percutaneous transcatheter ablation of atrial fibrillation. Circulation. 2004b;109:2724-6.
82. Pappone C, Oreto G, Rosanio S, et al. Atrial electroanatomic remodeling after circumferential radiofrequency pulmonary vein ablation: Efficacy of an anatomic approach in a large cohort of patients with atrial fibrillation. Circulation. 2001;104:2539-44.
83. Pappone C, Radinovic A, Manguso F, et al. Atrial fibrillation progression and management: A 5-year prospective follow-up study. Heart Rhythm. 2008;5:1501-7.
84. Pappone C, Rosanio S, Augello G, et al. Mortality, morbidity, and quality of life after circumferential pulmonary vein ablation for atrial fibrillation: Outcomes from a controlled nonrandomized long-term study. J Am Coll Cardiol. 2003;42:185-97.
85. Pappone C, Santinelli V, Manguso F, et al. Pulmonary vein denervation enhances long-term benefit after circumferential ablation for paroxysmal atrial fibrillation. Circulation. 2004a;109:327-34.
86. Purerfellner H, Martinek M, Aichinger J, et al. Quality of life restored to normal in patients with atrial fibrillation after pulmonary vein ostial isolation. Am Heart J. 2004;148:318-25.
87. Rostock T, Rotter M, Sanders P, et al. Fibrillating areas isolated within the left atrium after radiofrequency linear catheter ablation. J Cardiovasc Electrophysiol. 2006;17:807-12.
88. Rostock T, Rotter M, Sanders P, et al. High-density activation mapping of fractionated electrograms in the atria of patients with paroxysmal atrial fibrillation. Heart Rhythm. 2006;3:27-34.
89. Rostock T, Steven D, Hoffmann B, et al. Chronic Atrial Fibrillation Is a Biatrial Arrhythmia: Data from Catheter Ablation of Chronic Atrial Fibrillation Aiming Arrhythmia Termination Using a Sequential Ablation Approach. Circ Arrhythmia Electrophysiol. 2008;1:344-53.
90. Roy D, Talajic M, Nattel S, et al. Rhythm control versus rate control for atrial fibrillation and heart failure. N Engl J Med. 2008;358:2667-77.
91. Sacher F, Monahan KH, Thomas SP, et al. Phrenic nerve injury after atrial fibrillation catheter ablation: characterization and outcome in a multicenter study. J Am Coll Cardiol. 2006;47:2498-503.
92. Sanders P, Berenfeld O, Hocini M, et al. Spectral analysis identifies sites of high-frequency activity maintaining atrial fibrillation in humans. Circulation. 2005;112:789-97.
93. Sanders P, Hocini M, Jais P, et al. Complete isolation of the pulmonary veins and posterior left atrium in chronic atrial fibrillation. Long-term clinical outcome. Eur Heart J. 2007;28:1862-71.
94. Sanders P, Jais P, Hocini M, et al. Electrophysiologic and clinical consequences of linear catheter ablation to transect the anterior left atrium in patients with atrial fibrillation. Heart Rhythm. 2004;1:176-84.

95. Sarabanda AV, Bunch TJ, Johnson SB, et al. Efficacy and safety of circumferential pulmonary vein isolation using a novel cryothermal balloon ablation system. J Am Coll Cardiol. 2005;46:1902-12.
96. Schauerte P, Scherlag BJ, Pitha J, et al. Catheter ablation of cardiac autonomic nerves for prevention of vagal atrial fibrillation. Circulation. 2000;102:2774-80.
97. Scherlag BJ, Yamanashi W, Patel U, et al. Autonomically induced conversion of pulmonary vein focal firing into atrial fibrillation. J Am Coll Cardiol. 2005;45:1878-86.
98. Schwartz JF, Pellersels G, Silvers J. A catheter-based curative approach to atrial fibrillation in humans. Circulation. 1993;90:I-335.
99. Seow SC, Lim TW, Koay CH, et al. Efficacy and late recurrences with wide electrical pulmonary vein isolation for persistent and permanent atrial fibrillation. Europace. 2007;9:1129-33.
100. Sharifov OF, Zaitsev AV, Rosenshtraukh LV, et al. patial distribution and frequency dependence of arrhythmogenic vagal effects in canine atria. J Cardiovasc Electrophysiol. 2000;11:1029-42.
101. Singh BN, Connolly SJ, Crijns HJ, et al. Dronedarone for maintenance of sinus rhythm in atrial fibrillation or flutter. N Engl J Med. 2007;357:987-99.
102. Singh BN, Singh SN, Reda DJ, et al. Amiodarone versus sotalol for atrial fibrillation. N Engl J Med. 2005;352:1861-72.
103. Spach MS, Miller WTr, Dolber PC, et al. The functional role of structural complexities in the propagation of depolarization in the atrium of the dog. Cardiac conduction disturbances due to discontinuities of effective axial resistivity. Circ Res. 1982;50:175-91.
104. Stewart S, Hart CL, Hole DJ, et al. Population prevalence, incidence, and predictors of atrial fibrillation in the Renfrew/Paisley study. Heart. 2001;86:516-21.
105. Stewart S, Hart CL, Hole DJ, et al. A population-based study of the long-term risks associated with atrial fibrillation: 20-year follow-up of the Renfrew/Paisley study. Am J Med. 2002;113:359-64.
106. Stewart S, Murphy NF, Walker A, et al. Cost of an emerging epidemic: an economic analysis of atrial fibrillation in the UK. Heart. 2004;90:286-92.
107. Takahashi Y, Jais P, Hocini M, et al. Shortening of fibrillatory cycle length in the pulmonary vein during vagal excitation. J Am Coll Cardiol. 2006;47:774-80.
108. Takahashi Y, O'Neill MD, Hocini M, et al. Effects of stepwise ablation of chronic atrial fibrillation on atrial electrical and mechanical properties. J Am Coll Cardiol. 2007;49:1306-14.
109. Tan AY, Li H, Wachsmann-Hogiu S, et al. Autonomic innervation and segmental muscular disconnections at the human pulmonary vein-atrial junction: Implications for catheter ablation of atrial-pulmonary vein junction. J Am Coll Cardiol. 2006;48:132-43.
110. Van Gelder IC, Hagens VE, Bosker HA, et al. A comparison of rate control and rhythm control in patients with recurrent persistent atrial fibrillation. N Engl J Med. 2002;347:1834-40.
111. Verma A, Novak P, Macle L, et al. A prospective, multicenter evaluation of ablating complex fractionated electrograms (CFEs) during atrial fibrillation (AF) identified by an automated mapping algorithm: Acute effects on AF and efficacy as an adjuvant strategy. Heart Rhythm. 2008;5:198-205.
112. Verma A, Patel D, Famy T, et al. Efficacy of adjuvant anterior left atrial ablation during intracardiac echocardiography-guided pulmonary vein antrum isolation for atrial fibrillation. J Cardiovasc Electrophysiol. 2007;18:151-6.
113. Verma A, Wazni OM, Marrouche NF, et al. Pre-existent left atrial scarring in patients undergoing pulmonary vein antrum isolation: An independent predictor of procedural failure. J Am Coll Cardiol. 2005;45:285-92.

114. Weerasooriya R, Jais P, Hocini M, et al. Effect of catheter ablation on quality of life of patients with paroxysmal atrial fibrillation. Heart Rhythm. 2005;2:619-23.
115. Willems S, Klemm H, Rostock T, et al. Substrate modification combined with pulmonary vein isolation improves outcome of catheter ablation in patients with persistent atrial fibrillation: A prospective randomized comparison. Eur Heart J. 2006;27:2871-8.
116. Wright M, Haissaguerre M, Knecht S, et al. State of the art: Catheter ablation of atrial fibrillation. J Cardiovasc Electrophysiol. 2008;19:583-92.
117. Wyse DG, Waldo AL, DiMarco JP, et al. A comparison of rate control and rhythm control in patients with atrial fibrillation. N Engl J Med. 2002;347:1825-33.
118. Yoshida K, Ulfarsson M, Tada H, et al. Complex electrograms within the coronary sinus: time- and frequency-domain characteristics, effects of antral pulmonary vein isolation, and relationship to clinical outcome in patients with paroxysmal and persistent atrial fibrillation. J Cardiovasc Electrophysiol. 2008;19:1017-23.

Chapter

6

Idiopathic Ventricular Fibrillation: Electrophysiological Mechanisms, Mapping and Ablation

Emmanuel Catez, Matthew Wright, Thierry Verbeet, José Castro-Rodriguez, Marielle Morissens, Emmanuel Tran-Ngoc, Béatrice Peperstraete, Valentin Tatnga, Gabriella Vivian Flores, Christophe Janssen, Nathalie Ngo Mandag, Bilel, Pierre Decoodt, Sébastien Knecht

Abstract. Basic mechanisms implicated in idiopathic ventricular fibrillation such as triggering sources, arrhythmia perpetuation, crucial role of the Purkinje system have been discussed. Electrocardiographic and endocardial characterisics of the triggering VPBs and catheter ablation for idiopathic ventricular fibrillation were studied in the patients. Notably, ipsilateral intraventricular conduction delay was the only independent predictor of success because once this occurs it masks ipsilateral Purkinje potentials in sinus rhythm. Conversely, the frequency of VPB at the time of electrophysiological study and a higher frequency of prior events did not predict adverse outcome in this study. Ablation of idiopathic ventricular fibrillation, targeted to its ventricular premature beats triggers is feasible and results in an excellent long-term outcome.

Keywords. Ventricular fibrillation, catheter ablation, electrocardiogram.

INTRODUCTION

Ventricular fibrillation (VF) is the main cause of sudden cardiac death (Wever et al 1993), which is responsible for almost 500000 deaths per year in the US alone (Silvia et al 1997, Zipes and Wellens 1998). The vast majority of VF patients have an underlying cardiac disease which is often unrecognized (Chugh et al 2000). However, in about 10% of the VF patients, no underlying cardiac abnormality can be evidenced (Silvia et al 1997, Belhassen and Viskin 1993). This so-called idiopathic VF is proportionally more encountered in younger patients, therefore creating even more dramatic emotional situation.

At least 30% of patients with idiopathic VF will suffer from a recurrence of VF, syncope or cardiac arrest at 3 years from the first episode (Champagne et al 2005, Mewis et al 1998). Therefore, insertion of an implantable cardiac-defibrillator (ICD) therapy remains the gold standard for either primary or secondary VF prevention. Nevertheless, as ICD does not prevent VF to occur, an invasive catheter ablation strategy has to be envisaged in ICD patients with recurrent clinical events. The catheter ablation approach for VF patients is mainly based on results from studies depicting the key role played by the Purkinje network in idiopathic VF mechanisms (Berenfeld et al 1998, Haïssaguerre et al 2002, Gray et al 1995).

This review will focus on the underlying mechanisms of idiopathic VF and mapping and ablation of this arrhythmia during different clinical substrates.

BASIC MECHANISMS IMPLICATED IN IDIOPATHIC VENTRICULAR FIBRILLATION

As for every arrhythmia, VF occurrence implicates a trigger and a substrate which allows for the perpetuation if the arrhythmia.

Triggering Sources

VF may be triggered by short coupling ventricular premature beats (VPB) occurring during the vulnerable period of the ventricle (Haïssaguerre et al. 2002a, Storstein 1949). Different mechanisms have been involved, like triggered activity (due to after-depolarization phenomenon) or automaticity (Tabereaux et al 2007, Dosdall et al 2007, Dosdall et al 2008). These mechanisms have been shown to involve different structures of the ventricle: The myocardial tissue and the Purkinje fibers (Tabereaux et al 2007, Dosdall et al 2007, Dosdall et al 2008). At a molecular level, aberrant cell to cell coupling through deficient gap junction channels—a process called gap junction remodeling - is observed in many forms of human heart disease and can be responsible for malignant ventricular rhythm disorders and sudden cardiac death (Morley et al 2005). Some data indicate that electrical properties of the cell membrane predisposing tissue to VF could be directly determined by abnormal calcium release from sarcoplasmic reticulum (Saitoh et al 1989, Walker et al 2003).

Arrhythmia Perpetuation

Reentry is the main cause VF perpetuation, although automatic mechanisms have also been described (Haïssaguerre et al, 2002a, Haissaguerre et al 2002b). A reentry happens when the propagation of an electrical wave through the ventricle breaks and forms a functional reentry. Some waves propagating outward from the primary reentry may lead to additional wave breaks and finally to fibrillation (Weiss et al 2005). Several promoting factors who act synergistically to promote wave break and fibrillation have been described: Tissue heterogeneity exacerbated by electrical and structural remodeling from cardiac (in particular ischemic) disease; dynamic factors related to cellular properties of the cardiac action potential which generate wave instability and wave break even in "normal" heart tissue. These factors are mainly linked to membrane voltage (V_m) (electrical restitution of action potential duration and conduction velocity, short term cardiac memory, and electronic currents) and Ca_i cycling properties (Weiss et al 2005).

Crucial Role of the Purkinje System

Even if triggering sources have been described in the ventricular myocardium like in the right ventricular outflow track, the Purkinje system has been shown to be the most important source for triggering VF.

The Purkinje system has been first described in 1839 by Jan Evangelista Purkinje, a Czech anatomist and physiologist. He demonstrated that the Purkinje system was able to conduct electrical impulses from the atrioventricular node to all parts of both cardiac ventricles. We know now that the Purkinje network, localized endocardially in the human heart, consists of a single branch on the right that penetrates a limited portion of the right ventricle, and 2 larger branches on the left that ramify more intricately to supply a greater area of the left ventricle area (Myerburg et al 1970, Lazzara et al 1974, Myerburg et al 1970, Lazzara and Yeh 1974). Many clinical and animal studies have shown that this Purkinje system was notably implicated in the idiopathic VF mechanisms, by triggering and also maintaining the arrhythmia (Berenfeld et al 1998, Haïssaguerre et al. 2002a, Haissaguerre et al 2002b, Friedman et al 1973, Moise et al 1997, Haissaguerre et al 2002, Nogami et al 2005, Tabereaux et al 2009).

In experiments performed in canine hearts, multielectrode mapping of the endocardial left ventricle have shown an important activity of Purkinje fibers during the first 10 minutes of VF and a focal initiating mechanism for VF in 34% of cases, of which 42% arose from Purkinje fibers. In this study, evidence also suggested reentrant mechanisms implicating the Purkinje fibers in VF maintenance (Sasyniuk and Mendez 1971). In another study using a 3-dimensional model, Berenfeld (Berenfeld et al 1998) also showed that reentry involving the Purkinje-muscle junction may be a mechanism of focal subendocardial activation and a trigger for VF. He showed that Purkinje-muscle reentry may be important during VF, at least at the initial stage of the arrhythmia (Berenfeld et al 1998). Interestingly, in this 3-dimensional model, reentry was terminated when the Purkinje system was disconnected from the muscle before it reached a steady state, confirming its crucial role.

Animal studies and 3D model implicating the Purkinje system for idiopathic VF have been confirmed in human electrophysiological and ablation studies (Haïssaguerre et al. 2002a, Haissaguerre et al 2002b).

ELECTROCARDIOGRAPHIC AND ENDOCARDIAL CHARACTERISTICS OF THE TRIGGERING VPBS

Ectopy arising from the Purkinje system produces a characteristic 12-lead ECG pattern; VPBs originating in the right Purkinje system typically have a uniform left bundle branch block pattern with left superior axis. VPBs originating in the left Purkinje system produce more variable 12-lead ECG patterns, reflecting the more complex and extended Purkinje arborization on the left. VPBs originating from the right ventricular outflow tract (RVOT) have the classical aspect with a left bundle branch block pattern and a inferior axis.

The QRS duration of VPBs is shorter when originating from the left than the right Purkinje system (130 ± 24 ms vs. 162 ± 19 ms, p = 0.002), but the QRS duration of VPBs are not significantly different between VPBs originating from the left Purkinje system and the right ventricular outflow track (130±24 ms vs. 150 ± 16ms respectively, p = 0.11) (Knecht et al 2009). Furthermore, as compared to RVOT, VPBs originating from the Purkinje system have a shorter coupling (280 ± 26 vs. 355 ± 30ms; p = 0.01) and a higher prevalence of spontaneous polymorphic VPBs (18/5 vs. 1/3; p = 0.06) (Haissaguerre et al 2002b).

During sinus rhythm, the location of the Purkinje network is indicated by initial sharp potentials (<10 ms in duration) preceding the QRS complex by ≤15 ms. Such electrograms are distinct from earlier electrograms (>15 ms prior to the QRS) that are taken to indicate proximal Purkinje fascicle activation. The absence of a Purkinje potential at the site of earliest activation indicates the ventricular myocardium as the origin of the VPB.

During premature beat, the earliest Purkinje potential precedes the local muscle activation by a conduction interval of 38 ± 28 ms, with a greater precocity in the left than in the right ventricle (46 ± 29 versus 19 ± 10ms, P = 0.04) (Haissaguerre et al 2002b). At the same site, differing conduction times can be associated with varying morphologies, suggesting either changes in ventricular activation route or origin from another part of Purkinje system.

During VPB, conduction delay from the Purkinje network to the myocardium are shorter in the right than left ventricle, with variable conduction delays and dissociated Purkinje potentials in some patients (Macle et al 2002).

Patients with idiopathic VF triggered from the Purkinje system are older as compared to RVOT (43 ± 14 vs. 27 ± 8 years, p = 0.02) while patients with RVOT VF have more frequent ectopic beats but fewer episodes of VF. Moreover whereas 25% of Purkinje VF cases have a family history of sudden cardiac death, this has not yet been described for RVOT VF patients.

CATHETER ABLATION FOR IDIOPATHIC VENTRICULAR FIBRILLATION

The initial study that investigated the feasibility of VF ablation studied a population with idiopathic VF ((Haïssaguerre et al 2002a). Patients were recruited from six centres with recurrent VF. None of the patients enrolled had evidence of known electrophysiological abnormalities (Long or Short QT, Brugada Syndrome) or structural heart disease based on established criteria. All patients enrolled had frequent ventricular ectopy, with a mean of over 9000 ventricular ectopics per day, which allowed endocardial mapping of the ventricular ectopics. Surface ECG leads and bipolar intracardiac electrograms were filtered at 30-500 Hz and recorded simulataneously. Using between two and four intracardiac catheters the site of earliest activation of the ventricular ectopics responsible for initiation of VF (from previous ECGs) was mapped. In 12 of the 16 patients an initial sharp potential (<10 ms duration) was observed before a larger and slower ventricular electrogram. This potential represented a Purkinje component, and when present before ventricular ectopy suggested that the source of the ectopy originated form the Purkinje system. In the four remaining patients the site of earliest activation was not preceded by the early sharp potential but the larger slower potential, suggesting that the origin of these ventricular ectopics was from the myocardium itself, and these were all mapped to the right ventricular outflow tract (RVOT).

Radiofrequency ablation was targeted to the site of earliest activation of the ectopic beats with a mean of nine applications when the origin was from the distal Purkinje fibres and six when the origin was ventricular myocardium. In 13 patients the procedure was successful resulting in a dramatic reduction in the number of ventricular ectopic beats to a mean of 29 per day. During follow up of a mean of 32 months none of these 13 patients had a recurrence of VF. In the 3 patients who continued to have frequent premature beats even after the ablation two went onto have defibrillating shocks for VF, delivered by their ICD.

In another multicentre study, comprising of five tertiary electrophysiology centres, 27 patients were recruited following resuscitation from recurrent idiopathic VF (Haissaguerre et al 2002b). Ventricular ectopics were present at the time of the procedure and could be mapped in 24 of the patients. The site of earliest ventricular activation was mapped to the RVOT in four patients whereas in the remaining 20 patients ventricular ectopy was preceded by a Purkinje potential. The three remaining patients who did not have ventricular ectopy at the time of the procedure had ablation based upon previously recorded ectopic beats. With a mean of 24 months of follow up 24 of the 27 patients did not experience syncope, VF or sudden death, and three patients had a recurrence of either VF or ventricular tachycardia.

Long-term Follow-up after Idiopathic VF Catheter Ablation

In a multicentre study, we studied 38 patients from 6 different centers after idiopathic VF ablation. The median duration of radiofrequency energy delivered, fluoroscopy and total ablation procedural time were 14 min, 28 min and 135 min, respectively. 30 patients (81%) had clinical VPB at the time of the procedure while 8 patients (19%) did not. Clinical VPBs triggering VF arose from the right Purkinje system in 16 patients, the left Purkinje in 14 patients, in both the left and right Purkinje system in 3 patients and in the myocardium in 5 patients (including the right ventricular outflow track in 4 patients). A mean of 1.7 ± 2.0 VPB morphologies were targeted per patient. When VPB were present at the time of the procedure, catheter ablation was successful in abolishing VPB in all patients.

Following ablation, one patient developed transient left bundle branch block. Six other patients developed nonspecific intraventricular conduction defects not meeting formal criteria for a bundle branch block.

During a median follow up of 63 months (IQ range 40 to 80), 7/38 patients (18%) experienced a recurrence of VF. This occurred after a median of 24 months

(IQ range 1 to 60). VF recurrence was detected by the ICD and did not lead to syncope or clinical sudden cardiac arrest in any of the patients. Ablation was repeated in 5 of these 7 patients (1 patient had 2 repeat procedures). Four of these 5 patients had other VPB morphologies as compared to the initial procedure, while one patient had the same clinical VPB recurrence triggering VF. These 5 patients had no subsequent recurrence of VF or documented VPBs for 28 months (IQ range 24 to 72 months).

Two patients with VF recurrence were not reablated. In these 2 patients, clinical VPB morphology triggering VF recurrence could not be analyzed as there was no 12 lead ECG of the events. Of these 2 patients, one was treated with quinidine. This had been ineffective prior to ablation and was stopped without medical advice after ablation; following reinitiation of quinidine there have been no VF recurrences (for 6 months). The second non re-ablated patient had a single asymptomatic short run of polymorphic VT 2 years after the ablation, which terminated spontaneously (without ICD therapy) and which did not recur for 5 years.

Prior to ablation, 12 patients (32%) experienced electrical storm 3 months (IQ range 1 to 6 months) beforehand while, after ablation, only 3 patients (8% of all patients) had a recurrence of electrical storm ($p=0.03$) that occurred 1, 48 and 60 months postablation.

Three patients experienced clinical recurrence of the initial clinical VPB following the initial ablation procedure, which did not result in malignant ventricular arrhythmia. One symptomatic patient has been reablated without recurrence of VPB, and the 2 other patients never experienced malignant ventricular arrhythmia recurrence on verapamil and quinidine therapy despite persistence of VPB.

Ablation significantly reduced the number of significant events (confirmed VF/VT or sudden death) from (4 (IQ range 3 to 9) before ablation to 0 (total range 0 to 4, $p=0.01$) after wards.

After a mean follow-up of 52±28 months after the last procedure, 36/38 patients are free from VF after a mean of 1.28±0.6 procedures. Five of the 38 patients (13%) are currently on antiarrhythmic therapy, including 2 who experienced VF recurrence and 2 with VPB recurrence.

Notably, ipsilateral intraventricular conduction delay was the only independent predictor of success because once this occurs it masks ipsilateral Purkinje potentials in sinus rhythm. Conversely, the frequency of VPB at the time of electrophysiological study and a higher frequency of prior events did not predict adverse outcome in this study.

CONCLUSION

Ablation of idiopathic ventricular fibrillation, targeted to its ventricular premature beats triggers is feasible and results in an excellent long-term outcome. Short coupled VPB triggering VF originates predominantly from the Purkinje system and the right ventricular outflow track.

ACKNOWLEDGEMENTS

The authors acknowledge financial support from the Department of Health via the National Institute for Health Research (NIHR) comprehensive Biomedical Research Centre award to Guy's and St Thomas' NHS Foundation Trust in partnership with King's College London and King's College Hospital NHS Foundation Trust.

BIBLIOGRAPHY

1. Belhassen B, Viskin S. Idiopathic Ventricular Tachycardia and Fibrillation. J Cardiovasc Electrophysiol. 1993;4(3):356-68.
2. Berenfeld O, Jalife J. Purkinje-Muscle Reentry as a Mechanism of Polymorphic Ventricular Arrhythmias in a 3-Dimensional Model of the Ventricles. Circ Res. 1998;82(10):1063-77.
3. Champagne J, Peter Geelen P, Philippon F, Brugada P. Recurrent events in patients with idiopathic ventricular fibrillation, excluding patients with the Brugada syndrome. BMC Med 2005;10.1186/1741-7015-3-1.
4. Chugh SS, Kelly KL, Titus JL. Sudden Cardiac Death With Apparently Normal Heart. Circulation. 2000;102(6):649-54.
5. Dosdall DJ, Cheng K-A, Huang J, Allison JS, Allred JD, Smith WM, Ideker RE. Transmural and endocardial Purkinje activation in pigs before local myocardial activation after defibrillation shocks. Heart Rhythm. 2007;4(6):758-65.
6. Dosdall DJ, Tabereaux PB, Kim JJ, Walcott GP, Rogers JM, Killingsworth CR, et al. Chemical ablation of the Purkinje system causes early termination and activation rate slowing of long-duration ventricular fibrillation in dogs. Am J Physiol Heart Circ Physiol. 2008;295:883-9.
7. Friedman PL, Stewart JR, Wit AL. Spontaneous and Induced Cardiac Arrhythmias in Subendocardial Purkinje Fibers Surviving Extensive Myocardial Infarction in Dogs. Circulation Research. 1973;33(5):612-26.
8. Gray R, Jalife J, Panfilov A, Baxter W, Cabo C, Davidenko J, AM P. Mechanism of cardiac fibrillation. Science. 1995;270(5239):1224-5.
9. Haïssaguerre M, Shah DC, Jaïs P, Shoda M, Kautzner J, Arentz T, et al. Role of Purkinje conducting system in triggering of idiopathic ventricular fibrillation. The Lancet. 2002a;359(9307):677-8.
10. Haissaguerre M, Shoda M, Jais P, Nogami A, Shah DC, Kautzner J, et al. Mapping and Ablation of Idiopathic Ventricular Fibrillation. Circulation. 2002b;106(8):962-7.
11. Knecht S, Sacher F, Wright M, Hocini M, Nogami A, Arentz T, et al. Long-term follow-up of idiopathic ventricular fibrillation ablation: A multicenter Study. Journal of the American College of Cardiology. 2009;54(6):522-8.
12. Lazzara R, Yeh BK, Samet P. Functional anatomy of the canine left bundle branch. The American Journal of Cardiology. 1974;33(5):623-32.
13. Lazzara R, Yeh BK, PS. Functional anatomy of the canine left bundle branch. Am J Cardiol. 1974;33:623-32.
14. Macle L, Shah DC, Jaïs P, Haïssaguerre M. Accessory Pathway Automaticity After Radiofrequency Ablation. J Cardiovasc Electrophysiol. 2002;13(3):285-7.
15. Mewis C, Kühlkamp V, Spyridopoulos I, Bosch RF, Seipel L. Late Outcome of Survivors of Idiopathic Ventricular Fibrillation. The American Journal of Cardiology. 1998;81(8):999-1003.
16. Moise NS, Gilmour RF JR, Riccio ML. An Animal Model of Spontaneous Arrhythmic Death. Journal of Cardiovascular Electrophysiology. 1997;8(1):98-103.
17. Morley GE, Danik SB, Bernstein S, Sun Y, Rosner G, Gutstein DE, Fishman GI. Reduced intercellular coupling leads to paradoxical propagation across the Purkinje-ventricular junction and aberrant myocardial activation. PNAS. 2005;102(11):4126-9.

18. Myerburg RJ, Stewart JW, Hoffman BF. Electrophysiological Properties of the Canine Peripheral A-V Conducting System. Circulation Research. 1970;26(3):361-78.
19. Nogami A, Sugiyasu A, Kubota S, Kato K. Mapping and ablation of idiopathic ventricular fibrillation from the Purkinje system. Heart rhythm: The official journal of the Heart Rhythm Society. 2005;2(6):646-9.
20. Saitoh H, Bailey JC, Surawicz B. Action potential duration alternans in dog Purkinje and ventricular muscle fibers. Further evidence in support of two different mechanisms. Circulation. 1989;80(5):1421-31.
21. Sasyniuk BI, Mendez C. A. Mechanism for Reentry in Canine Ventricular Tissue. Circulation Research. 1971;28(1):3-15.
22. Silvia G. Priori, Fondazione S. Maugeri, Policlinico S. Matteo and Piazzale Golgi. Survivors of Out-of-Hospital Cardiac Arrest With Apparently Normal Heart: Need for Definition and Standardized Clinical Evaluation. Circulation. 1997;95(1):265-72.
23. Storstein O. Adams-Stokes attacks caused by ventricular fibrillation in a man with otherwise normal heart. Acta Med Scand. 1949;133(6):437-41.
24. Tabereaux PB, Walcott GP, Rogers JM, Kim J, Dosdall DJ, Robertson PG, et al. Activation Patterns of Purkinje Fibers During Long-Duration Ventricular Fibrillation in an Isolated Canine Heart Model. Circulation. 2007;116(10):1113-9.
25. Tabereaux PB, Dosdall DJ, Ideker RE. Mechanisms of VF maintenance: Wandering wavelets, mother rotors, or foci. Heart Rhythm. 2009;6(3):405-15.
26. Walker ML, Wan X, Kirsch GE, Rosenbaum DS. Hysteresis Effect Implicates Calcium Cycling as a Mechanism of Repolarization Alternans. Circulation. 2003;108(21):2704-9.
27. Weiss JN, Qu Z, Chen P-S, Lin S-F, Karagueuzian HS, Hayashi H, et al. The Dynamics of Cardiac Fibrillation. Circulation. 2005;112:1232-40.
28. Wever EF, Hauer RN, Oomen A, Peters RH, Bakker PF, Robles de Medina EO. Unfavorable outcome in patients with primary electrical disease who survived an episode of ventricular fibrillation. Circulation. 1993;88(3):1021-9.
29. Zipes DP, Wellens HJJ. Sudden Cardiac Death. Circulation. 1998;98(21):2334-51.

Chapter

7

Blood Cholinesterase Level and QTc Interval in Patients with Organophosphate Poisoning

Ahmet Baydin, Turker Yardan, Ali Kemal Erenler

Abstract. Organophosphate compounds are predominant group of insecticides used for pest control in many parts of the world. Organophosphates inhibit both true cholinesterase and pseudocholinesterase. Organophosphates cause poisoning as a result of the excessive accumulation of acetylcholine at the cholinergic synapses due to inhibition of acetylcholinesterase. In the literature, it has been reported that there have been electrocardiographic abnormalities, including QT interval prolongation in most patients with organophosphate poisoning. In this paper, our aim is emphasize relationship between blood cholinesterase levels and QTc interval after organophosphate intoxication in the light of recent reports.

Keywords. Intoxication, organophosphate, QTc-interval, cholinesterase, cardiac toxicity.

INTRODUCTION

There are thousands of published reports about organophosphate (OP) poisoning in the literature and it is a recognized fact that these substances are highly toxic. Furthermore, poisoning related to these substances is being seen in developing countries at an increasing rate. Among anticholinesterase agents, OP compounds are possibly the most widely used insecticides. Organophosphates are usually esters, amides or thiol derivates of phosphoric acid (Karalliedde et al 2003, Kamanyire and Karalliedde 2004). They form a large family of about 50,000 chemical agents with biological properties that have important and sometimes unique implications for man. The first potent synthetic OP was synthesized by Clermont in 1854 and further OP development occurre d in the late 1930s and early 1940s. Modern investigations of OP compounds began in 1932 when Lange and Krueger recorded the synthesis of dimethyl and diethyl phosphorus fluoridates. Unfortunately, in addition to their development as agricultural pesticides, their clinical effects would lead to their use in chemical warfare as potential nerve agents (Karalliedde and Senanayake 1989). In 1932, Lange and Krueger reported choking and blurred vision following inhalation of organic phosphorus compounds. This report inspired Schrader, a German chemist, to investigate these agents, initially as pesticides, and later as chemical warfare. During this research, Schrader and coworkers synthesized hundreds of compounds, including the popular pesticide parathion and a chemical warfare agent.

OP compounds are, at present, the predominant insecticides group used for pest control in many parts of the world (Balali-Mood and Shariat 1998). The term "pesticides" is a general term encompassing many chemicals, primarily in the classes of insecticides (organophosphates, organochlorines, carbamates and pyrethroides) and herbicides. OP pesticides are easily available due to the inadequate regulations in controlling their sale. This easily availability has resulted in a gradual increase in accidental and suicidal poisonings they bring about, mainly in developing countries (Hayes et al 1978, Saadeh et al 1996, Guven et al 1997, Sungur and Guven 2001). According to the annual World Health Organization report, one million accidental poisonings and two million suicide attempts with insecticides occur worldwide, and of these, approximately 200,000 result in death (Chaudhry et al 1998, Singh and Sharma 2000).

Despite the wide-spread use of pesticides and the many studies that have been conducted to investigate the clinical findings, diagnosis, treatment and prognosis of the poisoning, little information exists in the literature about the relationship between blood cholinesterase levels and corrected Q-T (QTc) interval in patients with OP poisoning. In this chapter, our aim is to emphasize the relationship between blood cholinesterase levels and QTc interval after OP intoxication in accord with recent reports.

PHARMACOKINETICS OF ORGANOPHOSPHATE INSECTICIDES

The organophosphates are popular insecticides. In many third-world countries, OP pesticides are one of the most important causes of both occupational and suicidal poisonings. Especially in the regions where highly toxic OP compounds are easily available, deaths due to intentional poisonings are more common than those due to accidental poisonings (Eddleston et al 2002, Yurumez et al 2007). The increase in accidental OP poisoning as well as the rise in the number of cases of attempted suicides using organophosphates is due primarily to the widespread use of these compounds in agriculture. Poisonings may occur after oral ingestion, absorption via the skin or mucous membranes and by inhalation. It sometimes occurs by injection (Heath and Vale 1992, Sungur and Guven 2001, Yurumez et al 2007).

Poisoning with organophosphates is considered as one of the most common acute intoxications. Peroral ingestion with suicidal intent constitutes the majority of the OP poisoning cases (Kara et al 2002, Karki et al 2004, Baydin et al 2007, Yurumez et al 2007). The modes of exposure include dermal, gastrointestinal, inhalational, and intravenous routes. Routes other than peroral are rarely seen (Hayes et al 1978, Sungur and Guven 2001, Yurumez et al 2007). The primary target for organophosphates is the cholinesterase enzymes. Alles and Hawes revealed for the first time in 1940, that cholinesterase enzymes are located within the blood of mammals and that there are at least two enzymes capable of enhancing hydrolysis of acetylcholine; one located mostly within the erythrocytes and the other essentially within the plasma. In the following years, this view was accepted, and the term "true cholinesterase" was used to refer to the cholinesterase located in erythrocytes, while "pseudocholinesterase" referred to that in plasma. Currently, it is assumed that true cholinesterase, or acetylcholinesterase (AChE) is located in erythrocytes and nerve tissue and that pseudocholinesterase, or plasma cholinesterase, is located in blood serum and the liver, heart, pancreas, and brain.

OP insecticides inhibit both true cholinesterase (acetylcholinesterase) and pseudocholinesterase (Wang et al 1998, Rusyniak and Nanagas 2004). The bond between OP and cholinesterase is not reversible without intervention. This property causes OP to act as an irreversible cholinesterase inhibitor. This inhibition occurs as a result of the covalent binding of phosphate radicals to the active site of the cholinesterase enzyme, thereby converting cholinesterase enzyme into an inert protein such as acetic acid, and choline (Chuang et al 1996, Lotti 2001). Acetylcholine accumulation caused by the organophosphate-induced inhibition of cholinesterase is responsible for this toxic effect. The massive accumulation of acetylcholine initially stimulates and then paralyzes the transmission in cholinergic synapses. Some OP insecticides inhibit pseudocholinesterase more than true cholinesterase while others do the opposite (Wilson et al 1997, Eddleston et al 2005). The inhibition of AchE leads to the accumulation of acetylcholine, the neurotransmitter at all ganglia in the autonomic nervous system and at many synapses in the brain and skeletal neuromuscular junctions, at some postganglionic nerve endings of the sympathetic nervous system and adrenal medulla. The role of pseudocholinesterase in the body is yet to be fully identified, but it is known to be involved in the hydrolysis of many therapeutic agents (e.g. suxamethonium, esmolol, procaine, and cocaine).

Most organophosphates are highly lipid-soluble agents and are well absorbed by all routes of exposure, including the skin, conjunctiva, and respiratory and gastrointestinal routes. Generally, absorption is the fastest after inhalation and the slowest after percutaneous exposure. The effector organ dysfunction is local at first and rapidly spreads to become generalized. The onset, severity and duration of poisoning are dependent on the dose, route of exposure, physicochemical properties of the OP (e.g. lipid solubility), rate of metabolism, and whether the organophosphorylated cholinesterase ages rapidly (Karalliedde et al 2003). Vale reported in 1998 that OP insecticides were typically lipophilic and stored in fat tissue and that their serum half-lives varied from minutes to hours. Lipophilic organophosphates may be protected from metabolism by fat storage, obviously prolonging their elimination half-life (Davies et al 1975, Karalliedde and Senanayake 1989, Gallo and Lawryk 1991). Gadoth and Fisher (1978) reported that cholinergic crisis may recur in patients with OP poisoning when fat stores of unmetabolized organic phosphorus agents are mobilized. Reports involving patients with OP poisoning have described an illness with cholinergic symptoms developed shortly after exposure. Although cases of poisoning with OP compounds are considered and approached as acute illnesses that manifest peak toxicity within 24 hours after ingestion or exposure, there are reports about compounds like fenthion that claim onset of cholinergic crisis may delay 5 days and recur in 24 days. The reason for this delay can be associated with the long-lasting activity of such compounds (Merrill and Mihm 1982).

Organic phosphorus insecticides are thought to be metabolized by various mixed functional oxidases in the liver and intestinal mucosa, but the exact pathways are not yet well understood (Sultatos et al 1984). Inactive metabolites of these compounds are excreted in the urine (Gallo and Lawryk 1991).

PATHOPHYSIOLOGY OF ORGANOPHOSPHATE INSECTICIDES

Exposure to organophosphates may be acute, chronic or subchronic. In acute exposure, the main mechanism of toxicity of organophosphates is their irreversible binding to the enzyme AchE and inhibition of its activity, which results in accumulation and prolonged effect of acetylcholine, consequently followed by acute muscarinic and nicotinic effects. In chronic and subchronic exposure, in addition to cholinesterase inhibition, induction of oxidative stress has been reported as the main mechanism of toxicity (Akhgari et al 2003, Abdollahi et al 2004, Ranjbar et al 2005).

Acetylcholine is a major neurotransmitter in the central, autonomic and somatic nervous systems. Acetylcholine released from cholinergic nerve terminals is disposed of solely through hydrolysis by AchE. In fact, differently from other neurotransmitters (e.g., noradrenaline), it is the product of acetylcholine hydrolysis by AchE, choline, that is taken up by the presynaptic terminal (Robey and Meggs 2000). The enzyme AchE hydrolyzes the neurotransmitter acetylcholine to two inactive fragments, choline and acetic acid. OP compounds bind to both types of cholinesterase covalently at their anionic binding site for acetylcholine, changing them into enzymatically inactive proteins (Bardin et al 1994). As a result of the cholinesterase inhibition by organophosphates, the acetylcholine accumulates at nerve synapses and neuromuscular junctions, resulting in overstimulation of acetylcholine receptors. This initial overstimulation is followed by paralysis of cholinergic synaptic transmission in the central nervous system (CNS), in autonomic ganglia and in somatic nerves (O'Malley 1997, Robey and Meggs 2000, Goel and Aggarwal 2007). OP pesticides inhibit esterase enzymes, especially AchE in synapses and on red cell membranes, and pseudocholinesterase in plasma. While the inhibition of pseudocholinesterase does not seem to cause clinical features, AchE inhibition results in the accumulation of acetylcholine and overstimulation of acetylcholine receptors in the synapses of autonomic nervous system, CNS, and neuromuscular junctions (Eddleston et al 2008). Organophosphates bind irreversibly to the active serine residue of AchE and subsequently disturb the nerve impulse transmission in both the peripheral and CNS (Cherian et al 2005). Although differences between OP insecticides were reported in 1977, acute OP poisonings are frequently considered as a homogeneous entity in most textbooks, reviews and research articles. However, the cause of these differences has not been clearly identified (Eddleston et al 2005).

Cholinesterase activity in red blood cells is low in the newborn and in patients with leukemia and multiple myeloma. Cholinesterase activity is elevated whenever the proportion of reticulocytes and young erythrocytes in the blood is increased, as in thalassemia major and hereditary spherocytosis. Plasma cholinesterase activity is depressed in allergic diseases, protein and calorie malnutrition, decompensated heart disease, liver disease (malignant metastases, hepatitis, and cirrhosis), obstructive jaundice, malignant neoplasm, and pregnancy (Wills JH 1972, Cahill-Morasco et al 1998).

CLINICAL FEATURES OF ORGANOPHOSPHATE POISONING

In OP poisoning, clinical findings depend on the specific agent involved, degree of exposure, type of exposure, and quantity absorbed. Most victims of acute poisoning become symptomatic within 30 minutes to 3 hours of exposure, and nearly all are symptomatic within 24 hours (Namba et al 1970). However, patients suffering massive ingestions can become symptomatic as quickly as 5 minutes following ingestion (Lokan and James 1981). Highly fat-soluble compounds, however, may cause recurrent or delayed symptoms and signs on redistribution from adipose tissue. Toxicity is produced by the rapid absorption of the compound through the gastrointestinal and respiratory tracts and skin. OP agents such as malathion are associated with local irritation of the skin and respiratory tract with resulting dermatitis and wheezing, respectively, without evidence of systemic absorption. A few cases of persistent reactive airways disease independent of cholinesterase inhibition have been reported (Deschamps et al 1994).

Clinical findings of OP poisoning derive from excessive stimulation of muscarinic and nicotinic cholinergic receptors by acetylcholine in the central and autonomic nervous systems, and at skeletal neuromuscular junctions. Due to the widespread distribution of cholinergic neurons in the central and peripheral nervous systems, the signs and symptoms involve various organ systems, such as the gastrointestinal system, CNS, skeletal muscles, respiratory system, and cardiovascular system, other organs, and metabolic effects (Table 7.1). Patients with OP poisoning usually present with nonspecific gastrointestinal symptoms of vomiting, emesis and abdominal pain. Subsequent clinical manifestations are multisystemic and involve muscarinic, nicotinic and central receptor stimulation. Muscarinic receptor stimulation by acetylcholine leads to salivation, lacrimation, urinary incontinence, defecation, gastrointestinal cramps and emesis, diaphoresis, miosis, bronchospasm or bronchorrhea, hypotension, bradycardia, and QT prolongation with development of various types of arrhythmias. Aaron et al (1990) reported that the severity of symptoms in acute OP poisoning parallels the degree of AchE activity. Predisposing factors for the development of most of the cardiac complications occur when hypoxemia, acidosis and electrolyte derangements are present (Robey and Meggs 2000, Karki et al 2004).

Table 7.1: Signs and symptoms of organophosphate poisoning [Modified from Bardin et al. Arch Intern Med 1994;154:1433-41].

Muscarinic	Nicotinic	Central receptors
Cardiovascular	**Cardiovascular**	Anxiety
Bradycardia	Tachycardia	Ataxia
Hypotension	Hypertension	Absent reflexes
Respiratory	**Musculoskeletal**	Convulsions
Rhinorrhea	Weakness	Coma
Bronchorrhea	Fasciculations	Circulatory collapse
Rronchospasm	Cramps	Cheyne-Stoke respiration
Cough	Paralysis	Dysarthria
Gastrointestinal		Insomnia
Increased salivation		Respiratory depression
Nausea and vomiting		Restlessness
Abdominal pain		Tremor
Diarrhea		
Faecal incontinence		
Genitourinary		
Urinary incontinence		
Ocular		
Blurred vision		
Increased lacrimation		
Miosis		
Others		
Excessive sweating		

In patients with OP poisoning, a sequential triphasic illness occurs. In many of these patients, the only phase that can be observed is the cholinergic phase. In 20% of the patients, this cholinergic phase progresses to the intermediate syndrome (IS). Both the cholinergic phase and IS are associated with a high mortality risk. Cases other than mild ones should be managed in intensive care units (ICU). Organophosphate-induced delayed polyneuropathy, also known as the final phase, sets in 7-21 days after exposure and may not be preceded by either the cholinergic phase or the IS (Kamanyire and Karaliedde 2004).

The cardiovascular manifestations also reflect mixed effects on the autonomic nervous system. Increased sympathetic tone is often initially present, and most patients manifest a sinus tachycardia and sometimes hypertension (Ludomirsky et al 1982). As toxicity becomes more severe, bradycardia with a prolonged PR interval and varying degrees of AV blocks occur degrees occur because of excessive parasympathetic tone, and possibly because of reduced coronary blood flow (Namba et al 1971, Ludomirsky et al 1982). Unequal sympathetic stimulation of myocardial cells and interactions with potassium channels and the Na^{+}/Ca^{++} exchanger in the myocardial cell membrane are likely responsible for the occasional prolonged QTc interval (Clark RF 2002). This prolongation in the QTc interval can be associated with polymorphic ventricular tachycardia (Ludomirsky et al 1982, Kiss and Fazegas 1983, Wang et al 1998). In 1993, Agarwal stated that bradycardia or tachycardia might occur with severe poisoning (Agarwal SB 1993). Nicotinic stimulation at neuromuscular junctions results in muscle fasciculation, cramps, weakness, and paralysis. Miosis and muscle fasciculations are considered reliable signs of OP poisoning. Respiratory muscle paralysis results in acute respiratory failure and death.

Acetylcholine is the presynaptic neurotransmitter at nicotinic receptors in the sympathetic ganglia and adrenal medulla. Stimulation of sympathetic ganglia leads to pallor, mydriasis, hypertension, and tachycardia. Heart rate and blood pressure can be potentially misleading findings, as an increase or decrease can occur in both vital signs. CNS manifestations include headache, dizziness, tremor, restlessness, anxiety, confusion, convulsion, and coma.

The Intermediate Syndrome (IS)

This syndrome was first described in 1974 by Wadia et al as Type II paralyses, and was subsequently characterized and termed as "intermediate syndrome" by Senanayake and Karalliedde in 1987. Since then, there have been numerous reports of the syndrome. IS is characterized clinically by weakness in the proximal limb muscles, the flexor muscles of the neck, and/or respiratory muscles. At present, the exact pathogenesis of the IS is unknown, but is likely due to alteration in the function and activity of the nicotinic receptors at the neuromuscular junction (Kamanyire and Karalliedde 2004). One of the earliest manifestations in these patients is the presence of marked weakness of flexion of the neck and inability to lift the head from the pillow. Usually, extraocular muscle supplier cranial nerves are involved. Cranial nerves VII and X are affected less frequently (Peter and Cherian 2000). In this syndrome, Senanayake also described various degrees of cranial nerve palsies, particularly in cranial nerves innervating the extraocular muscles. IS can develop within the first 96 hours after acute OP poisoning (Karalliedde L 1999). While Karalliedde stated that IS develops in 96 hours after OP poisoning. Yardan et al (2007) reported that IS might delay up to 114 hours. Difficulty in breathing may progress to respiratory failure following paralysis of the diaphragm and other muscles of respiration. Complete recovery occurs within 4–21 days after appropriate ventilatory care. Some patients have attributed the IS to either inadequate or delayed oxime therapy (Benson et al 1992). The predictors of IS have been a common interest of the researches. In one study, Aygun et al (2007) investigated the muscle enzyme creatine kinase in this regard but no significant correlation was found.

Organophosphate-induced Delayed Polyneuropathy (OPIDP)

OPIDP is a sensory-motor distal axonopathy that usually occurs after ingestion of large doses of OP insecticides (Lotti et al 1984). Unlike the IS, OPIDP usually occurs 2-3 weeks after the acute poisoning episode and predominantly affects the long nerves in the nervous system causing symmetrical weakness of peripheral muscles in the hands and feet, with a variable degree of sensory impairment. At present, the phosphorylation of an enzyme in nerve tissue, the neuropathy target esterase, is considered responsible for the dysfunction. High-dose methyl prednisolone has been shown to be beneficial in experimental animals (Baker and Stanec 1985).

Other Sequelae of Exposure

Workers occupationally exposed to organophosphates with a decrease in serum and red blood cell cholinesterase activity had a greater frequency of upper respiratory tract infection (Hermanowicz and Kossman 1984). In one study, after exposure to occupational organophosphates, influenza-like symptoms were observed in 23 patients (Murray et al 1992). In 1979, Kiss and Fazekas reported pancreatitis and hyperamylasemia after oral or dermal exposure. They also reported that hyperamylasemia was closely related to the clinical severity and the presence of shock. Acute pancreatitis (Roeyen et al 2008), pseudopancreatic cyst (Rizos et al 2004), personality changes (Dahlgren et al 2004), neuroleptic malignant-like syndrome (Ochi et al 1995), depression, and confusion may be seen as sequelae following ingestion of the poison in some patients.

MECHANISMS OF CARDIOVASCULAR TOXICITY IN ORGANOPHOSPHATE POISONING

There are many reports in the literature about the effects of the cholinesterase inhibitors. One of these reports by Blandizzi et al in 2001 stated that as a cholinesterase inhibitor, phosphamidon causes direct mechanical and electrophysiological effects in an isolated rat heart. They also reported that high concentrations of phosphamidon caused a significant prolongation of the Q-T interval, indicating that it has a potent cardiotoxic effect. It was also reported by Smith et al in an animal assay in 2001 that as OP pesticides inhibit AchE and cause cholinergic stimulation in the CNS and peripheral tissues, oxotremorine also caused elevation in blood pressure, heart rate and cardiac contractility. In another study with dichlorvos, Parveen and Kumar (2001) observed inhibition in heart AchE activity in intoxicated rats.

Organophosphates frequently have harmful effects on heart and may cause multiple cardiac abnormalities, such as cardiac rhythm or conduction abnormalities, pulmonary edema, and fatality. These abnormalities are potentially preventable if they are diagnosed early and treated adequately. Organophosphates may cause an alteration in blood pressure, heart rate and cardiac rhythm. These components of the hemodynamic system are susceptible to the toxic effects of organophosphates. Cardiac toxicity due to organophosphates may be shown by the development of (a) Hemodynamic instability (i.e. hypotension, hypertension), (b) Heart failure and pulmonary edema, (c) Cardiac conduction abnormalities, or (d) Dysrhythmia. Therefore, continuation of adequate tissue perfusion depends on cardiac rhythm, cardiac contractility, and vascular resistance in addition to volume status.

Hypotension may be caused by intravascular volume depletion as a result of vomiting, diarrhea, or excessive secretions, or to a reduction in cardiac output due to negative inotropic and chronotropic effects of the organophosphates (Morita et al 1995). Hypertension and sinus tachycardia, which may be seen in OP poisoning, are nicotinic effects (Clark RF 2002). Congestive cardiac failure (Fazekas and Kiss 1980), heart failure and pulmonary edema (Karki et al 2004), cardiac conduction abnormalities (Ludomirsky et al 1982) and dysrhythmias (Luzhnikov et al 1975) were also reported as other cardiac effects.

Organophosphates interfere with the destruction of acetylcholine by binding to the AchE enzyme and cause the accumulation of acetylcholine in the synaptic space. Hammer et al in 1986 stated that the accumulated acetylcholine interacts with muscarinic M2 receptors in the heart. Levy and Martin (1991) reported that acetylcholine exerts a direct negative chronotropic effect on the sinoatrial node, a negative dromotropic effect on AV conduction, and a direct negative inotropic effect both in atrial and ventricular tissues in the presence of a sympathetic tone. Shadnia et al (2009) stated that cholinergic innervations of the heart result in both negative chronotropy and negative inotropy that slows myocardial conduction or repolarization. The cardiac effect of OP poisoning is characterized by the profound upsurge in sympathetic tone expressed as sinus tachycardia, and the robust increase in parasympathetic tone displayed by ST/T segment changes, abnormal AV conduction, and arrhythmias. Although intensively studied over the last decades, the mechanisms of organophosphate-induced cardiac toxicity are not fully understood. The cardiac toxicity associated with OP poisoning is caused by more than one mechanism. Possible mechanisms include (1) Over activity of cholinergic or nicotinic receptors causing hemodynamic alterations, (2) Direct toxic effect of the compound on the myocardium, (3) Acidosis, (4) Hypoxemia, (5) Electrolyte abnormalities, and (6) High-dose atropine therapy (Kiss and Fazekas 1979; Brill et al 1984; Klingelhofer and Sander 1997; Karki et al 2004; Taira et al 2006). Pesticides may also induce oxidative stress, leading to generation of free radicals and alteration in antioxidants, oxygen free radicals, the scavenging enzyme system, and lipid peroxidation. In addition, oxidative stress in the heart cells may be the cause of myocardial damage that may result in several conduction problems (Abdollahi et al 2004). However, unequal sympathetic stimulation of myocardial cells and interactions with potassium channels and the Na^{+}/Ca^{++} exchanger in the myocardial cell membrane are probably responsible for the occasional prolonged QTc interval (Clark RF 2002).

Thirty years ago, Ludomirsky et al first described three phases of cardiac toxicity after OP poisoning as follows: Phase 1. A brief initial period of increased sympathetic tone; hypertension and sinus tachycardia occur in this phase. These are considered nicotinic effects. Phase 2. A prolonged phase characterized by sinus bradycardia and hypotension. These effects are thought to be due to extreme parasympathetic overflow, usually accompanied by electrocardiographic ST/T segment changes and AV conduction disturbances of varying degrees. Phase 3. Characteristics of this phase include Q-T interval prolongation, polymorphic ventricular tachycardia and sudden death are.

According to Ranjbar et al (2005), antioxidant capacity reduces in acute and chronic OP intoxication, and this reduction causes myocardial damage (via free oxygen radicals). Abdollahi et al (2004) reported that various conduction abnormalities can be observed after damage to the myocardium by free oxygen radicals.

Organophosphates can reduce cardiac inotropy or contractility, with a resulting decrease in cardiac ejection fraction and cardiac output, a decrease in blood pressure, and development of heart failure and cardiogenic pulmonary edema. Therefore, patients with organophosphate-induced cardiovascular toxicity should receive aggressive hemodynamic support. A change in hemodynamic stability may be either by direct toxic effects on the heart or secondary to development of metabolic abnormalities (especially acidemia, hypoxia and electrolyte imbalance). Standard noninvasive hemodynamic assessment may not accurately define the nature of the cardiac deterioration and the intravascular volume status. Therefore, invasive hemodynamic monitoring (i.e. pulmonary artery catheters and transesophageal echocardiography) may be needed to determine the correct pathophysiological cause. Every effort must be made to support the patient's vital functions until the poison can be eliminated or removed. In these patients, supportive care with ventilation, oxygenation, and fluid and electrolyte repletion will usually improve the cardiac status. If the patient is bradycardic, an electrical pacemaker may be required.

ELECTROCARDIOGRAPHIC ABNORMALITIES RELATED TO ORGANOPHOSPHATE POISONING

Changes on electrocardiography (ECG) may occur in patients after acute or chronic exposure to OP insecticides and vary from nonspecific to life-threatening ventricular dysrhythmia. It is reported that the electrocardiographic changes due to OP poisoning demonstrate themselves as disturbances in heart rate, rhythm and intraventricular conduction. In particular, conduction abnormalities in the electrocardiogram may be an indicator of cardiac toxicity in OP poisoning. Common sense regarding the timing of the presentation of the electrocardiographic abnormalities observed in OP poisoning would dictate that they may be seen as early as the first day after intoxication. However, these changes have been reported to also occur up to 2-3 months later (Chhabra et al 1970). The current knowledge about cardiac toxic effects of organophosphates is for the most part based on limited publications, studies and case reports.

After exposure to a toxic dose of OP insecticide, plasma cholinesterase activity is rapidly reduced. Some authors reported that reduction in plasma cholinesterase activity after organophosphate poisoning correlates with the severity of the intoxication and possibility of arrhythmia development (Luzhnikov et al 1975, Kiss and Frazekas 1979, Chuang et al 1996). In addition, Kiss and Fazekas (1979) reported that administration of atropine in high doses has been implicated in the development of ventricular arrhythmias. On the other hand, Karki et al (2004) and Ludomirsky et al (1982) claimed in their studies that there was no such correlation between high-dose atropine administration and arrhythmia development.

Therefore, studies on the cardiac effects of organophosphate insecticides have been inconclusive, and have sometimes produced conflicting results.

Changes on ECG following organophosphate poisoning as reported by some authors have included sinus tachycardia, sinus bradycardia, AV block, ST-T wave changes, Q-T interval prolongation, and ventricular arrhythmias (Ludomirsky et al 1982, Brill et al 1984, Saadeh et al 1997, Wang et al 1998, Karki et al 2004). On the other hand, many authors have reported that electrocardiographic abnormalities may be severe in the presence of underlying cardiac disease, electrolyte abnormalities, metabolic acidosis, or hypoxia (Roth et al 1993, Klasaer et al 1996, Saadeh et al 1997, Van Mieghem et al 2004). Anand et al stated that electrocardiographic changes seen in OP intoxication could improve with the correction of underlying electrolyte abnormalities, acidosis and hypoxemia. Therefore, the ECG is a useful tool for evaluating arrhythmias produced by organophosphates and may show possible cardiac toxicity in OP poisoning.

Although the frequency of abnormal electrocardiographic findings in patients with OP insecticide poisoning may vary, published reports within the last 40 years cite sinus tachycardia, nonspecific ST-T wave changes, and prolongation of the Q-T interval as the more commonly seen rhythm disturbances in these patients (Saadeh et al 1997, Karki et al 2004, Venetz et al 2009, Yurumez et al 2009, Shadnia et al 2009). Other electrocardiographic changes are seen less frequently. Furthermore, abnormalities in electrocardiographic patterns and arrhythmias that developed after OP administration were observed in experimental studies in dogs (Das et al 1985) and rats (Allon et al 2005). Prolongation of the Q-T interval was recorded in rats for up to 3 months (Abraham et al 2001) and 5 months (Allon et al 2005) after exposure to acute OP administration.

Electrocardiographic changes resulting from exposure to OP insecticides were first reported by Chhabra et al (1970). They reported 35 patients who had ingested Diazole (malathion) in attempted suicides. Electrocardiographic changes, observed in 37% of the patients, included intraventricular conduction disturbances in the acute phase and ST/T changes (detected even at 2 months' follow-up). In 1975, Luzhnikov et al published 183 cases of severe intoxication with organophosphates admitted to the hospital in Moscow. Various arrhythmias and conduction disturbances were observed in 18.5% of the patients in that report. All patients with arrhythmias had a prolonged Q-T interval that was correlated with the severity of intoxication and decrease in cholinesterase activity in the blood. In 1979, Kiss and Fazekass reported 168 patients who were intoxicated by the organophosphates methyl parathion and dimethoate. In 72.4%, the main cause of exposure was suicide attempt. In about 80% of the patients intoxicated by the organophosphates, prolongation of the Q-T interval and ST-T changes were observed. These electrocardiographic changes correlated with the severity of intoxication.

The Q-T interval represents the duration of ventricular depolarization and subsequent repolarization processes (Lanjevar et al 2004). Generally the Q-T interval is dependent on the heart rate (the faster the heart rate, the shorter the Q-T interval), and alterations in the heart rate make measurement of the Q-T interval difficult. Therefore, the QTc interval must be considered in order to identify the accurate duration of the Q-T interval in different heart rates. Currently, the widely used formula for measuring QTc interval is the one developed by Bazett. Modern computer-based ECG machines can easily calculate a QTc, but this correction may not aid in the detection of patients at increased risk of arrhythmia.

Prolonged Q-T intervals are based on a QTc of >440 ms. In general populations, a prolonged QTc interval has been associated with aging, female sex, arterial hypertension, underlying coronary artery disease, and diabetes and impaired glucose tolerance (Cardoso et al 2003). In 1982, Ludomirsky et al reported 15 patients who were intoxicated with organophosphates. In that study, the authors observed Q-T prolongation in 14 patients and malignant tachyarrhythmia in 6 patients with QTc longer than 0.58 seconds. They noted that prolongation of the Q-T interval could be seen from 5 hours up to 5 days following exposure. Finkelstein et al (1989) described 53 cases of OP intoxication who needed artificial ventilation, ICU monitoring and treatment. They reported 22 of their patients (41.5%) who presented with cardiac arrhythmias: 27% of them had asymptomatic prolonged Q-T interval while 37% had ventricular tachycardia and/or torsades de pointes. Cardiac arrhythmias were found in all of the patients who were treated with high doses of both atropine and obidoxime. In a large study in 1996, Chuang et al reported 223 patients with OP intoxication. Ninety-seven patients (43.5%) had QTc prolongation. They noted that prolongation of the Q-T interval is accompanied by respiratory failure and high mortality. Respiratory failure is the most important cause of death in patients with OP poisoning, for many reasons, including excessive secretions, aspirations of gastric contents, pneumonia, paralysis of the respiratory muscles, CNS depression, and sepsis (Robey and Meggs 2000; Grmec et al 2004). Respiratory failure may be considered an important indicator of severe OP poisoning. In the previous studies, it was reported that respiratory failure was seen in 47% (Saadeh et al 1996), 75% (Sungur and Guven 2001), and 40% (Baydin et al 2007) of cases. Baydin et al observed and reported lower blood cholinesterase levels and significant QTc prolongation on ECG in patients with severe respiratory failure. However, with respect to QTc interval and blood cholinesterase levels, there was no statistically significant difference between the patients with and without respiratory failure. They concluded that these findings may at the least indicate that the presence of QTc interval prolongation might be a warning criterion for respiratory failure. Chuang et al stated that there is a correlation between severity of intoxication, decrease in cholinesterase activity in blood and prolongation of QTc (as reported by Luzhnikov et al in 1975). In 1997, Saadeh et al reported 47 patients with OP and carbamate intoxication. 43.5% of their patients had QTc prolongation and 41% had ST-T wave alterations, but they could not determine blood cholinesterase levels in these patients. In a retrospective study with 20 patients, Baydin et al reported QTc prolongation in 35.4% of patients and declared a negative correlation between plasma cholinesterase levels and the prolongation of QTc. Anand et al (2009), in their analysis of 36 patients with OP intoxication, determined that the most common change in ECG was sinus tachycardia (in 72.2% of patients). They noted that sinus tachycardia was likely more common because of atropine administration, sympathetic overstimulation and dehydration.

Kiss and Fazekas (1979) and Sungurtekin et al reported that nonspecific ST-T wave alterations may be due to transient myocardial ischemia (Brill et al 1984), myocardial ion dysregulation, direct myocardial toxicity, and parasympathetic overstimulation.

Dessertenne was the first to report torsades de pointes arrhythmia, in 1966. Torsades de pointe is an electrocardiographic pattern of continuously changing morphology of the QRS complexes. Torsades de pointe requires an initiating impulse that spreads through the myocardial tissue and a branch point with unequal refractory periods. The presence of a prolonged QTc interval on the ECG may indicate the possible existence of conditions within the myocardium that favor occurrence of reentry dysrhythmias. It is maintained by some investigators that torsades pointes type arrhythmia can be seen after OP poisoning (Lyzhnikov et al 1975, Ludomirshy et al 1982). Besides poisoning with OP insecticides, the risk of torsades de pointes is increased with hypokalemia, hypomagnesemia, hypocalcemia, severe bradycardia, high-grade atrioventricular (AV) block, myocarditis, autonomic neuropathy, and impaired ventricular function (Ludomirsky et al 1982, Zareba et al 1994, Soroker et al 1995, Villa et al 1995, Khan IA 2002). The other clinical conditions known to predispose to torsades de pointes include drugs, intracranial hemorrhage, air encephalography, hypothyroidism and anorexia nervosa (Di Pasquale et al 1988, Kearney et al 1993, Fredlund and Olsson 1983, Surawicz and Knoebel 1984).

CONCLUSION

In conclusion, usage of OP compounds either as agricultural pesticides or as chemical warfare agents gives rise to their importance for public health. In the diagnosis and prognosis, in addition to clinical appearance, pseudocholinesterase levels and the relationship with ECG findings must be considered. Physicians must remember that ECG changes may vary from sinus tachycardia/bradycardia to life-threatening arrhythmias. Prolongation of the QTc interval may be an indicator of such fatal and late occurring arrhythmias.

BIBLIOGRAPHY

1. Aaron CK, Goldfrank LR, Bresnitz EA, Kirsten RH, Howland MA. Insectisides: Organophosphates and Carbamates in Goldfrank's Toxicologic Emergency, X. Section, 4. Edition, USA: Appleton and Lange. 1990; pp.679-89.
2. Abdollahi M, Ranjbar A, Shadnia S, Nikfar S, Rezaie A. Pesticides and oxidative stress: a review. Med Sci Monit. 2004;10:141-7.
3. Abraham S, Oz N, Sahar R, Kadar T. QTc Prolongation and Cardiac Lesions Following Acute Organophosphate Poisoning in Rats Proc West Pharmacol Soc. 2001;44:185-6.
4. Agarwal SB. A clinical, biochemical, neurobehavioral, and sociopsychological study of 190 patients admitted to hospital as a result of acute organophosphorus poisoning. Environ Res. 1993;62:63-70.
5. Akhgari M, Abdollahi M, Kebryaeezadeh A, Hosseini R, Sabzevari O. Biochemical evidence for free radical-induced lipid peroxidation as a mechanism for subchronic toxicity of malathion in blood and liver of rats. Hum Exp Toxicol. 2003;22:205-11.

6. Allon N, Rabinovitz I, Manistersky E, Weismann BA, Grauer E. Acute and Long-Lasting Cardiac Changes Following a Single Whole-Body Exposure to Sarin Vapor in Rats. Toxicol Sci. 2005;87:385-90.
7. Anand S, Singh S, Saikia UN, Bhalla A, Sharma YP, Singh D. Cardiac abnormalities in acute organophosphate poisoning. Clinical Toxicology. 2009;47:230-5.
8. Aygun D, Erenler AK, Karatas AD, Baydin A. Intermediate syndrome following acute organophosphate poisoning: correlation with initial serum levels of muscle enzymes. Basic Clin Pharmacol Toxicol. 2007;100:201-4.
9. Baker T, Stanec A. Methylprednisolone treatment of an organophosphorus induced delayed neuropathy. Toxicol Appl Pharmacol. 1985;79:348-52.
10. Balali-Mood M, Shariat M. Treatment of organophosphate poisoning. Experience of nerve agents and acute pesticide poisoning on the effects of oximes. J Physiol Paris. 1998;92:375-8.
11. Bardin PG, van Eeden SF, Moolman JA, Foden AP, Joubert JR. Organophosphate and Carbamate Poisoning. Arch Intern Med. 1994;154:1433-41.
12. Baydin A, Aygun D, Yazici M, Karataş A, Deniz T, Yardan T. Is there a relationship between the blood cholinesterase and QTc interval in the patients with acute organophosphate poisoning? Int J Clin Pract. 2007;61:927-30.
13. Benson B, Tolo D, McIntire M. Is the intermediate syndrome in organophosphate poisoning the result of insufficient oxime therapy? J Toxicol Clin Toxicol. 1992;30:347-9.
14. Blandizi C, De Paolis B, Colucci R, Di Paolo A, Danesi R, Del Tacca M. Acetylcholinesterase blockade does not account for the adverse cardiovascular effects of the antitumor drug irinotecan : a preclinical study. Toxicol Appl Pharmacol. 2001;177:149-56.
15. Brill DM, Maisel AS, Prabhu R. Polymorphic ventricular tachycardia and other complex arrhythmias in organophosphate insecticide poisoning. J Electrocardiol. 1984;17: 97-102.
16. Cahil-Morasco R, Hoffman RS, Goldfrank LR. The effects of nutrition on plasma cholinesterase activity and cocaine toxicity in mice. J Toxicol Clin Toxicol. 1998;36:667-72.
17. Cardoso CR, Salles GF, Deccache W. QTc interval prolongation is a predictor of future strokes in patients with type 2 diabetes mellitus. Stroke. 2003;34:2187-94.
18. Chaudhry R, Lall SB, Baijayantimal M, Dhawan B. A foodborne outbreak of organophosphate Poisoning. BMJ. 1998;17:268-9.
19. Cherian MA, Roshini C, Peter JV, Cherian AM. Oximes in Organophosphorus Poisoning. Indian J Crit Care Med. 2005;9:155-63.
20. Chhabra ML, Sepaha GC, Jain SR, Bhagwat ER, Khadikar ID. ECG and necropsy changes in organophosphorus compound (malathion) poisoning. Indian J Med Sci. 1970;24:424-9.
21. Chuang FR, Jang SH, Lin JL, Chern MS, Chen JB, Hsu KT. QTc prolongation indicates a poor prognosis in patients with organophospahte poisoning. Am J Emerg Med. 1996;14: 451-3.
22. Clark RF. Insecticides: Organic Phosphorus Compounds and Carbamates. In: Goldfrank LR, Flomenbaum NE, Lewin NA, Howland MA, Hoffman RS, Nelson LS (eds). Goldfrank's Toxicologic Emergencies. 7th ed. New York, NY: McGraw-Hill. 2002;pp1346-60.
23. Dahlgren JG, Takhar HS, Ruffalo CA, Zwass M. Health effects of diazinon on a family. J Toxicol Clin Toxicol. 2004;42:579-91.
24. Das PK, Bhattacharya TK, Gambhir SS. Role of the cholinergic system in the modulation of ventricular arrhythmias induced by subepicardial epinephrine in the dog. Adv Myocardiol. 1985;6:349-65.
25. Davies JE, Barquet A, freed VH, Haque R, Morgade C, Sonneborn RE, Vaclavek C. Human Pesticide Poisonings by a Fat-Soluble Organophosphate Insecticide. Arch Environ Health. 1975;30:608-13.
26. Deschamps D, Questel F, Baud FJ, Gervais P, Dally S. Persistent asthma after acute inhalation of organophosphate insecticide. Lancet. 1994;344:1712.
27. Di Pasquale G, Pinelli G, Andreoli A, Manini GL, Grazi P, Tognetti F. Torsade de pointes and ventricular flutter-fibrillation following spontaneous cerebral subarachnoid hemorrhage. Int J Cardiol. 1988;18:163-72.

28. Eddleston M, Buckley NA, Eyer P, Dawson AH. Management of acute organophosphorus pesticide poisoning. Lancet. 2008;371:597-607.
29. Eddleston M, Eyer P, Worek F, Mohamed F, Senarathna L, Meyer L, et al. Differences between organophosphorus insecticides in human self-poisoning: a prospective cohort study. Lancet. 2005;366:1452-59.
30. Eddleston M, Karalliedde L, Buckley N, Fernando R, Hutchinson G, Isbiter G, et al. Pesticide poisoning in the developing world-a minimum pesticides list. Lancet. 2002;360:1163-67.
31. Fazekas T, Kiss Z. Organophosphate cardiomyopathy. Congestive cardiomyopathy caused by long-term organic phosphoric acid ester exposure (author's transl). Z Kardiol. 1980;69:584-6.
32. Finkelstein Y, Kushnir A, Raikhlin-Eisenkraft B, Taitelman U. Antidotal therapy of severe acute organophosphate poisoning: a multihospital study. Neurotoxicol Teratol. 1989;11:593-6.
33. Fredlund BO, Olsson SB. Long QT interval and ventricular tachycardia of "torsade de pointe" type in hypothyroidism. Acta Med Scand. 1983;213:231.
34. Gadoth N, Fisher A. Late onset of neuromuscular block in organophosphorus poisoning. Ann Intern Med. 1978;88:654-5.
35. Gallo MA, Lawryk NJ. Organic phosphorus pesticides. In: Hayes WJ, Laws ER, eds: Handbook of Pesticide Toxicology. San Diego, CA, Academic Press. 1991;pp.917-1090.
36. Goel A, Aggarwal P. Pesticide poisoning. Natl Med J India. 2007;20:182-91.
37. Grmec S, Mally S, Klemen P. Glasgow Coma Scale score and QTc interval in the prognosis of organophosphate poisoning. Acad Emerg Med. 2004;11:925-30.
38. Guven M, Unluhizarci K, Goktas Z, Kurtoglu S. Intravenous organophosphate injection: an unusual way of intoxication. Hum Exp Toxicol. 1997;16:279-80.
39. Hammer R, Giraldo E, Schiavi GB, Monferini E, Ladinsky H. Binding profile of a novel cardioselective muscarine receptor antagonist, AF-DX 116, to membranes of peripheral tissues and brain in the rat. Life Sci. 1986;38:1653-62.
40. Hayes MM, Van der Westhuizen NG, Gelfand M. Organophosphate poisoning in Rhodesia. S Afr Med J. 1978;54:230-4.
41. Heath AJW, Vale JA. Clinical presentation and diagnosis of acute organophosphate insecticide and carbamate poisoning. In Clinical and Experimental Toxicology of Organophosphates and Carbamates. ed. Ballantyne, B. & Marrs, T.C. 1992;pp.513-9. Oxford: Butterworth-Heinemann.
42. Hermanowicz A, Kossman S. Neutrophil function and infectious disease in workers occupationally exposed to phosphoorganic pesticides: role of mononuclear-derived chemotactic factor for neutrophils. Clin Immunol Pathol. 1984;33:13-22.
43. Kamanyire R, Karalliedde L. Organophosphate toxicity and occupational exposure. Occupational Medicine. 2004;54:69-75.
44. Kara IH, Guloglu C, Karabulut A, Orak M. Sociodemographic, Clinical, and Laboratory Features of Cases of Organic Phosphorus Intoxication who Attended the Emergency Department in the Southeast Anatolian Region of Turkey. Environ Res. 2002;88:82-8.
45. Karalliedde L, Edwards P, Marrs TC. Variables influencing the toxicity of organophosphates in humans. Food Chem Toxicol. 2003;41:1-13.
46. Karalliedde L, Senanayake N. Organophosphorus insecticide poisoning. Br J Anaesth. 1989;63:736-50.
47. Karalliedde L. Organophosphorus poisoning and anaesthesia. Anaesthesia. 1999;54:1073-88.
48. Karki P, Ansari JA, Bhandary S, Koirala S. Cardiac and electrocardiographical manifestations of acute organophosphate poisoning. Singapore Med J. 2004;45:385-9.
49. Kearney P, Reardon M, O'Hare J. Primary hyperparathyroidism presenting as torsades de pointes. Br Heart J. 1993;70:473.

50. Khan IA. Mechanisms of syncope and Stokes–Adams attacks in bradyarrhythmias: asystole and torsade de pointes. Cardiology. 2002; pp.98.
51. Kiss Z, Fazekas T. Arrhythmia in organophosphate poisonings. Acta Cardiol. 1979;34:323-30.
52. Kiss Z, Fazekas T. Organophosphates and torsade de pointes ventricular tachycardia. Journal of the Royal Society of Medicine. 1983;76:984-5.
53. Klasaer AE, Scalzo AJ, Blume C, Johnson P, Thompson MW. Marked hypocalcemia and ventricular fibrillation in two pediatric patients exposed to a fluoride-containing wheel cleaner. Ann Emerg Med. 1996;28:713-8.
54. Klingelhofer J, Sander D. Cardiovascular consequences of clinical stroke. Baillieres Clin Neurol. 1997;6:309-35.
55. Lanjewar P, Pathak V, Lokhandwala Y. Issues in QT interval measurement. Indian Pacing Electrophysiol J. 2004;4:156-61.
56. Levy MN, and Martin P. Parasympathetic control of the heart. In: Randall WC, (ed). Nervous Control of Cardiovascular Function. New York, Oxford University Pres, 1984.
57. Lokan R, James R. Rapid death by mevinphos poisoning while under observation. Forensic Sci Int. 1981;22:179-82.
58. Lotti M, Becker CE, Aminoff MJ. Organophosphate polyneuropathy: pathogenesis and prevention. Neurology. 1984;34:658-62.
59. Lotti M. Clinical toxicology of anticholinesterase agents in humans. In: Krieger RI, Doull J, eds. Handbook of pesticide toxicology. Volume 2. Agents, 2nd edition. San Diego: Academic Press. 2001:1043-85.
60. Ludomirsky A, Klein HO, Sarelli P, Becker B, Hoffman S, Taitelman U, et al. Q-T prolongation and polymorphous "torsades de pointes" ventricular arrhythmias associated with organophophorus insecticide poisoning. Am J Cardiol. 1982;49:1654-8.
61. Luzhnikov EA, Savina AS, Shepelev VM. On the pathogenesis of cardiac rhythm and conductivity disorders in cases of acute insecticides poisoning. Kardiologiya (U.S.S.R.). 1975;15:126-9.
62. Merrill DG, Mihm FG. Prolonged toxicity of organophosphate poisoning. Crit Care Med. 1982;10:550-1.
63. Morita H, Yanagisawa N, Nakajima T, Shimizu M, Hirabayashi H, Okudera H, et al. Sarin poisoning in Matsumoto, Japan. Lancet. 1995;346:290-3.
64. Murray VS, Wiseman HM, Dawling S, Morgan I, House IM. Health effects of organophosphate sheep dips. Br Med J. 1992;305:1090.
65. Namba T, Greenfield M, Brob D. Malathion poisoning: A fatal case with cardiac manifestations. Arch Environ Health. 1970;21:533-41.
66. Namba T, Nolte CJ, Jackrel J, Grob D. Poisoning due to organophosphate insecticides. Acute and chronic manifestations. Am J Med. 1971;50:475-92.
67. Ochi G, Watanabe K, Tokuoka H, Hatakenaka S, Arai T. Neuroleptic malignant-like syndrome: a complication of acute organophosphate poisoning. Can J Anaesth. 1995;42:1027-30.
68. O'Malley M. Clinical evaluation of pesticide exposure and poisonings. Lancet. 1997;349:1161-6.
69. Parven M, Kumar S. Effect of DDVP on the histology and AChE kinetics of the heart muscles of Rattus norvegicus. J Environ Biol. 2001;22:257-61.
70. Peter JV, Cherian AM. Organic insecticides. Anaest Intensive Care. 2000;28:11-21.
71. Ranjbar A, Solhi H, Mashayekhi FJ, Susanabdi A, Rezaie A, Abdollahi M. Oxidative stress in acute human poisoning with organophosphorus insecticides; a case control study. Environmental Toxicology and Pharmacology. 2005;20:88-91.
72. Rizos E, Liberopoulos E, Kosta P, Efremidis S, Elisaf M. Carbofuran-induced acute pancreatitis. JOP. 2004;5:44-7.

73. Robey WC, Meggs WJ. Insecticides, Herbicides, Rodentyicides. In: Tintinalli J.E., Kelen G.D., Stapczynski J.S. (eds). Emergency medicine: a comprehensive study guide. 5th ed. New York: McGraw Hill; 2000;pp.1174-82.
74. Roeyen G, Chapelle T, Jorens P, de Beeck BO, Ysebaert D. Necrotizing pancreatitis due to poisoning with organophosphate pesticides. Acta Gastroenterol Belg. 2008;71:27-9.
75. Roth A, Zellinger I, Arad M, Atsmon J. Organophosphates and the heart. Chest. 1993;103:576-82.
76. Rusyniak DE, Nanagas KA. Organophosphate Poisoning. Semin Neurol. 2004;24:197-204.
77. Saadeh AM, Farsakh NA, Ali MK. Cardiac manifestations of acute carbamate and organophosphate poisoning. Heart. 1997;77:461-4.
78. Saadeh AM, al-Ali MK, Farsakh NA, Ghani MA. Clinical and sociodemographic features of acute carbamate and organophosphate poisoning: a study of 70 adult patients in north Jordan. J Toxicol Clin Toxicol. 1996;34:45-51.
79. Shadnia S, Okazi A, Akhlaghi N, Sasanian G, Abdollahi M. Prognostic Value of Long QT Interval in Acute and Severe Organophosphate Poisoning. J Med Toxicol. 2009;5:196-9.
80. Singh S, Sharma N. Neurological syndromes following organophosphate poisoning. Neurol India. 2000;48:308-13.
81. Smith EC, Padnos B, Cordon CJ. Peripheral versus central muscarinic effects on blood pressure, cardiac contractility, heart rate, and body temperature in the rat monitored by radiotelemetry. Pharmacol Toxicol. 2001;89:35-42.
82. Soroker D, Ezri T, Szmuk P, Merlis P, Epstein M, Caspi A. Perioperative torsade de pointes ventricular tachycardia induced by hypocalcemia and hypokalemia. Anesth Analg. 1995;80:630-3.
83. Sultatos LG, Shao M, Murphy SD. The role of hepatic biotransformation in mediating the acute toxicity of the phosphorothioate insecticide chlorpyrifos. Toxicol Appl Pharmacol 1984;73:60-8.
84. Sungur M, Guven M. Intensive care management of organophosphate insecticide poisoning. Crit Care. 2001;5:211-15.
85. Sungurtekin H, Guissen E, Balci C. Evaluation of several clinical scoring tools in organophosphate poisoned patients. Clin Toxicol. 2006;44:121-6.
86. Surawicz B, Knoebel SB. Long QT: good, bad and indifferent. J Am Coll Cardiol. 1984;4:398-413.
87. Taira K, Aoyama Y, Kawamata M. Long QT and ST-T change associated with organophosphate. Environ Toxicol Pharmacol. 2006;22:40-5.
88. Van Mieghem C, Sabbe M, Knockaert D. The clinical value of the ECG in noncardiac conditions. Chest. 2004;125:1561-76.
89. Venetz P, Vanek P, Bonetti PO. Electrocardiographic repolarisation abnormalities after acute organophosphate poisoning. Kardiovaskulare Medizin. 2009;12:129-31.
90. Villa A, Foresti V, Confalonieri F. Autonomic neuropathy and prolongation of QT interval in human immunodeficiency virus infection. Clin Auton Res. 1995;5:48-52.
91. Wadia RS, Sadagopan C, Amin RP, Sardesai HV. Neurological manifestations of organophosphorous insecticide poisoning. J Neurol Neurosurg Psychiatr. 1974;37: 841-7.
92. Wang MH, Tseng CD, Bair SY. Q-T interval prolongation and pleomorphic ventricular tachyarrhythmia ('Torsade de pointes') in organophosphate poisoning: report of a case. Hum Exp Toxicol. 1998;17:587-90.
93. Wills JH. The measurement and significance of changes in the cholinesterase activities of erythrocytes and plasma in man and animals. CRC Critical Reviews in Toxicology. 1972;1:153-202.
94. Wilson BW, Sanborn JR, O'Malley MA, Henderson JD, Billitti JR. Monitoring the pesticide-exposed worker. Occup Med. 1997;12:347-63.

95. Yardan T, Baydin A, Aygun D, Karatas AD, Deniz T, Doganay Z. Late-onset Intermediate Syndrome Due to Organophosphate Poisoning. Clinical Toxicology. 2007;45:733-4.
96. Yurumez Y, Durukan P, Yavuz Y, Ikizceli I, Avsarogullari L, Ozkan S, Akdur O, Ozdemir C. Acute organophosphate poisoning in university hospital emergency room patients. Intern Med. 2007;46:965-9.
97. Yurumez Y, Yavuz Y, Saglam H, Durukan P, Ozkan S, Akdur O, Yucel M. Electrocardiographic Findings of Acute Organophosphate Poisoning. J Emerg Med. 2009;36:39-42.
98. Zareba W, Moss AJ, le Cessie S, Hall WJ. T wave alternans in idiopathic long QT syndrome. J Am Coll Cardiol. 1994;23:1541-6.

Chapter

8

Are There Sex Differences in Serum Troponin in Cardiac Surgery?

C Javierre, A Ricart, E Farrero, L Carrió,
D Rodríguez-Castro, H Torrado, JL Ventura

Abstract. Objective 1: To determine whether there are sex-based differences in serum troponin I (TnI) after cardiac surgery with cardiopulmonary bypass (CPB), excluding patients with perioperative myocardial infarction (AMI) with ST changes (STEMI).
Objective 2: To determine whether there are sex-based differences in TnI in conjunction with the incidence and characteristics of AMI after cardiac surgery with CPB.
Design: Prospective, observational, cohort study.
Setting: Tertiary, cardiac surgery intensive care unit (ICU) at a university hospital.
Interventions: None.
Measurements and main results: Serum TnI was measured in samples obtained at ICU admission and 6, 12, 24 and 48 h later. Study 1 was based on 761 consecutive patients (444 men and 317 women), while Study 2 was based on 2,038 consecutive patients (1,276 men and 762 women).
Study 1: In the whole sample of 761 patients without AMI/STEMI (444 men and 317 women) there were no significant sex differences in the TnI peak (7.7 ± 5.9 mcg/L in men versus 8.5 ± 6.7 mcg/L in women; p = ns).
The characteristics and results of the different sex subgroups were:

a. Coronary bypass: 165 men, 38 women. Age, Parsonnet score, APACHE III, incidence of renal failure, intraaortic balloon use and the lengths of cardiopulmonary bypass, mechanical ventilation and ICU stay were similar in the two groups. Body mass index (BMI), red-cell transfusion needs and the use of noradrenaline were significantly higher in women, while dobutamine requirements were higher in men. Mortality: 3 men (1.6%) versus 0 women (p = ns).
The TnI peak was slightly, but significantly, higher in men (6.2 ± 4.9 versus 4.5 ± 2.6 mcg/L; $p < 0.05$).

b. Valve surgery: 279 men, 279 women. Some significant differences were found: Women were older than men and had higher Parsonnet score and greater transfusion needs. The other recorded parameters were similar. Mitral prosthesis: 62 men, 125 women ($p < 0.05$). Mitral valvuloplasty: 24 men, 7 women ($p < 0.05$). Aortic prosthesis: 162 men, 103 women ($p < 0.05$). Mitral and aortic prosthesis: 31 men, 44 women ($p < 0.05$). TnI peaks were similar for both sexes in each valve subgroup. Mortality: 3 men (1%) versus 11 women (3.4%) ($p < 0.05$).
The TnI peak did not show any significant differences between the sexes (men 7.9 ± 6.0 mcg/L versus 8.5 ± 6.5 mcg/L in women; p = ns).

Study 2: After applying the exclusion criteria to the initial sample of 2434 patients we were left with 2038 consecutive patients undergoing cardiac surgery with CPB, in whom we determined new AMI: 1) According to ECG criteria (STEMI = ST myocardial infarction); and 2) Non-STEMI, according to their TnI peak and concentration at 48 h and clinical evolution.

This group comprised 1276 men and 762 women and we studied three subgroups: 1) without AMI (1126 men [88.2% of all men] and 720 women [94.4% of all women]); 2) with STEMI (77 men [6.0% of all men] and 14 women [1.8% of all women]); and 3) with non-STEMI (73 men [5.7% of all men] and 29 women [3.8% of all women]). Here the sex differences were highly significant. The TnI peak was 10.4 ± 23.6 mcg/L in the first group, 62.8 ± 117.5 mcg/L in the second and 63.8 ± 107.1 mcg/L in the third, the differences being significant ($F = 145.3$; $p < 0.001$) between the first group with respect to the second and third groups. There were no sex differences in either the whole sample or in patients without AMI. However, there were significant sex differences in patients with AMI (due to the large difference in the TnI peak in the STEMI group) (Table 8.1).

In these three groups the percentage of men and women was similar in the whole group and in the subgroups of valve surgery, CABG and both surgeries. As regards the Parsonnet score there were no significant sex differences in either the whole sample or in the patients with AMI. APACHE II and III scores were higher in the group with AMI, but without sex differences. ICU stay was longer in women than in men. It was also longer in patients with AMI and longer in women with AMI than in men with AMI. ICU and in hospital mortality showed no sex differences in patients without AMI, those with AMI, in patients with STEMI or in those with non-STEMI. Patients with AMI had higher in-hospital mortality than did patients without AMI (13.6% and 4.5%, respectively; $p < 0.01$).

Conclusion:

Study 1: No clinically relevant sex-based differences were found in the TnI peaks after cardiac surgery without AMI. Therefore, there is no reason to change the myocardial damage stratification in a sex-specific manner.

Study 2: This confirms the lack of TnI sex differences after cardiac surgery when AMI is not present, but shows a significant difference between men and women in the TnI peak and curve after cardiac surgery when an AMI occurs. The TnI curves reveal a highly-significant sex difference in the STEMI and non-STEMI groups. Men have a higher percentage of AMI (11.7% versus 5.6%), of STEMI (6.0% versus 1.8%) and of non-STEMI (5.7% versus 3.8%). These differences do not seem to be based on previous differences between the patients and had important repercussions in terms of mortality, there being sex differences in the time of ICU stay but not in the mortality in any subgroup.

Keywords. Gender differences, troponin I, cardiac surgery, prosthetic valves, coronary artery bypass graft.

INTRODUCTION

There is growing medical interest in the study of differences between the two sexes as regards physiological and clinical variables (Crabbe et al 2003,Ricart et al 2008, Blacker et al 2009, Ciambrone and Kaski 2009, Kwon et al 2009, Mason and MacLeod 2009, Ennker et al 2009, Alehagen et al 2009, Combes et al 2009). Serum cardiac-specific TnI is a biomarker that improves diagnosis and risk stratification for patients with acute coronary syndromes (Antman et al 1996) and after coronary artery bypass grafting (CABG) (Gensini et al 1998). Higher TnI levels are correlated with increased mortality rates in patients admitted to the ICU after both non-cardiac surgery (Relos et al 2003) and cardiac surgery (Fellahi et al 2003, Adabag et al 2007). Specifically, the higher the value of the cardiac biomarker after the procedure, the greater the damage to the myocardium, irrespective of the mechanism of injury (Alpert et al 2000).

Differences between men and women on several cardiac variables have been reported (Carey et al 1995, Edwards et al 1998, Christakis et al 1995, Abramov et al 2000, Aldea et al 1999, Jacobs et al 1998, Koch et al 2003, Mickleborough et al 1995). CABG postoperative mortality is reported to be higher in women. Furthermore, some studies show statistically significant sex differences in hospital outcome, both adjusted and unadjusted for risk, whereas other reports found no such differences with adjusted mortality rates (Jacobs et al 1998). Neither the various guidelines nor text books in the field contain references to possible differences between men and women in biomarkers after myocardial infarction or cardiac surgery (Fellahi et al 2003, Alpert et al 2000, Edwards et al 1998, Edwards et al 2005, Edmunds et al 1996).

One interesting study, comparing a sample of 17 males with 17 matched females, found a 3-fold higher serum TnI peak after cardiac surgery with cardiopulmonary bypass (CPB) but without perioperative myocardial infarction (AMI). As a possible explanation, the authors suggested a different perioperative activation of the inflammatory response to cardiopulmonary bypass. They recommended studies in a larger number of patients to assess these findings, which, if confirmed, would have a major bearing on the interpretation of TnI for diagnosis and risk stratification in males and females (Schwarzenberger et al 2003).

We also sought to determine whether there are any sex-based differences in the TnI curve after cardiac surgery when an AMI occurs, as we are unaware of research into the possible sex-related differences in this regard. The worst outcomes observed in women after cardiac surgery in some studies are attributed to the higher presence of risk variables, rather than to an intrinsic sex difference, and they do not focus on specific TnI differences (Mickleborough et al 1995, McGee et al 1998, Hussain et al 1998, Aldea et al 1999, Ott et al 2001). We considered both AMI/STEMI, according to classical ECG criteria (Alpert et al 2000), and AMI/non-STEMI, defined as a troponin I peak>20 ng/ml (Benoit et al 2000), the time when the TnI peak occurs and TnI at 48 h (Selvanayagam et al 2005), ST changes and clinical criteria.

THE AIMS OF THE PRESENT STUDIES

1. To analyze the possibility of sex-based differences in peak TnI in a large sample after cardiac surgery with cardiopulmonary bypass (CPB) but without AMI/ STEMI (Study 1) (Ricart et al 2009).
2. To analyze the possibility of sex-based differences in TnI peak and curve and the incidence and outcome of AMI (STEMI and non-STEMI) after cardiac surgery with CPB (Study 2) (unpublished data).

Inclusion Criteria

Consecutive patients undergoing elective cardiac surgery with CPB in a tertiary university hospital. For Study 1 only patients with valve surgery or CABG were included, while for Study 2 we also considered a subgroup with both surgical procedures.

Exclusion Criteria

- **Study 1:** Emergency cardiac surgery or presurgery procedures, CABG and valve replacement in the same surgical intervention, reoperation procedures, AMI according to classical ECG criteria (Alpert et al 2000).
- **Both studies:** Treatments with tamoxifen or gonadotropin-releasing hormone agonists, or a history of hyperprolactinemia, recent head trauma, stroke or cerebral tumors. Patients who, for any reason, underwent nonprotocolized procedures for anesthesia or surgery were also excluded, as were patients undergoing surgery other than CABG or valve surgery.

The studies were approved by the Ethics Committee of the Bellvitge University Hospital (University of Barcelona).

Study 1

A cohort of 875 consecutive patients underwent cardiac surgery with CPB (514 men and 361 women) between February 2004 and June 2006. Of these, 114 (70 men and 44 women) were excluded on the basis of the abovementioned exclusion criteria. The final sample thus comprised 761 patients (444 men and 317 women).

Study 2

A cohort of 2,434 consecutive patients underwent cardiac surgery with or without CPB between February 2004 and April 2009. After applying the exclusion criteria the sample comprised 2,038 patients (1,276 men and 762 women).

Gender, age, Parsonnet score, APACHE II and III scores, incidence of AMI (STEMI and non-STEMI), TnI curve and peak of this curve, stay in ICU and in-hospital mortality were all recorded in both studies.

ANESTHETIC MANAGEMENT

The anesthesia protocol used fentanyl and midazolam for induction, rocuronium or cisatracurium for myorelaxation, and midazolam, propofol and remifentanyl for anesthesia maintenance. Inhaled anesthesia was not used.

All patients received the same standardized anesthetic regime and were extubated in the ICU according to standard criteria (Reyes et al 1997).

SURGICAL AND CARDIOPULMONARY BYPASS MANAGEMENT

All operations followed the same protocol for surgical procedure, sternotomy and cardiopulmonary bypass without sex-based differences.

Myocardial protection consisted of intermittent anterograde and/or retrograde administration of cold blood cardioplegia (Abboplegisol®) mixed with blood at a ratio of 1:4.

BLOOD SAMPLING AND SPECIMEN PROCESSING

All blood samples were obtained from a central venous catheter.

Serum TnI samples were obtained immediately after surgery upon ICU admission, and then 6, 12, 24 and 48 h later, this being usual practice in our ICU. The samples were measured with a Dimension RxL analyzer (Dade Behring, Newark, DE, USA).

The TnI measurement method was a one-step enzyme immunoassay based on the "sandwich" principle, using two monoclonal antibodies specific to cardiac TnI that recognize different epitopes. The detection limit, calculated as the lowest concentration of TnI that can be distinguished from 0, was 0.17 ug/L. The myocardial injury cut-off used in our laboratory was 0.20 ug/L.

STATISTICAL METHODS

Data are reported as mean ±SD, with p values <0.05 considered significant. Non-significant values are recorded as **ns**.

The homogeneity of the quantitative samples was analyzed by means of the one-sample Kolmogorov-Smirnov test. To evaluate the differences between groups (male and female) for patient characteristics (e.g. APACHE II and III, Parsonnet score, BMI, etc.) and for the quantitative samples with a normal distribution (e.g. CPB time, etc.) the unpaired Student's t test was used. For the main troponin peak values (whole coronary bypass and valve surgery) showing nonnormal distribution, we compared groups via the log transformation of data. To compare the quantitative samples without a normal distribution, the Mann-Whitney U test was used.

The differences in TnI evolution across the five measurements (admission to ICU and 6, 12, 24 and 48 h later) were analyzed with ANOVA for repeated measurements.

The Chi-squared test was used to compare the male and female groups for nonparametric samples (e.g. mortality).

Study 1

In the whole sample of 761 patients (444 men and 317 women) there were no sex differences in either the TnI peak or the TnI curve (Figure 8.1).

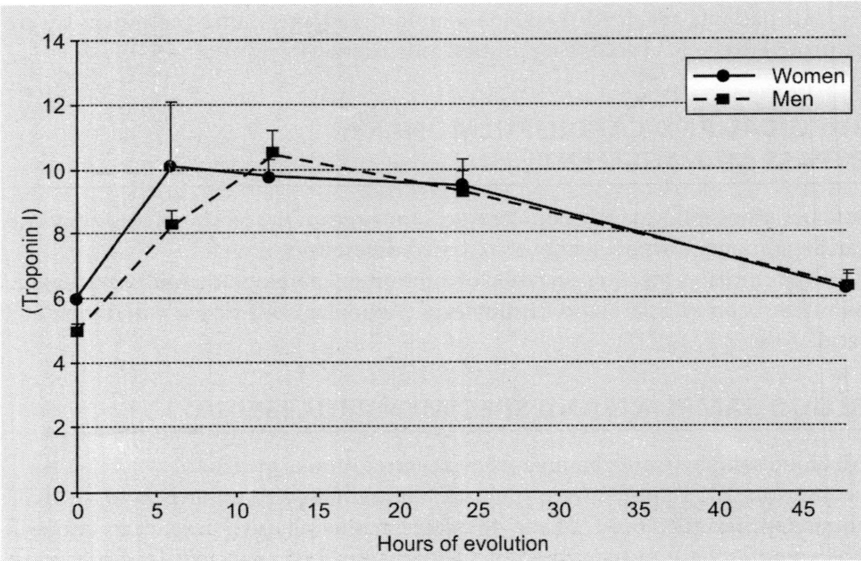

Figure 8.1: Troponin I curves in both groups (444 men and 317 women)

a. Coronary Bypass

Here we studied 165 men and 38 women. Three men (1.6%) but no women died during the postoperative period (p = ns).

1. Postoperative peaks of TnI: Men 6.4 ± 4.9 vs. women 4.5 ± 2.6 ug/L ($p < 0.01$). The peak was recorded at the third evaluation, 12 h after admission in both sexes.
   TnI peak logarithm: Men 1.61 ± 0.69 vs. women 1.35 ± 0.54; t = 1.38, $p < 0.05$.
   TnI curves are shown in Figure 8.2.
2. Patient characteristics: Age (years) 63.9 ± 8.9 men and 65.1 ± 8.5 women; BMI (kg/m^2) 28.0 ± 3.4 men and 29.7 ± 4.7 women; Parsonnet score 6.1 ± 3.8 men and 6.3 ± 3.4 women; APACHE III score 44.3 ± 13.6 men and 46.2 ± 14.8 women.
3. There were no differences between men and women in length of cardiopulmonary bypass, time spent on mechanical ventilation or length of stay in ICU.

b. Valve Surgery

Here we studied 279 men and 279 women. Three men (1%) died during the postoperative period, compared with 11 women (3.4%) ($p < 0.05$).

1. Postoperative peaks of TnI: Men 7.9 ± 6.0 vs. women 8.5 ± 6.5 ug/L (ns). The peak was recorded at the third evaluation, 12 h after admission.
   In both sexes the TnI peak was significantly higher in patients with double prosthesis (mitral and aortic) and significantly lower in those with aortic prosthesis ($p < 0.05$). Patients with mitral prosthesis or valvuloplasty showed no differences between these two conditions, but were significantly different from the other two groups ($p < 0.05$).
   TnI curves are shown in Figure 8.3.

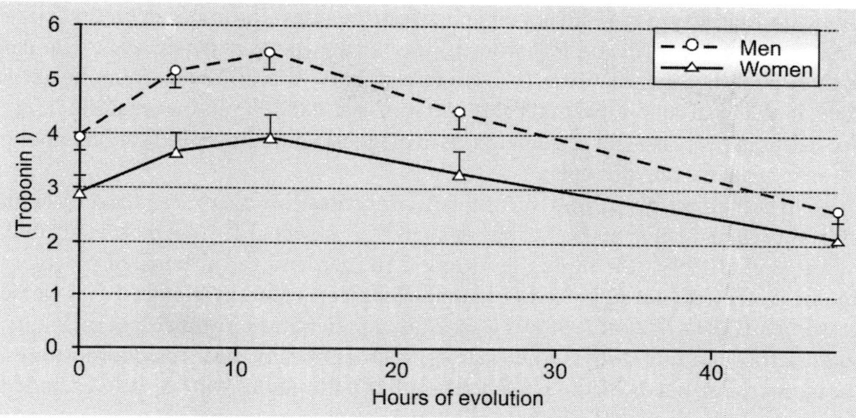

Figure 8.2: Coronary bypass. Troponin I curves (ug/L). N = 165 men and 38 women (Adapted from Ricart et al, Crit Care Med. 2009;37:2210-5).

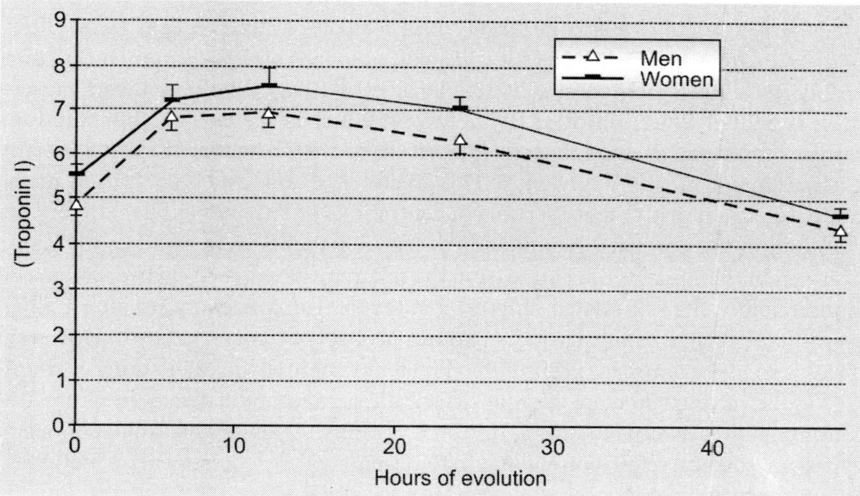

Figure 8.3: Valve surgery. Troponin I curves (ug/L). N = 279 men and 279 women (Adapted from Ricart et al, Crit Care Med. 2009;37:2210-5).

2. Patient characteristics: Age (years) 62.7 ± 12.7 men and 66.5 ± 10.4 women; BMI (kg/m^2) 27.3 ± 4.4 men and 27.8 ± 4.6 women; Parsonnet score 11.9 ± 6.9 men and 13.7 ± 6.3 women; APACHE III score 46.9 ± 17.9 men and 49.8 ± 17.6 women.
3. There were no differences between men and women in length of cardiopulmonary bypass, time spent under mechanical ventilation or length of ICU stay.

The slight, but significant, differences found in TnI serum concentration after CABG should have no clinical relevance, since mortality and the lengths of mechanical ventilation and stay in ICU did not differ between the sexes. The imbalance found in the CABG group (81% men and 19% women) was not a surprise, as the figures are similar to those published in recent years (Kokkonen et al 2005, Patel et al 2006, Toumpulis et al 2006, Puskas et al 2007, Edwards et al 2005, Guru et al 2006, Humphries et al 2007). The debate about the reason for sex differences in diagnosis and surgery indications among coronary patients remains open.

Furthermore, given that serum TnI concentration correlates directly with mortality (Fellahi et al 2003, Adabag et al 2007, Carey et al 1995, Alpert et al 2000, Edwards et al 1998), the higher level found in men and the absence of mortality among women do not support the claim that clinical evolution after CABG is worse in women (Edwards et al 1998), at least among patients at a lower risk of mortality, such as those in our study. Other factors, such as obesity, transfusion, inotropes, vasoconstrictor needs or the presence of other pathologies, which were excluded from this study, are probably responsible for the differences.

At all events, men had significantly higher TnI peaks and curves after CABG. The different postoperative TnI peaks may be due to differences in body composition between women and men. Men's hearts account for 0.45% of their total weight, while women's hearts account for 0.4% (Kitzman et al 1988). Lean body mass in women is 77% of total weight compared with 85% in men (Jackson and Pollock 2004, Jackson et al 1980, Hense et al 1998). Therefore, heart muscle mass is related to lean body mass, not to fat mass, as are oxygen consumption, cardiac output and exercise capacity (Morrow et al 1995, Chantler et al 2005, Stefani 2006). If men have approximately 8-12% greater lean body and heart muscle mass, this is consistent with higher serum concentrations of TnI after similar surgery. In addition, in the coronary group studied, female patients were significantly more overweight than males, thus increasing the relative difference in myocardial mass. Consequently, the sex-related difference in serum TnI concentration after CABG seems to be related to muscle mass and can probably be corrected by it. However, if this is so in the coronary group, why does it not apply to the valve surgery group?

In the valve group there were no statistically significant differences in serum TnI concentrations between the sexes and, in clinical terms, the lengths of cardiopulmonary bypass, mechanical ventilation and stay in ICU were similar. Requirements of inotropes, intraaortic balloon or vasoconstrictors were also similar.

The valve group showed significantly higher serum TnI concentration figures than the coronary group in both sexes, as described elsewhere (Gensini et al 1998, Fellahi et al 2007, Sánchez, et al 2001). We believe that this could be due to the aortotomy (for aortic valve), atrial myotomy (for mitral valve) or the myocardial injury at the ring level that surgeons perform in order to place the prosthesis.

Other differences in the valve group were that patients with double aortic and mitral prosthesis showed significantly higher TnI peak than did patients who underwent only mitral surgery; furthermore, mitral patients showed significantly higher TnI peak than did aortic patients. This is probably due to differences in the technique, as explained in the preceding paragraph.

The greater incidence of mitral or double valve surgery in women may partially explain why, without reaching statistical significance, the TnI peak is slightly higher in women. Nevertheless, despite the lack of significant differences in TnI peak, the mortality rate was significantly higher among women than men.

In the group studied, women had greater transfusion needs, were older than men and had higher mortality risks as measured by the Parsonnet score. These characteristics are of greater importance than the TnI peak in assessing mortality. Conceivably, if our first hypothesis is correct and TnI can be corrected by heart muscle mass (or lean body mass), women would have nearly 10% lower serum TnI concentrations than men after similar procedures for valve surgery. However, they had an 8% higher TnI peak. This idea may appear speculative, yet the data show that similar levels of TnI are associated with higher mortality in women. Rather than state that "the higher the troponin peak, the greater the mortality" it would, perhaps, be more accurate to say "the higher the troponin peak/lean body mass ratio, the greater the mortality".

At all events, it is clear that factors such as obesity, age, Parsonnet score, transfusion needs or other gender characteristics play a major role in mortality, regardless of the small differences in serum TnI concentration.

The relatively low rates of mortality are not surprising, as patients with a higher risk of mortality – For instance, those with emergency surgery, perioperative myocardial infarction, coronary insufficiency added to valvulopathy, and so on – were excluded from the study.

The results of a previous study (Schwarzenberger et al 2003) indicating a 300% higher value in men than in women after cardiac surgery may have been due to the small sample size; it could also be the result of perioperative myocardial infarction, often without electrocardiographic necrosis *q* waves after cardiac surgery (Ponce et al 2001, Svedjeholm et al 1998) in some men, which may have raised the serum TnI concentrations to pathological levels. Our new study, with a much larger sample and more serial determinations, seems to clarify the doubts raised by Schwarzenberger et al (Schwarzenberger et al 2003).

Study 1

Study 1 does have certain limitations. First, it was performed in low-risk patients and further studies are therefore required to determine whether the results are applicable to high-risk patients.

Second, the matching process used in this study was not designed to assess the effect on the TnI peak of the different factors recorded (transfusion needs, use of noradrenaline or dobutamine, mitral or aortic surgery, etc.), but rather to identify differences between the sexes in TnI peak.

Study 2

After applying the exclusion criteria to the initial cohort of 2,434 consecutive patients, the sample consisted of 2,038 patients: 1,276 men and 762 women. Of these, 1,165 patients (595 men and 570 women) were in subgroup A (valve surgery), 563 (455 men and 108 women) in subgroup B (coronary artery bypass grafting, CABG) and 140 (104 men and 36 women) in subgroup C (both types of surgery).

There were no significant differences in the percentage of the two sexes in these three subgroups.

The total sample was also considered according to AMI and STEMI, there again being three groups. Group 1, comprising 1,845 patients (88.3% of all men and 94.4% of all women), had no evidence of AMI; Group 2, with 91 patients (77 men, 6.0% of all men, and 14 women, 1.8% of all women), suffered a STEMI; and Group 3, including 102 patients (73 men, 5.7% of all men, and 29 women, 3.8% of all women), suffered a non-STEMI. These sex differences were highly significant ($p < 0.001$). There were also other statistically significant differences between these three groups:

- TnI peak in the non-AMI group was 10.4 ± 23.6 mcg/L, compared to 62.8 ± 117.5 mcg/L in Group 2 and 63.8 ± 107.1 mcg/L in Group 3 ($p < 0.001$);
- Number of hours postsurgery when the TnI peak occurred was 10.9 ± 9.0 h in Group 1, 17.0 ± 9.6 h in Group 2 and 16.5 ± 8.7 h in Group 3 ($p < 0.001$);
- TnI at 48 h was 4.4 ± 5.6 ng/ml in Group 1, 24.6 ± 28.6 ng/ml in Group 2 and 25.3 ± 34.6 ng/ml in Group 3 ($p < 0.001$). These TnI concentrations and evolution confirm the AMI in groups 2 and 3. These results are consistent with new imaging studies which found that when an AMI occurs in cardiac surgery the TnI peak occurs later and the TnI at 48 h is the other best sign of myocardial necrosis (Wagner et al 2003, Selvanayagam et al 2005).

The non-AMI group showed no evidence of TnI curve sex differences (Figure 8.4), thus confirming the results of Study 1. There were sex differences in the TnI peak when an AMI occurs, due to the large differences between men and women in the STEMI group (Table 8.1).

As regards the Parsonnet score there were no significant sex differences in either the whole sample or in patients with AMI. The APACHE II and III score was higher in the group with AMI, but without sex differences. ICU stay was longer in women than in men, longer in patients with AMI than in those without, and longer in women with AMI than in men with AMI. ICU and in-hospital mortality revealed no sex differences in patients without AMI, those with AMI, in patients with STEMI or those with non-STEMI. Patients with AMI had higher in-ICU and in-hospital mortality than did patients without AMI (Table 8.1).

The lack of sex-based Parsonnet differences supports the argument that the observed differences are not due to the differences in the presurgical evaluation. The absence of Parsonnet differences between patients with and without AMI, makes evident the lack of sensitivity of this score in detecting a propensity to perioperative AMI. The higher APACHE II and III scores in patients with AMI illustrates the sensitivity of these scores in detecting important physiologic changes as a product of AMI. The longer ICU stays among women may be a sex difference that is not correlated with the variables studied. We do not believe that the longer stay and mortality among patients with AMI merits further comment.

The minor appearance of AMI in women makes evident their greater resistance to this condition, as occurs generally with acute coronary syndromes (Barrett-Connor 1997, Wexler 1999). However, this protection does not seem so important for perioperative non-STEMI, which is very frequent perioperatively and very often subendocardial (Blacker et al 2009, Wagner et al 2003, Landesberg et al 2009), a

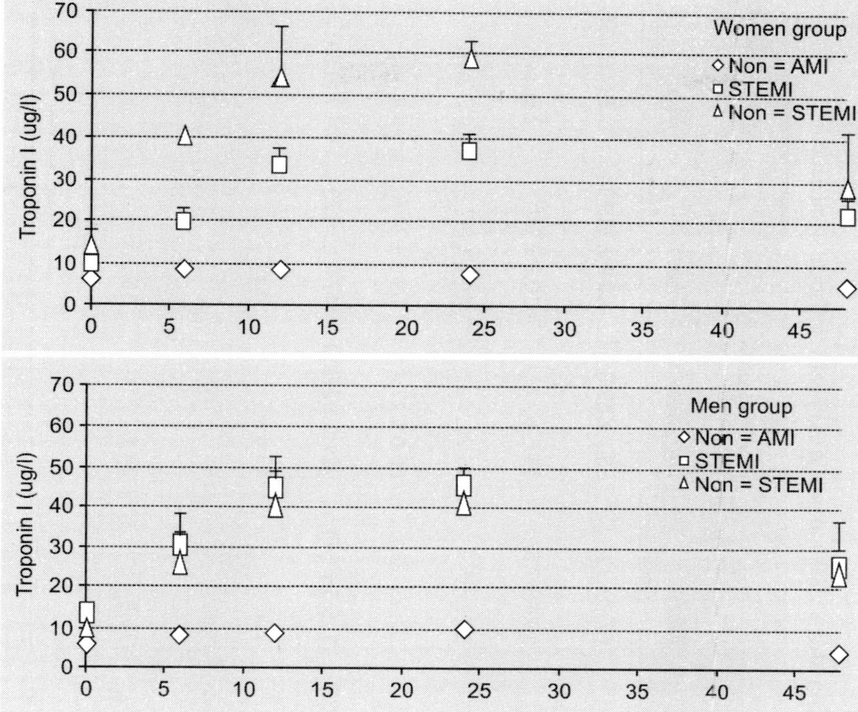

Figure 8.4: Study 2: 2,038 patients (1,276 men and 762 women). Patients with and without AMI (STEMI and non-STEMI). In AMI patients there were significant differences between men and women ($p < 0.05$).

finding that may indicate a lower level of protection at this level. For the diagnosis of AMI after cardiac surgery the elevated TnI criterion obtained from magnetic resonance imaging (Selvanayagam et al 2005) seems an important step forward in the diagnosis of this often difficult-to-diagnose condition.

A possible limitation of Study 2 is that there are no clear guidelines to determine the AMI/non-STEMI (some without stable ST changes and others with left bundle branch block or permanent pacemaker stimulation masking the possible ST repercussions). Another potential limitation is that the study does not take into consideration the long-term mortality, a limitation common to many important studies.

CONCLUSION

Study 1

This study of patients undergoing cardiac surgery with cardiopulmonary bypass found no substantial sex-based differences for TnI. Therefore, there is no point in changing diagnosis or risk stratification in a sex-specific manner.

Table 8.1: Values for men and women in three groups (non AMI, STEMI and non STEMI) with statistical significance

	Non-AMI		STEMI		Non-STEMI		Statistical
	Women	**Men**	**Women**	**Men**	**Women**	**Men**	**F(p)**
Troponin I (ug/L)	11.1 ± 31.6	9.9 ± 12.4	38.5 ± 18.1	67.2 ± 127.1	66.2 ± 69.8	62.9 ± 119.1	3.1 (< 0.05)
Parsonnet	13.1 ± 6.8	10.5 ± 7.2	8.1 ± 4.0	10.0 ± 7.5	13.6 ± 7.4	10.3 ± 7.7	2.5 (ns)
APACHE II	12.6 ± 4.2	11.6 ± 4.2	13.3 ± 2.4	12.7 ± 6.1	15.2 ± 7.1	14.6 ± 6.7	0.2 (ns)
APACHE III	50.8 ± 17.7	47.2 ± 16.6	60.2 ± 15.0	52.9 ± 22.1	66.0 ± 27.4	59.9 ± 24.8	0.4 (ns)
Hores UCI	124.1 ± 146.6	112.2 ± 135.0	289.2 ± 290.9	165.5 ± 144.5	227.2 ± 272.0	174.2 ± 179	4.1 (0.02)
Exitus UCI %	3.0	2.5	14	10.7	13.8	8.2	
		ns		ns		ns	
Exitus hospital %	4.7	3.6	20.9	15.3	24.1	15.2	
		ns		ns		ns	

Study 2

The results show:

1. That in cardiac surgery there is a higher risk of AMI in men than in women, especially for STEMI.
2. In cardiac surgery, men and women differ as regards the TnI values in the AMI.
3. A longer ICU stay in women, both with and without AMI.
4. Similar ICU and in-hospital mortality in men and women, both in the group without AMI and also in the STEMI and non-STEMI groups.

There is no potential conflict of interest relevant to this article.

ACKNOWLEDGEMENTS

We acknowledge the assistance of J. Valero PhD in the analyses, of JM. Roses MD in offering statistical supervision, and of the top level nursing team of the ICU in which we work.

BIBLIOGRAPHY

1. Abramov D, Tamariz MG, Sever JY, Christakis GT, Bhatnagar G, Heenan AL, et al. The influence of gender on the outcome of coronary artery bypass surgery. Ann Thorac Surg. 2000;70:800-6.
2. Adabag AS, Rector T, Mithani S, Harmala J, Ward HB, Kelly RF, et al. Prognostic significance of elevated cardiac troponin I after heart surgery. Ann Thorac Surg. 2007;83:1744-50.
3. Aldea GS, Gaudiani JM, Shapira OM, Jacobs AK, Weinberg J, Cupples AL, et al. Effect of gender on postoperative outcomes and hospital stays after coronary artery bypass grafting. Ann Thorac Surg. 1999;67:1097-103.
4. Alehagen U, Ericsson A, Dahlström U. Are there any significant differences between females and males in the management of heart failure? Gender aspects of an elderly population with symptoms associated with heart failure. J Card Fail. 2009;15:501-7.
5. Alpert JS, Thygesen K, Antman E, Bassand JP. Myocardial infarction redefined-a consensus document of The Joint European Society of Cardiology/American College of Cardiology Committee for the redefinition of myocardial infarction. J Am Coll Cardiol. 2000;36:959-69.
6. Antman EM, Tanasijevic MJ, Thompson B, Schactman M, McCabe CH, Cannon CP, et al. Cardiac-specific troponin I levels to predict the risk of mortality in patients with acute coronary syndromes. N Engl J Med. 1996;335:1342-9.
7. Barrett-Connor E. Differences in coronary heart disease. Circulation. 1997;95:252-64.
8. Benoit MO, Paris M, Silleran J, Fiemeyer A, Moati N. Cardiac Troponin I. Its contribution to the diagnosis of perioperative myocardial infarction and various complications of cardiac surgery. Crit Care Med. 2001;29:1880-6.
9. Blacker SD, Wilkinson DM, Rayson MP. Gender differences in the physical demands of British Army recruit training. Mil Med. 2009;174:811-6.
10. Carey JS, Cukingnan RA, Singer LK. Health status after myocardial revascularization: Inferior results in women. Ann Thorac Surg. 1995;59:112-7.
11. Chantler PD, Clements RE, Sharp L, George KP, Tan LB, Goldspink DF. The influence of body size on measurements of overall cardiac function. Am J Heart Cir Physiol. 2005;289:H2059-65.

12. Christakis GT, Weisel RD, Buth KJ, Fremes SE, Rao V, Panagiotopoulos KP, et al. Is body size the cause for poor outcomes of coronary artery bypass operations in women? J Thorac Cardiovasc Surg. 1995;110:1344-58.
13. Ciambrone G, Kaski JC. Gender differences in the treatment of chronic ischemic heart disease: Prognostic implications. Fundam Clin Pharmacol 2009;30.
14. Combes A, Luyt CE, Trouillet JL, Nieszkowska A, Chastre J. Gender impact on the outcomes of critically ill patients with nosocomial infections. Crit Care Med. 2009;37:2506-11.
15. Crabbe DL, Dipla K, Ambati S, Zafeiridis A, Gaughan JP, Houser SR, et al. Gender differences in postinfarction hypertrophy in end-stage failing hearts. J Am Coll Cardiol. 2003;41:300-6.
16. Edmunds LH, Clark RE, Cohn LH, Grunkemeier GL, Miller DC, Weisel RD. Guidelines for reporting morbidity and mortality after cardiac valvular operations. The American Association for Thoracic Surgery, Ad Hoc Liaison Committee for Standardizing Definitions of Prosthetic Heart Valve Morbidity. Ann Thorac Surg. 1996;62:932-5.
17. Edwards FH, Carey JS, Grover FL, Bero JW, Hartz RS. Impact of gender on coronary bypass operative mortality. Ann Thorac Surg. 1998;66:125-31.
18. Edwards FH, Ferraris VA, Shahian DM, Peterson E, Furnary AP, Haan CK, et al. Society of Thoracic Surgeons. Gender-specific practice guidelines for coronary artery bypass surgery: Perioperative management. Ann Thorac Surg. 2005;79:2189-94.
19. Edwards ML, Albert NM, Wang C, Apperson-Hansen C. 1993-2003 gender differences in coronary artery revascularization: Has anything changed? J Cardiovasc Nurs. 2005;20:461-7.
20. Ennker IC, Albert A, Pietrowski D, Bauer K, Ennker J, Florath I. Impact of gender on outcome after coronary bypass surgery. Asian Cardiovasc Thorac Ann. 2009;17:253-8.
21. Fellahi JL, Gué X, Richomme X, Monier E, Guillou L, Riou B. Short- and long-term prognostic value of postoperative cardiac troponin I concentration in patients undergoing coronary artery bypass grafting. Anesthesiology. 2003;99:270-4.
22. Fellahi JL, Hedoire F, Le Manach Y, Monier E, Guillou L, Riou B. Determination of the threshold of cardiac troponin I associated with an adverse postoperative outcome after cardiac surgery: A comparative study between coronary artery bypass graft, valve surgery, and combined cardiac surgery, Crit Care Med. 2007;11:R106.
23. Gensini GF, Fusi C, Conti AA, Calamai GC, Montesi GF, Galanti G, et al. Cardiac troponin I and Q-wave perioperative myocardial infarction after coronary artery bypass surgery. Crit Care Med. 1998;26:1986-90.
24. Guru V, Fremes SE, Austin PC, Blackstone EH, Tu JV. Gender differences in outcomes after hospital discharge from coronary artery bypass grafting. Circulation. 2006;113:507-16.
25. Hense HW, Gneiting B, Muscholl M, Broeckel U, Kuch B, Doering A, et al. The associations of body size and body composition with left ventricular mass: Impacts for indexation in adults. J Am Coll Cardiol. 1998;32:451-7.
26. Humphries KH, Gao M, Pu A, Lichtenstein S, Thompson CR. Significant improvement in short-term mortality in women undergoing coronary artery bypass surgery (1991 to 2004). J Am Coll Cardiol. 2007;49:1552-8.
27. Hussain KM, Kogan A, Estrada AQ, Konstandy G, Foschi A, Dadkhah S. Referral pattern and outcome in men and women undergoing coronary artery bypass surgery: A critical. Angiology. 1998;49:243-50.
28. Jackson A, Pollock M, Ward A. Generalized equations for predicting body density of women. Med Sci Sports Exer. 1980;12:175-81.
29. Jackson AS, Pollock M. Generalized equations for predicting body density of men. 1978. Br J Nutr. 2004;91:161-8.

30. Jacobs AK, Kelsey SF, Brooks MM, Faxon DP, Chaitman BR, Bittner V, et al. Better outcome for women compared with men undergoing coronary revascularization: A report from the bypass angioplasty revascularization investigation (BARI). Circulation. 1998;98:1279-85.
31. Kitzman DW, Scholz DG, Hagen PT, Ilstrup DM, Edwards WD. Age-related changes in normal human hearts during the first 10 decades of life. Part II (Maturity): A quantitative anatomic study of 765 specimens from subjects 20 to 99 years old. Mayo Clin Proc. 1988;63:137-46.
32. Koch CG, Khandwala F, Nussmeier N, Blackstone EH. Gender profiling in coronary artery bypass grafting. J Thorac Cardiovasc Surg. 2003;126:2044-51.
33. Kokkonen L, Järvinen O, Majahalme S, Virtanen V, Pehkonen E, Mustonen J, et al. Atrial fibrillation in elderly patients after coronary artery bypass grafting; gender differences in outcome. Scand Cardiovasc J. 2005;39:293-8.
34. Kwon DH, Halley CM, Popovic ZB, Carrigan TP, Zysek V, Setser R, et al. Gender differences in survival in patients with severe left ventricular dysfunction despite similar extent of myocardial scar measured on cardiac magnetic resonance. Eur J Heart Fail. 2009;11:937-44.
35. Landesberg G, Beattie WS, Mosseri M, Jaffe AS, Alpert JS. Perioperative myocardial infarction. Circulation. 2009;119:2936-44.
36. Mason SA, MacLeod KT. Cardiac action potential duration and calcium regulation in males and females. Biochem Biophys Res Commun. 2009;388:565-70.
37. McGee WA, Eggerstedt JM, Mancini MC. Coronary artery bypass surgery in women. J La State Med Soc. 1998;150:81-4.
38. Mickleborough LL, Takagi Y, Maruyama H, Sun Z, Mohamed S. Is sex a factor in determining operative risk for aortocoronary bypass graft surgery? Circulation. 1995;92(9 Suppl):1180-4.
39. Morrow J, Jackson A, Disch J, Mood D. In "Measurement and Evaluation in Human Performance". Chapter 8: Physical Assessment in Adults. Edit. Human Kinetics, Champaign, USA. 1995.
40. Ott RA, Gutfinger DE, Alimadadian HF. Conventional coronary artery bypass grafting: Why women take longer to recover. J Cardiovasc Surg. 2001;42:311–5.
41. Patel S, Smith JM; Engel AM. Gender differences in outcomes after off-pump coronary artery bypass graft surgery. Am Surg. 2006;72:310-3.
42. Ponce G, Romero JL, Hernández G, Padrón A, Cabrera E, Abad C. The non Q wave myocardial infarction in conventional valvular surgery. Diagnosis with cardiac troponin I. Rev Esp Card. 2001;54:1175-82.
43. Puskas JD, Kilgo PD, Kutner M, Pusca SV, Lattouf O, Guyton RA. Off-pump techniques disproportionately benefit women and narrow the gender disparity in outcomes after coronary artery bypass surgery. Circulation. 2007;116:I192-9.
44. Relos RP, Hasinoff IK, Beilman GJ. Moderately elevated serum troponin I concentrations are associated with increased morbidity and mortality rates in surgical intensive care unit patients. Crit Care Med. 2003;31:2598-603.
45. Reyes A, Vega G, Blancas R, Morató B, Moreno JL, Torrecilla C, et al. Early vs conventional extubation after cardiac surgery with cardiopulmonary bypass. Chest. 1997;112:193-201.
46. Ricart A, Farrero E, Ventura JL, Javierre C, Carrió L, Rodríguez D, et al. Are there sex-based differences in serum troponin I after cardiac surgery? Crit Care Med. 2009;37:2210-5.
47. Ricart A, Pagés T, Viscor G, Leal C, Ventura Farré JL. Sex-linked differences in pulse oxymetry. Br J Sports Med. 2008;42:620-1.
48. Schwarzenberger JC, Sun LS, Pesce MA, Heyer EJ, Delphin E, Almeida GM, Wood M. Sex-based differences in serum cardiac troponin I, a specific marker for myocardial injury, after cardiac surgery. Crit Care Med. 2003;31:689-93.
49. Selvanayagam JB, Pigott D, Balacumaraswami L, Petersen SE, Neubauer S, Taggart DP. Relationship of irreversible myocardial injury to troponin I and creatine kinase-MB elevation after coronary artery bypass surgery: Insights from cardiovascular magnetic resonance imaging. J Am Coll Cardiol. 2005;45:62931

50. Stefani RT. The relative power output and relative lean body mass of World and Olympic male and female champions with implications for gender equity. J Sports Sci. 2006;24:1329-39.
51. Svedjeholm R, Dahlin LG, Lundberg C, Szabo Z, Kägedal B, Nylander E, Olin C, Rutberg H. Are electrocardiographic Q-wave criteria reliable for diagnosis of perioperative myocardial infarction after coronary surgery? Eur J Cardiothorac Surg. 1998;13:655-61.
52. Sánchez, JM. García, R. Aragonés, M. Delgado, MD. Matas, A. Vera. La troponina I como predictor de la morbilidad tras cirugía cardíaca con circulación extracorpórea. Medicina Intensiva. 2001;25:257-62.
53. Toumpulis IK, Anagnostopoulos CE, Balaram SK, Rokkas CK, Swistel DG, Ashton RC Jr, et al. Assessment of independent predictors for long-term mortality between women and men after coronary artery bypass grafting: Are women different from men? J Thorac Cardiovasc Surg. 2006;131:343-51.
54. Wagner A, Mahrholdt H, Holly TA, Elliot MD, Regerfus M, Parker M, et al. Contrast enhanced MRI and routine single photon emission computed tomography (SPECT) perfusion imaging for detection of subendocardial myocardial infarcts: An imaging study. Lancet. 2003;361:374-9.
55. Wexler LF. Studies of acute coronary syndromes in women-Lessons for everyone. NEJM. 1999;341:275-6.

Chapter

9

Angiomyogenesis for Myocardial Repair

Vien Khach Lai, Khawaja Husnain Haider, Muhammad Ashraf

Abstract. The heart cell therapy using stem cells has emerged as a potential treatment modality for ischemic cardiomyopathy. More than a decade long experimental animal studies and clinical trials have shown the safety and feasibility of this approach. The strategy is based on the principle to supplement the inadequate intrinsic repair mechanism of the heart through stem cell transplantation. The transplanted cells undergo milieu dependent myogenic differentiation to compensate for the colossal cardiomyocyte loss resulting from ischemic injury with resultant reduction in infarct size, attenuated left ventricular remodeling and preserved global cardiac function. More recent studies have shown that in vitro manipulation of stem cells to achieve angiogenesis augments their therapeutic potential for better prognosis via improved regional blood flow in the infarcted myocardium. This review summarizes our current knowledge about combined angiomyogenic approach using stem cells for myocardial repair.

Keywords. Cardiomyogenesis, angiogenesis, gene delivery, stem cells.

INTRODUCTION

Ischemic heart disease is the leading cause of morbidity and death worldwide and its incidence is on the rise and becoming a true pandemic. Despite recent advancements in pharmacological management and surgical interventions, which led to improved prognosis and better survival rates, 1 in 4 men and 1 in 3 women in the USA die within a year after myocardial infarction diagnosis (Mackay and Mensah 2006). The coronary artery occlusion leads to compromised regional blood flow with a resultant loss of functioning cardiomyocytes, which are replaced by poorly vascularized scar tissue. Despite the presence of a pool of resident cardiac stem cells, an outside intervention is required to support the inadequate intrinsic repair mechanism of the heart. Amongst the large portfolio of therapies to combat ischemic heart disease investigated during the last decade, the heart cell therapy and angiogenic protein/gene therapy have emerged as potential approaches for myocardial repair and represent a paradigm shift in cardiovascular treatment strategies. The underlying mechanism of stem cells based cardiac repair largely remains contentious; it is considered as multifactorial and also varies with the type of the cells used in the procedure. It involves myogenic transdifferentiation of stem cells (Kajstura et al 2005, Rota et al 2007), paracrine release of growth factors (Gnecchi et al 2008, Baraniak and McDevitt 2010, Matsuura et al 2009) which provide cue for recruitment and homing-in of stem and progenitor cells to participate in the repair process besides improving regional blood flow via angiogenesis (Uemura et al. 2006, Templin et al 2009).

The basic criterion for choice of stem cells for the heart cell therapy is: Autologous availability without ethical issues, ease of propagation in vitro and, pluri- to multilineage potential to adopt cardiac phenotype. Even though search for an ideal stem cell type remains an area of intense investigation, bone marrow derived stem cells and skeletal myoblasts are two of the most extensively studied cell types for their cardiac reparability in experimental animal studies (Kajstura et al 2005, Jain et al 2001, Tambara et al 2003, He et al 2005, Brasselet et al 2005) as well as in clinical trial (Siminiak et al 2004, Smits et al 2003, Menasche et al 2001, Beeres et al 2007, Stamm et al 2007) with encouraging results. Nevertheless, neomyogenesis alone can only occur at very low rate and may be less meaningful for the improvement of cardiac function in the absence of regional blood flow restoration in the infarcted myocardium. To this end, stem cell therapy warrants to be combined with angiogenic therapy which is anticipated to be more effective therapeutic intervention as compared to the use of either of the strategies as monotherapy. We here focus on the beneficial effects of myoangiogenesis which comprises essential neovascularization to bring in oxygen and nutrients to support the transplanted/mobilized cells and the newly formed myocardium.

CARDIOMYOGENESIS

The adult mammalian heart has always been considered as a postmitotic organ, given that cardiomyocytes possess only limited ability to reenter into cell cycle, and the heart has a relatively constant number of cardiomyocytes throughout the lifespan of a human being since shortly after birth. This long-standing dogma has been challenged by Bergmann and colleagues who observed that adult human cardiomyocytes has the been ability of self-renewal, with a gradual decrease from 1% turnover annually at the age of 25 to 0.45% at the age of 75 and less than 50% of total cardiomyocytes are exchanged during a normal life span (Bergmann et al 2009). Furthermore, the pioneering work of Anversa et al. have shown the existence of resident stem and progenitor cells in the heart which participate in the repair process in the event of myocardial injury (Nadal-Ginard et al 2005). More importantly, resident cardiac stem and progenitor cells were shown to have the capability to adopt all the phenotypes required for *de novo* myocardial regeneration (Beltrami et al 2003). The investigators have successfully isolated and purified resident cardiac stem and progenitor cells from various species and shown that these cells can be propagated *in vitro* for re-engraftment in the injured myocardium, without compromising their differentiation potential (Dawn et al 2005).

Subsequent to the studies showing transplantability of bone marrow cells and their ability to undergo milieu dependent differentiation (Liechty et al 2000), Orlic et al. were the first to report that cardiac muscles can be regenerated using bone marrow derived stem cells in a mouse model of myocardial infarction. During acute phase subsequent to coronary ligation, Lin^- $c\text{-}kit^+$ cells were injected in the contracting wall bordering the infarct region (Orlic et al 2001). Nine days after treatment, newly formed myocardium from the transplanted cells was observed to constitute more than 68% of the infarcted left ventricle. These results indicated that the locally delivered bone marrow cells possessed the ability of de novo myocardial regeneration and ameliorated infarct size expansion. Similar results were obtained when bone marrow stem cells were mobilized and homed-into the infracted myocardium (Tomita et al 2004, Orlic et al 2001, Barile et al 2009). These results established the possibility that the infarcted heart is repairable using stem cell engraftment approach and paved the way for subsequent studies which showed encouraging results in both small as well as large experimental animal models. The success story of bone marrow stem cell transplantation for myocardial repair is not without controversies. Some investigators have failed to duplicate reparability of bone marrow stem cells in the infarcted heart and have reported failure of bone marrow stem cells to adopt cardiac phenotype (Murry et al 2004, Balsam et al 2004). Even the intrinsically mobilized bone marrow cells have been reported to contribute only meagerly towards regeneration of the infarcted myocardium (Fukuhara et al 2005). Moreover, there are also some reports which have issued a note of caution about the bone marrow stem cells due to their plastic and malleable nature. Transplantation of unselected bone marrow cells into the acutely infarcted myocardium caused significant intramyocardial calcification in the periinfarct area or normal myocardium (Yoon et al 2004). Similarly, transplantation of undifferentiated mesenchymal stem cells has been shown to develop into fibroblastic scar tissue (Wang et al 2001). These results underscore the importance of regulating cellular differentiation of adult stem cells in therapeutic applications. Obviously, these data have intrigued the exploration of interventions with therapeutic implications that can be used to support unwanted differentiation ability of the unselected the healing process in cardiac pathologies. Besides the use of bone marrow cells, stem/progenitors stem cells from different origins are being assessed for myocardial repair (Table 9.1).

With the recent modifications in National Institutes of Health policy on the use of embryonic stem (ES) cells, there is a rejuvenated interest to explore the possibility of ES cells for use in the heart cell therapy (Zhang et al 2008, Foldes et al 2008). In comparison with the adult stem cells, ES cells are pluripotent and have unlimited self-renewal capacity *in vitro* in undifferentiated state (Mummery et al 2007). ES cells have been successfully programmed to adopt cardiac phenotype in vitro as well as post engraftment in experimental animal studies. ES cell are being considered as an excellent source of cardiomyocytes for *in vitro* (Farokhpour et al 2009, Abdul Kadir et al 2009) as well as transplantation studies (van Laake et al 2009,

Table 9.1: Experimental animal studies with various stem cells

Experimental studies	Subjects	Observed benefits
Human ESC	Human to rats	No improvement
ESC derived cardiomyocyte:	Human to rats	Functional improvement
EPCs	Mice	Angiogenesis, functional enhancement
EPCs	Pigs	Angiogenesis, functional preservation
HSCs	Mice	No difference
HSCs	Mice	No difference
BMC	Mice	Regeneration
BMC	Dogs	Functional improvement, infarct size reduction
MSC	Human to mice	Myogenesis
Side population cell	Mice	Angiomyogenesis
MAPCs	Rats	Angiomyogenesis,Functional improvement
Lin-/C-kit^{+}	Rats	Angiomyogenesis
Sca1^{+} cells	Mice	Myogenesis
Cord blood progenitors	Human to mice	Angiogenesis
iPS cells	Human to mice	Functional improvement
Mauritz	Mice	*In vitro* myocardial regeneration
Adipose stromal stem cells[1]	Mice	*In vitro* cardiac-like cell development
Spermatogonial stem cells	Mice	*In vitro* cardiac cell transdifferentiation

BMS= bone marrow stem cells; EPCs = endothelial progenitor cells; HSCs = hematopoietic stem cells; iPS cells = induced pluripotent stem cells.

van Laake et al 2007, Dai et al 2007, Singla et al 2006). However, teratogenicity, immunorejection of the cell graft over time and ethical issues regarding their use remain the biggest unresolved issues (Caspi et al 2007, Leor et al 2007). In this notion, the recent advancement in developing of induced pluripotent stem (iPS) cells, which possess culture characteristics such as unlimited self-renewal in undifferentiated state *in vitro* and multilineage differentiation features similar to ES cells. However, iPS cells have the added advantages of availability without ethical issues and autologous origin thus eliminating the problem of immuno-rejection thus allowing the establishment of new approach in cardiac regeneration (Park et al 2008). Since the inception of this concept that somatic cells can be reprogrammed to achieve pluripotency by overexpression of a combination of transcription factors (Oct3/4, Sox2, Klf4 and c-Myc) (Takahashi and Yamanaka 2006), several labs have successfully reported iPS cells generation from somatic cells of different tissues (Takahashi et al 2007, Park et al 2008, Kim et al 2008). Moreover, the methods of iPS cells generation have been refined to make the cells clinically safer by reducing the number of transcription factors, without viral integration and methods to achieve their overexpression in the somatic cells (Stadtfeld et al 2008, Qin et al 2008, Okita et al 2008, Huangfu et al 2008, Lowry et al 2008). More recent *in vivo* studies in experimental animal models have shown that iPS cells engraftment into the infarcted myocardium could successfully preserve left ventricular contractile function in the failing heart and attenuate infarct size expansion (Martinez-Fernandez et al 2009, Nelson et al 2009).

In the clinical settings, most studies have used bone marrow derived mononuclear cells and their subpopulations (Table 9.2). Metaanalyses of clinical trials clearly shows only a meager improvement of approximately 3% in left ventricular function in the subjects treated with bone marrow cells versus control group of patients (Lipinski et al 2007, Abdel-Latif et al 2007). Furthermore, bone marrow cell administration following an acute myocardial infarction suggests a dose-response association between injected number of cells and change in left ventricular ejection fraction, with an as yet undefined mechanism. It is therefore necessary to measure other parameters such as the reduction of infarct size or neovascularization in infracted area to elucidate the putative mechanism so that appropriate aims can be established.

Besides bone marrow cells, skeletal myoblasts which possess an inherent capacity of myogenic differentiation have been studied in the patients. Since the first-in-man use of skeletal myoblasts transplantation for myocardial repair (Siminiak et al 2004), clinical studies with skeletal myoblasts by different research groups have shown the safety and feasibility of their use in patients with ischemic cardiomyopathy (Menasche et al 2001, Menasche et al 2003, Dib et al 2005, Pagani et al 2003, Sim et al 2005). In fact, there is ample histological and immunohistological evidence which shows that the transplanted skeletal myoblasts differentiated into neofibers and formed islands of new muscle in the infarct and periinfarct regions (Pagani et al 2003, Hagege et al 2003). Despite their contribution to improved global cardiac function, lack of electrophysiological coupling with the host cardiomyocytes remains one of the major negatives for use of skeletal myoblasts for the heart cell therapy (Reinecke and Murry et al 2000, Niagara et al 2007). This inability of skeletal myoblasts to functionally couple with the host cardiomyocytes has been implied as the possible explanation for high incidence of arrhythmias in the patients receiving skeletal myoblasts (Fouts et al 2006). However, these arrhythmias were not fatal and were pharmacologically treatable. Studies are underway to overcome this deficiency of skeletal myoblasts to ensure their coupling with the host myocytes (Suzuki et al 2001).

Table 9.2: Clinical studies using stem cells and angiogenic growth factor protein/gene delivery

Clinical studies	Randomized/ controlled	Delivery routes	Intervention/ control	Observed benefits
BMC: BMMNCs	Yes	IC	22/22	No difference
BOOST trial	Yes	IC	30/30	No difference
Leuven trial	Yes, double blind	IC	33/34	No effect on LV function but limit infarct size
ASTAMI trial	Yes	IC	47/50	No difference
REPAIR-AMI trial	Yes	IC	101/103	Improve LV function
Ang	Yes	During CABG	21/21/20 IC/IM/control	No difference
MSC: Chen	Yes	IC	34/35	Improve left ventricular function
Subsets: CD133+:	Yes	IM/IC	20/20	Improve LV function
CD34+: REGENT trial	Yes		80/80/40 CD34+/BMC/ control	No difference
SkM: MAGIC trial	Yes, double blind	IM	34/33/30 High/low dose/placebo	No improvement, increased arrhythmias
VEGF gene: Kuopio Angiogenesis Trial (KAT)	Yes	IC	37/28/38 Ad/Pl/control	Amelioration of myocardial perfusion in the VEGF-Adv-treated patients
VEGF protein: VIVA trial	Yes, double blind	IC	59/56/63 High/ low dose/ placebo	No difference
Ad-VEGF	Yes, double blind	IM	32/35	Improvement in exercise treadmill test
VEGF plasmid (EUROINJECT-ONE)	Yes, double blind	IC	40/40	Slight improvement

Contd...

Contd...

Clinical studies	Randomized/ controlled	Delivery routes	Intervention/ control	Observed benefits
FGF-2 protein	Yes, double blind	IC	85/84/82/86 High/medium/ low dose/ placebo	No difference
FGF-2 protein	Yes, double blind	During CABG	8/8/8 High/low dose/placebo	May improve myocardial perfusion
Ad-FGF	Yes, double blind	IC	175/180/177 High/low dose/control	Potential improvement in exercise treadmill test

CABG= coronary artery bypass grafting; IC= intracoronary; IM= intramyocardial

ANGIOGENESIS

The process of angiogenesis in the biological system consists of a cascade of events, regulated by a delicately balanced cross-talk between numerous proangiogenic and antiangiogenic factors and cells (Sim et al 2002). Angiogenesis requires proliferation, activation and migration of endothelial cells and remodeling of extracellular matrix followed by maturation of the newly formed vascular structure with the formation of a layer of smooth muscle cells. Whereas angiogenesis involves the formation of new capillary structures from the preexisting vessels, arteriogenesis, which is equally complex phenomenon, and engages a wider variety of cell types, growth factors and signaling molecules. In contrast, vasculogenesis is the formation of fully formed vessels from endothelial cell precursors. Preclinical animal studies have vastly explored the potential use of angiogenic growth factors (recombinant proteins) or genes in combination with or without stem/progenitor cell engraftment to treat ischemic heart disease.

Angiogenesis by Angiogenic Growth Factors Treatment

In the response to ischemia, hypoxia-inducible factor-1α (HIF-1α), a dominative transcriptional activator of oxygen homeostasis, regulates the expression of several angiogenic mediators including vascular endothelial growth factor (VEGF), neuoropilin-1, angiopoietin-1 (Ang-1), angiopoietin-2 (Ang-2), Platelet derived growth factor (PDGF) and placental growth factor (PIGF), hepatocyte growth factor (HGF) (Banai et al 1994, Kelly et al 2003, Pugh et al 2003, Yamakawa et al 2003, Morishita et al 2004). VEGF is one of the main member in the angiogenic cascade and participates via direct recruitment, proliferation and maturation of precursor cells such as endothelial progenitor cells (EPCs) and monocytes (Fujiyama et al 2003, Shintani et al 2001). Chemo-attractant such as stromal cell derived factor-1α (SDF-1α) (Elmadbouh et al 2007, Askari et al 2003), cytokines such as granulocyte colony stimulating factor (G-CSF), granulocyte–monocyte colony stimulating factor (CS-CSF) (Takahashi et al 1999), stem cell factor (SCF) (Kanellakis et al 2006), erythropoietin (Westenbrink et al 2007), thymosin β4 (Smart et al 2007), insulin-like growth factor (IGF-1) and fibroblast growth factor (FGF) (Nabel et al 1993, Unger et al 1994) can also mobilize EPCs from the bone marrow and peripheral circulation to ischemic myocardium and remarkably promote new blood vessel formation in the injured areas, enhance perfusion, and lead to recovery of ischemic tissue (Pearlman et al 1995, Harada et al 1994). Of all these growth factors, the best studied for angiogenic activities are VEGF and FGF (Kalka et al 2000, Goncalves et al 2010, Dong et al 2009, Haigh 2008, Detillieux et al 2003). Both of these growth factor proteins can induce angiogenesis *in vivo* in ischemic tissues, but the relative advantage of either factor is unclear. Moreover, the association of VEGF and other cytokine supplements for angiogenesis in clinical settings is not certain. For example, the data from the treatment of VEGF in Ischemia for Vascular Angiogenesis (VIVA) placebo-controlled double-blind trial of 178 patients for ischemic coronary diseases represent its safety profile but do not support the effective notion of the treatments although there is a trend in symptom improvement (Henry et al 2003).

Angiogenesis Using Angiogenic Growth Factor Gene Delivery

Alternative to the recombinant angiogenic growth factor delivery to the heart is the delivery strategy involving plasmids encoding for the growth factor/s of interest. The anticipated therapeutic effect from transgene delivery to the infarcted myocardium is to achieve overexpression of proangiogenic growth factors for extended time duration to promote angiogenic response for improved regional blood flow in the ischemic myocardium. The success of an experimental or clinical gene delivery to the heart is dependent on the efficiency of gene transfer and expression which varies with the choice of delivery vectors besides other factors. Direct injection of angiogenic growth factor cDNA into the heart has shown improved cardiac performance, stimulated angiogenesis and reduced cardiomyocyte apoptosis, the uptake of the delivered cDNA by the cardiomyocytes is less efficient (Ruixing et al 2007, Ye et al 2007) and therefore, it requires an efficient delivery system. Despite low transfection efficiency and short-term expression, nonviral gene delivery systems are safer and flexible in terms of the plasmid DNA size which can be delivered (Muller et al 2006, Muller et al 2008). We have already shown the efficiency of liposomal and nano-particle based nonviral vector systems for transfection of skeletal myoblasts to overexpress SDF1α and VEGF encoding transgenes respectively (Elmadbouh et al 2007, Ye et al 2007a). The results from these studies highlighted the safety and effectiveness of the liposome and nanoparticle based nonviral vectors for gene delivery to the heart. Of all the gene delivery vectors, however, viral gene delivery systems have shown better transfection efficiency (Young et al 2006). Replication deficient adenoviral vectors carrying genes encoding various growth factors can penetrate into the host cells through receptors of Coxsackievirus. These are low risk vectors in terms of immunogenicity and have been designed to carry single or multiple growth factor genes (Haider et al 2004, Arsic et al 2003, Ye et al 2007b). Viral vector based delivery of angiogenic growth factors has been extensively studied in experimental animal models (Haider et al 2004, Arsic et al 2003, Takahashi et al 2003, Rissanen et al 2004). However, uncontrolled, longer-term sustained expression of angiogenic growth factors may not be without its unwanted effects. There are reports wherein uncontrolled overexpression of VEGF has led to angioma formation instead of normal functioning vascular structures (Carmeliet 2000, Schwarz et al 2000). The development of regulatable delivery vectors may therefore be required to ensure transgene activity only when it is required (Guo et al 2008). A more interesting approach of ischemia regulated preemptive angiogenic growth factor gene delivery is being adopted to ensure that episodes of ischemia may be alleviated by the delivery of ischemia sensitive VEGF gene expression (Dulak et al 2006). Similarly, VEGF gene delivery alone may be insufficient to develop stable and mature vascular structures and therefore may require the support of other growth factors such as Ang-1 which are known for their activity as maturation factors (Arsic et al 2003, Ye et al 2007b).

Angiogenesis by Stem/Progenitor Cell Engraftment

Cellular angiogenesis approach offer significant advantages over protein and gene-based strategies. Transplantation of stem/progenitor cells with inherent ability to express secretable angiogenic growth factors provide sustained release of multiple growth factors at the site of the cell graft (Zisa et al 2009, Nesselmann et al 2010). In addition to cardioprotection via stimulation of survival signaling in cardiomyocytes, the growth factors thus secreted provide cue to facilitate the recruitment of stem cells to participate in myocardial repair process via myogenic differentiation as well as by participation in angiogenesis (Lee et al 2009). Additionally, these transplanted cells provide the much needed cellular substrate which is required for the development new vascular structures and get incorporated into the newly formed vascular structures (Jiang et al 2006). There is evidence from myocardial infarction experiments to suggest that enhanced angiogenesis with increased regional myocardial perfusion to support the survival of hibernating native cardiomyocytes (Fukuhara et al 2005, Garbade et al 2009). To date, various strategies have been adopted based on engraftment of stem/progenitor cells either alone or in combination with angiogenic growth factor protein/gene delivery to promote angiogenic response in the ischemic myocardium.

Myocardial angiogenesis has been observed subsequent to transplantation of a variety of cell types (Matsuura et al 2009, Tomita et al 1999, Finney et al 2010, Sanberg et al 2009, Hung et al 2009, Leobon et al 2009, Yerebakan et al 2009). However, the ideal cell type to achieve optimal angiogenic response is still not established. Of all these cells, bone marrow derived mesenchymal stem cells have shown promise for cellular angiogenesis in experimental animal models (Tomita et al 2004, et al 2009). One of the postulated mechanism by which mesenchymal stem cells enhance angiogenic response in the heart is the release soluble factors that alter the endothelial nitric oxide and calcium levels of endothelial cells and may be important to facilitate crossing of the endothelial barrier (Ladage et al 2007).

EPCs are central to de novo formation of vascular structures (Eguchi et al 2007). Found both in human and animals, EPCs were first isolated from peripheral blood by Asahara et al as CD34+/VEGFR-2+ progenitors, EPC also extrude Flk-1, Tie-2, KDR, C-kit, Sca-1 and CD133 antigens (Asahara et al 1997). These markers can also be found in hematopoietic progenitors that make EPCs represent a heterogeneous population (Iwami et al 2004). The subpopulatios of EPCs share common properties and function, and they can proliferate *in vitro* and differentiate into endothelial cells and present the capacity to improve neovascularization *in vivo* and enhance vascular endothelium and ameliorate cardiac function (Asahara et al 1997, Asahara et al 1999) [35-38]. EPCs home to sites of neovascularization and differentiate into endothelial cells (ECs) *in situ* and contribute to vascular organogenesis and are considered as therapeutic agents to supply the potent origin of neovascularization under pathological conditions. *Ex vivo* expansion and use of a large number of EPCs has allowed vigorously the repair, and the formation of new vessels (Kawamoto et al 2001). The accumulation of transplanted/mobilized EPCs help increase the number of vessels in the targeted tissue and the cells also release various secreted factors to surrounding area that in turn induce mobilization, engraftment and maturation of EPCs from bone marrow and peripheral blood to the lesion. These released factors also represent an indirect mechanism of angiogenesis via paracrine and autocrine effects (Shi et al 1998, Hamada et al 2006, Jujo et al 2008). Various strategies have also been adopted to enhance angiogenic potential of EPCs. Transfection of EPCs with the HGF gene released high levels of soluble HGF protein which promoted the proliferative, migratory and angiogenic capabilities (Song et al 2009).

Stem Cell Based Gene Delivery for Myocardial Angiomyogenesis

An alternative to stem cell therapy and angiogenic protein/gene delivery to the heart as montherapies is to combine both these approaches for concomitant angiomyogenic repair of the heart. Genetic modulation of stem cells or their use with concomitant administration with angiogenic growth factors improves their therapeutic efficiency (Elmadbouh et al 2007, Ye et al 2007a, Ahmed et al 2010, Das et al 2009, Zhu et al 2009, Yau et al 2007, Tang et al 2009). Cell based therapeutic approaches combined with therapeutic gene delivery attenuates infarct size expansion and prevents deterioration of the myocardial function postinfarction and may even reverse established heart failure (Haider et al 2004, Yau et al 2005). We have previously shown that transplantation of native skeletal myoblasts resulted in myogenesis in the infarcted heart. However, their angiomyogenic potential was considerably improved upon genetic modulation of the cells using adenoviral vectors for angiogenic growth factors including VEGF and Ang-1 (Ye et al 2007, Haider et al 2004). Given the complex nature of angiogenic response, we developed a novel bicistronic vector which simultaneous encoded for the expression of VEGF and Ang-1. The vector was used for genetic modification of skeletal myoblasts prior to engraftment in a rabbit model of acute hind limb ischemia as well as porcine heart model of chronic myocardial infarction (Ye et al 2007b, Niagara et al 2004). Our multimodal therapeutic approach resulted in higher percentage of functionally competent and mature vascular structures as compared with VEGF delivery alone.

In order to avoid viral vector associated complications, we have also used nonviral vector based delivery of angiogenic genes to the heart. In one of our recently published study, we have combined nanoparticles developed from polyethyleneimine (PEI) for transfection of angiogenic growth factor genes into skeletal myoblasts and shown the safety and effectiveness of this approach (Ye et al 2007a). We have also combined stem cell based gene delivery of angio-competent molecules with survival signaling molecules. This two pronged strategy on the one hand improved the survival of transplanted stem cells postengraftment in the heart besides improving angiogenesis in the infarcted myocardium (Jiang et al 2006). Long-term histological studies and the heart function analysis showed that the functional benefits of the treatment were stable until 4 months of observation (Shujia et al 2008). Other research groups have also shown similar results. Yau and colleagues have reported the functional benefits of their multimodal therapeutic approach wherein they used mesenchymal stem cells genetically modified to cooverexpress VEGF and basic FGF. They observed a powerful synergistic effect of their multimodal treatment approach in terms of angiogenic effect, albeit, without affecting perfusion or functional benefits. In their quest for an optimal combination of angiogenic growth factors, the same group of researchers combined VEGF overexpression with IGF-1 transgene delivery to the infarcted heart (Yau et al 2005). In one of our recently concluded study, we observed that stem cell based IGF-1gene delivery to the heart resulted in higher SDF-1α expression at the site of the cell graft (Haider et al 2008). The elevated expression of SDF-1α, which is known for $CXCR4^+$ stem cell mobilization and also a designated retention factor of the mobilized cells, was accompanied by extensive mobilization of stem and progenitor cells in the infarcted myocardium. Despite these encouraging results, the approach of combined stem cell and angiogenic gene delivery needs to be optimized for its safer applications in the clinical perspective.

FUTURE DEVELOPMENT

Both gene therapy as well as stem cell engraftment has given encouraging results in the clinical settings, albeit with some limitations. Therefore, a combined strategy of using stem cells genetically modified to deliver transgene of interest will be advantageous in terms of exploiting best of these two strategies. On one hand it will enhance the effectiveness of stem cells by improving their survival, paracrine activity, angiogenic and differentiation potential, and at the same time, genetically modified stem cells will ensure localized and regulatable expression of the gene of interest with reduced the incidence of untoward effects of the transgene product. However, many procedures and issues require optimization and clarification before the combined strategy of angiogenesis and myogenesis can be fully understood and safely applied in the clinical settings. The selection of the stem cells for use as a carrier of the transgene of interest to the heart is an important determinant factor for the success of the procedure. These genetically modified cells will serve as a reservoir of the transgene product, the concentration of which will be stably maintained over extended time duration as long as the gene will continue to express. Moreover, the transplanted cells will differentiate to adopt myogenic phenotype. Likewise, in-depth studies are required to optimize the basic issues pertaining to cell engraftment such as the optimal number of cells, their off-the shelf availability, route of administration and time of injection after infarction episode. The consideration regarding the number of genetically modified cells may mean different from native cell engraftment approach. As a general rule, it is considered that the outcome of native stem cell transplantation is directly related to the number of the transplanted cells (Lai et al 2009). The same principle may not hold good for genetically modified cells as it may lead to unnecessarily higher level of transgene expression product at the site of the cell graft. The beneficial effects of genetically modified stem cell engraftment is hence a result of complex mechanism, and therefore needs careful optimization of the procedure in general and regarding the use of nonviral transfection of stem cells in particular. Immunogenicity of the cells other than from the autologous source and, which may get altered by viral vector transduction of the transgene, may significantly influence the survival of the transplanted cells post engraftment. The strategy to encapsulate the genetically modified stem cells may immunoisolate the cells after engraftment from their surrounding host tissue and help the cells escape host immune response during acute phase of engraftment (Springer et al 2000). Additionally, it is worthwhile to acknowledge the possibility that *ex vivo* delivery of a cocktail of growth factor transgenes can help to achieve the required functional goals. MicroRNAs, which are small noncoding RNAs, have been shown to regulate stem cell characteristics and functionality (Hime et al 2009). With the emerging role of microRNAs in stem cell differentiation and activation of the angiogenic program in endothelial cells, angiomyogenesis may be achieved by microRNA manipulation of stem cells prior to engraftment. Thus, targeting the expression of microRNAs may be a novel therapeutic approach for diseases involving excess or insufficient vasculature in general and for the ischemic heart in particular.

BIBLIOGRAPHY

1. Abdel-Latif A, Bolli R, Tleyjeh IM, Montori VM, Perin EC, Hornung CA, et al. Adult bone marrow-derived cells for cardiac repair: A systematic review and meta-analysis. Arch Intern Med. 2007;167:989-97.
2. Abdul Kadir SH, Ali NN, Mioulane M, Brito-Martins M, Abu-Hayyeh S, Foldes G, et al. Embryonic stem cell-derived cardiomyocytes as a model to study fetal arrhythmia related to maternal disease. J Cell Mol Med. 2009;13:3730-41.
3. Ahmed RP, Haider KH, Shujia J, Afzal MR, Ashraf M. Sonic Hedgehog gene delivery to the rodent heart promotes angiogenesis via iNOS/netrin-1/PKC pathway. PLoS One. 2010;5:e8576.
4. Arsic N, Zentilin L, Zacchigna S, Santoro D, Stanta G, Salvi A, et al. Induction of functional neovascularization by combined VEGF and angiopoietin-1 gene transfer using AAV vectors. Mol Ther. 2003;7:450-9.
5. Asahara T, Masuda H, Takahashi T, Kalka C, Pastore C, Silver M, et al. Bone marrow origin of endothelial progenitor cells responsible for postnatal vasculogenesis in physiological and pathological neovascularization. Circ Res. 1999;85:221-8.
6. Asahara T, Murohara T, Sullivan A, Silver M, van der Zee R, Li T, et al. Isolation of putative progenitor endothelial cells for angiogenesis. Science. 1997;275:964-7.

7. Askari AT, Unzek S, Popovic ZB, Goldman CK, Forudi F, Kiedrowski M, et al. Effect of stromal-cell-derived factor 1 on stem-cell homing and tissue regeneration in ischaemic cardiomyopathy. Lancet. 2003;362:697-703.
8. Balsam LB, Wagers AJ, Christensen JL, Kofidis T, Weissman IL, Robbins RC. Haematopoietic stem cells adopt mature haematopoietic fates in ischaemic myocardium. Nature. 2004;428:668-73.
9. Banai S, Shweiki D, Pinson A, Chandra M, Lazarovici G, Keshet E. Upregulation of vascular endothelial growth factor expression induced by myocardial ischaemia: implications for coronary angiogenesis. Cardiovasc Res. 1994;28:1176-9.
10. Baraniak PR, McDevitt TC. Stem cell paracrine actions and tissue regeneration. Regen Med. 2010;5(1):121-43.
11. Barile L, Cerisoli F, Frati G, Gaetani R, Chimenti I, Forte E, et al. Bone marrow-derived cells can acquire cardiac stem cells properties in damaged heart. J Cell Mol Med. 2009;1.1.
12. Beeres SL, Bax JJ, Dibbets-Schneider P, Stokkel MP, Fibbe WE, van der Wall EE, et al. Intramyocardial injection of autologous bone marrow mononuclear cells in patients with chronic myocardial infarction and severe left ventricular dysfunction. Am J Cardiol. 2007;100:1094-8.
13. Beltrami AP, Barlucchi L, Torella D, Baker M, Limana F, Chimenti S, et al. Adult cardiac stem cells are multipotent and support myocardial regeneration. Cell. 2003;114:763-76.
14. Bergmann O, Bhardwaj RD, Bernard S, Zdunek S, Barnabe-Heider F, Walsh S, et al. Evidence for cardiomyocyte renewal in humans. Science. 2009;324:98-102.
15. Brasselet C, Morichetti MC, Messas E, Carrion C, Bissery A, Bruneval P, et al. Skeletal myoblast transplantation through a catheter-based coronary sinus approach: an effective means of improving function of infarcted myocardium. Eur Heart J. 2005;26:1551-6.
16. Carmeliet P. VEGF gene therapy: Stimulating angiogenesis or angioma-genesis? Nat Med. 2000;6:1102-3.
17. Caspi O, Huber I, Kehat I, Habib M, Arbel G, Gepstein A, et al. Transplantation of human embryonic stem cell-derived cardiomyocytes improves myocardial performance in infarcted rat hearts. J Am Coll Cardiol. 2007;50:1884-93.
18. Dai W, Field LJ, Rubart M, Reuter S, Hale SL, Zweigerdt R, et al. Survival and maturation of human embryonic stem cell-derived cardiomyocytes in rat hearts. J Mol Cell Cardiol. 2007;43:504-16.
19. Das H, George JC, Joseph M, Das M, Abdulhameed N, Blitz A, et al. Stem cell therapy with overexpressed VEGF and PDGF genes improves cardiac function in a rat infarct model. PLoS One. 2009;4:e7325.
20. Dawn B, Stein AB, Urbanek K, Rota M, Whang B, Rastaldo R, et al. Cardiac stem cells delivered intravascularly traverse the vessel barrier, regenerate infarcted myocardium, and improve cardiac function. Proc Natl Acad Sci USA. 2005;102:3766-71.
21. Detillieux KA, Sheikh F, Kardami E, Cattini PA. Biological activities of fibroblast growth factor-2 in the adult myocardium. Cardiovasc Res. 2003;57:8-19.
22. Dib N, McCarthy P, Campbell A, Yeager M, Pagani FD, Wright S, et al. Feasibility and safety of autologous myoblast transplantation in patients with ischemic cardiomyopathy. Cell. Transplant 2005;14:11-9.
23. Dong H, Wang Q, Zhang Y, Jiang B, Xu X, Zhang Z. Angiogenesis induced by hVEGF165 gene controlled by hypoxic response elements in rabbit ischemia myocardium. Exp Biol Med (Maywood). 2009;234:1417-24.
24. Dulak J, Zagorska A, Wegiel B, Loboda A, Jozkowicz A. New strategies for cardiovascular gene therapy: regulatable pre-emptive expression of pro-angiogenic and antioxidant genes. Cell Biochem Biophys. 2006;44:31-42.
25. Eguchi M, Masuda H, Asahara T. Endothelial progenitor cells for postnatal vasculogenesis. Clin Exp Nephrol. 2007;11:18-25.

26. Elmadbouh I, Haider H, Jiang S, Idris NM, Lu G, Ashraf M. Ex vivo delivered stromal cell-derived factor-1alpha promotes stem cell homing and induces angiomyogenesis in the infarcted myocardium. J Mol Cell Cardiol. 2007;42:792-803.
27. Farokhpour M, Karbalaie K, Tanhaei S, Nematollahi M, Etebari M, Sadeghi HM, et al. Embryonic stem cell-derived cardiomyocytes as a model system to study cardioprotective effects of dexamethasone in doxorubicin cardiotoxicity. Toxicol *In Vitro*. 2009;23:1422-8.
28. Finney MR, Fanning LR, Joseph ME, Goldberg JL, Greco NJ, Bhakta S, et al. Umbilical cord blood-selected CD133(+) cells exhibit vasculogenic functionality *in vitro* and *in vivo*. Cytotherapy. 2010;12(1):67-78.
29. Foldes G, Harding SE, Ali NN. Cardiomyocytes from embryonic stem cells: Towards human therapy. Expert Opin Biol Ther. 2008;8:1473-83.
30. Fouts K, Fernandes B, Mal N, Liu J, Laurita KR. Electrophysiological consequence of skeletal myoblast transplantation in normal and infarcted canine myocardium. Heart Rhythm. 2006;3:452-61.
31. Fujiyama S, Amano K, Uehira K, Yoshida M, Nishiwaki Y, Nozawa Y, et al. Bone marrow monocyte lineage cells adhere on injured endothelium in a monocyte chemoattractant protein-1-dependent manner and accelerate reendothelialization as endothelial progenitor cells. Circ Res. 2003;93:980-9.
32. Fukuhara S, Tomita S, Nakatani T, Fujisato T, Ohtsu Y, Ishida M, et al. Bone marrow cell-seeded biodegradable polymeric scaffold enhances angiogenesis and improves function of the infarcted heart. Circ J. 2005;69:850-7.
33. Garbade J, Dhein S, Lipinski C, Aupperle H, Arsalan M, Borger MA, et al. Bone marrow-derived stem cells attenuate impaired contractility and enhance capillary density in a rabbit model of Doxorubicin-induced failing hearts. J Card Surg. 2009;24:591-9.
34. Gnecchi M, Zhang Z, Ni A, Dzau VJ. Paracrine mechanisms in adult stem cell signaling and therapy. Circ Res. 2008;103:1204-19.
35. Goncalves GA, Vassallo PF, Dos Santos L, Schettert IT, Nakamuta JS, Becker C, et al. Intramyocardial transplantation of fibroblasts expressing vascular endothelial growth factor attenuates cardiac dysfunction. Gene Ther. 2010;17:305-14.
36. Guo ZS, Li Q, Bartlett DL, Yang JY, Fang B. Gene transfer: the challenge of regulated gene expression. Trends Mol Med. 2008;14:410-8.
37. Hagege AA, Carrion C, Menasche P, Vilquin JT, Duboc D, Marolleau JP, et al. Viability and differentiation of autologous skeletal myoblast grafts in ischaemic cardiomyopathy. Lancet. 2003;361:491-2.
38. Haider H, Jiang S, Idris NM, Ashraf M. IGF-1-overexpressing mesenchymal stem cells accelerate bone marrow stem cell mobilization via paracrine activation of SDF-1alpha/CXCR4 signaling to promote myocardial repair. Circ Res. 2008;103:1300-8.
39. Haider H, Ye L, Jiang S, Ge R, Law PK, Chua T, et al. Angiomyogenesis for cardiac repair using human myoblasts as carriers of human vascular endothelial growth factor. J Mol Med. 2004;82:539-49.
40. Haigh JJ. Role of VEGF in organogenesis. Organogenesis. 2008;4:247-56.
41. Hamada H, Kim MK, Iwakura A, Ii M, Thorne T, Qin G, et al. Estrogen receptors alpha and beta mediate contribution of bone marrow-derived endothelial progenitor cells to functional recovery after myocardial infarction. Circulation. 2006;114:2261-70.
42. Harada K, Grossman W, Friedman M, Edelman ER, Prasad PV, Keighley CS, et al. Basic fibroblast growth factor improves myocardial function in chronically ischemic porcine hearts. J Clin Invest. 1994;94:623-30.
43. He KL, Yi GH, Sherman W, Zhou H, Zhang GP, Gu A, et al. Autologous skeletal myoblast transplantation improved hemodynamics and left ventricular function in chronic heart failure dogs. J Heart Lung Transplant. 2005;24:1940-9.

44. Henry TD, Annex BH, McKendall GR, Azrin MA, Lopez JJ, Giordano FJ, et al. The VIVA trial: Vascular endothelial growth factor in Ischemia for Vascular Angiogenesis. Circulation. 2003;107:1359-65.
45. Hime GR, Somers WG. Micro-RNA mediated regulation of proliferation, self-renewal and differentiation of mammalian stem cells. Cell Adh Migr. 2009;3:425-32.
46. Huangfu D, Osafune K, Maehr R, Guo W, Eijkelenboom A, Chen S, et al. Induction of pluripotent stem cells from primary human fibroblasts with only Oct4 and Sox2. Nat Biotechnol. 2008;26:1269-75.
47. Hung HS, Shyu WC, Tsai CH, Hsu SH, Lin SZ. Transplantation of endothelial progenitor cells as therapeutics for cardiovascular diseases. Cell Transplant. 2009;18:1003-12.
48. Iwami Y, Masuda H, Asahara T. Endothelial progenitor cells: Past, state of the art, and future. J Cell Mol Med. 2004;8:488-97.
49. Jain M, DerSimonian H, Brenner DA, Ngoy S, Teller P, Edge AS, et al. Cell therapy attenuates deleterious ventricular remodeling and improves cardiac performance after myocardial infarction. Circulation. 2001;103:1920-7.
50. Jiang S, Haider H, Idris NM, Salim A, Ashraf M. Supportive interaction between cell survival signaling and angiocompetent factors enhances donor cell survival and promotes angiomyogenesis for cardiac repair. Circ Res. 2006;99:776-84.
51. Jujo K, Ii M, Losordo DW. Endothelial progenitor cells in neovascularization of infarcted myocardium. J Mol Cell Cardiol. 2008;45:530-44.
52. Kajstura J, Rota M, Whang B, Cascapera S, Hosoda T, Bearzi C, et al. Bone marrow cells differentiate in cardiac cell lineages after infarction independently of cell fusion. Circ Res. 2005;96:127-37.
53. Kalka C, Masuda H, Takahashi T, Gordon R, Tepper O, Gravereaux E, et al. Vascular endothelial growth factor(165) gene transfer augments circulating endothelial progenitor cells in human subjects. Circ Res. 2000;86:1198-202.
54. Kanellakis P, Slater NJ, Du XJ, Bobik A, Curtis DJ. Granulocyte colony-stimulating factor and stem cell factor improve endogenous repair after myocardial infarction. Cardiovasc Res. 2006;70:117-25.
55. Kawamoto A, Gwon HC, Iwaguro H, Yamaguchi JI, Uchida S, Masuda H, et al. Therapeutic potential of ex vivo expanded endothelial progenitor cells for myocardial ischemia. Circulation. 2001;103:634-7.
56. Kelly BD, Hackett SF, Hirota K, Oshima Y, Cai Z, Berg-Dixon S, et al. Cell type-specific regulation of angiogenic growth factor gene expression and induction of angiogenesis in nonischemic tissue by a constitutively active form of hypoxia-inducible factor 1. Circ Res. 2003;93:1074-81.
57. Kim JB, Zaehres H, Wu G, Gentile L, Ko K, Sebastiano V, et al. Pluripotent stem cells induced from adult neural stem cells by reprogramming with two factors. Nature. 2008;454:646-50.
58. Ladage D, Brixius K, Steingen C, Mehlhorn U, Schwinger RH, Bloch W, et al. Mesenchymal stem cells induce endothelial activation via paracine mechanisms. Endothelium. 2007;14:53-63.
59. Lai VK, Linares-Palomino J, Nadal-Ginard B, Galinanes M. Bone marrow cell-induced protection of the human myocardium: Characterization and mechanism of action. J Thorac Cardiovasc Surg. 2009;138:1400-08 e1.
60. Lee BC, Hsu HC, Tseng WY, Chen CY, Lin HJ, Ho YL, et al. Cell therapy generates a favourable chemokine gradient for stem cell recruitment into the infarcted heart in rabbits. Eur J Heart Fail. 2009;11:238-45.
61. Leobon B, Roncalli J, Joffre C, Mazo M, Boisson M, Barreau C, et al. Adipose-derived cardiomyogenic cells: *In vitro* expansion and functional improvement in a mouse model of myocardial infarction. Cardiovasc Res. 2009;83:757-67.
62. Leor J, Gerecht S, Cohen S, Miller L, Holbova R, Ziskind A, et al. Human embryonic stem cell transplantation to repair the infarcted myocardium. Heart. 2007;93:1278-84.

63. Liechty KW, MacKenzie TC, Shaaban AF, Radu A, Moseley AM, Deans R, et al. Human mesenchymal stem cells engraft and demonstrate site-specific differentiation after in utero transplantation in sheep. Nat Med. 2000;6:1282-6.
64. Lipinski MJ, Biondi-Zoccai GG, Abbate A, Khianey R, Sheiban I, Bartunek J, et al. Impact of intracoronary cell therapy on left ventricular function in the setting of acute myocardial infarction: A collaborative systematic review and meta-analysis of controlled clinical trials. J Am Coll Cardiol. 2007;50:1761-7.
65. Lowry WE, Plath K. The many ways to make an iPS cell. Nat Biotechnol. 2008;26:1246-8.
66. Mackay J. Mensah GA. The atlas of heart disease and stroke. The World Health Organization. 2006;48-49.
67. Martinez-Fernandez A, Nelson TJ, Yamada S, Reyes S, Alekseev AE, Perez-Terzic C, et al. iPS programmed without c-MYC yield proficient cardiogenesis for functional heart chimerism. Circ Res. 2009;105:648-56.
68. Matsuura K, Honda A, Nagai T, Fukushima N, Iwanaga K, Tokunaga M, et al. Transplantation of cardiac progenitor cells ameliorates cardiac dysfunction after myocardial infarction in mice. J Clin Invest. 2009;119:2204-17.
69. Menasche P, Hagege AA, Scorsin M, Pouzet B, Desnos M, Duboc D, et al. Myoblast transplantation for heart failure. Lancet. 2001;357:279-80.
70. Menasche P, Hagege AA, Vilquin JT, Desnos M, Abergel E, Pouzet B, et al. Autologous skeletal myoblast transplantation for severe postinfarction left ventricular dysfunction. J Am Coll Cardiol. 2003;41:1078-83.
71. Morishita R, Aoki M, Hashiya N, Yamasaki K, Kurinami H, Shimizu S, et al. Therapeutic angiogenesis using hepatocyte growth factor (HGF). Curr Gene Ther. 2004;4:199-206.
72. Muller OJ, Katus HA, Bekeredjian R. Targeting the heart with gene therapy-optimized gene delivery methods. Cardiovasc Res. 2006;73(3):453-62.
73. Muller OJ, Ksienzyk J, Katus HA. Gene-therapy delivery strategies in cardiology. Future Cardiol. 2008;4:135-50.
74. Mummery C, van der Heyden MA, de Boer TP, Passier R, Ward D, van den Brink S, et al. Cardiomyocytes from human and mouse embryonic stem cells. Methods Mol Med. 2007;140:249-72.
75. Murry CE, Soonpaa MH, Reinecke H, Nakajima H, Nakajima HO, Rubart M, et al. Hematopoietic stem cells do not transdifferentiate into cardiac myocytes in myocardial infarcts. Nature. 2004;428:664-8.
76. Nabel EG, Yang ZY, Plautz G, Forough R, Zhan X, Haudenschild CC, et al. Recombinant fibroblast growth factor-1 promotes intimal hyperplasia and angiogenesis in arteries *in vivo*. Nature. 1993;362:844-6.
77. Nadal-Ginard B, Anversa P, Kajstura J, Leri A. Cardiac stem cells and myocardial regeneration. Novartis Found Symp. 2005;265:142-54; discussion 155-7, 204-11.
78. Nelson TJ, Martinez-Fernandez A, Yamada S, Perez-Terzic C, Ikeda Y, Terzic A. Repair of acute myocardial infarction by human stemness factors induced pluripotent stem cells. Circulation. 2009;120:408-16.
79. Nesselmann C, Li W, Ma N, Steinhoff G. Stem cell-mediated neovascularization in heart repair. Ther Adv Cardiovasc Dis. 2010;4:27-42.
80. Niagara MI, Haider H, Jiang S, Ashraf M. Pharmacologically preconditioned skeletal myoblasts are resistant to oxidative stress and promote angiomyogenesis via release of paracrine factors in the infarcted heart. Circ Res. 2007;100:545-55.
81. Niagara MI, Haider H, Ye L, Koh VS, Lim YT, Poh KK, et al. Autologous skeletal myoblasts transduced with a new adenoviral bicistronic vector for treatment of hind limb ischemia. J Vasc Surg. 2004;40:774-85.
82. Okita K, Nakagawa M, Hyenjong H, Ichisaka T, Yamanaka S. Generation of mouse induced pluripotent stem cells without viral vectors. Science. 2008;322:949-53.

83. Orlic D, Kajstura J, Chimenti S, Jakoniuk I, Anderson SM, Li B, et al. Bone marrow cells regenerate infarcted myocardium. Nature. 2001;410:701-5.
84. Orlic D, Kajstura J, Chimenti S, Limana F, Jakoniuk I, Quaini F, et al. Mobilized bone marrow cells repair the infarcted heart, improving function and survival. Proc Natl Acad Sci USA. 2001;98:10344-9.
85. Pagani FD, DerSimonian H, Zawadzka A, Wetzel K, Edge AS, Jacoby DB, et al. Autologous skeletal myoblasts transplanted to ischemia-damaged myocardium in humans. Histological analysis of cell survival and differentiation. J Am Coll Cardiol. 2003;41:879-88.
86. Park IH, Lerou PH, Zhao R, Huo H, Daley GQ. Generation of human-induced pluripotent stem cells. Nat Protoc. 2008;3:1180-6.
87. Park IH, Zhao R, West JA, Yabuuchi A, Huo H, Ince TA, et al. Reprogramming of human somatic cells to pluripotency with defined factors. Nature. 2008;451:141-6.
88. Pearlman JD, Hibberd MG, Chuang ML, Harada K, Lopez JJ, Gladstone SR, et al. Magnetic resonance mapping demonstrates benefits of VEGF-induced myocardial angiogenesis. Nat Med. 1995;1:1085-9.
89. Pugh CW, Ratcliffe PJ. Regulation of angiogenesis by hypoxia: Role of the HIF system. Nat Med. 2003;9:677-84.
90. Qin D, Gan Y, Shao K, Wang H, Li W, Wang T, et al. Mouse meningiocytes express Sox2 and yield high efficiency of chimeras after nuclear reprogramming with exogenous factors. J Biol Chem. 2008;283:33730-5.
91. Reinecke H, Murry CE. Transmural replacement of myocardium after skeletal myoblast grafting into the heart. Too much of a good thing? Cardiovasc Pathol. 2000;9:337-44.
92. Rissanen TT, Rutanen J, Yla-Herttuala S. Gene transfer for therapeutic vascular growth in myocardial and peripheral ischemia. Adv Genet. 2004;52:117-64.
93. Rota M, Kajstura J, Hosoda T, Bearzi C, Vitale S, Esposito G, et al. Bone marrow cells adopt the cardiomyogenic fate in vivo. Proc Natl Acad Sci USA. 2007;104:17783-8.
94. Ruixing Y, Dezhai Y, Hai W, Kai H, Xianghong W, Yuming C. Intramyocardial injection of vascular endothelial growth factor gene improves cardiac performance and inhibits cardiomyocyte apoptosis. Eur J Heart Fail. 2007;9:343-51.
95. Sanberg PR, Park DH, Kuzmin-Nichols N, Cruz E, Hossne NA Jr, Buffolo E, et al. Monocyte Transplantation for Neural and Cardiovascular Ischemia Repair. J Cell Mol Med.1.
96. Schwarz ER, Speakman MT, Patterson M, Hale SS, Isner JM, Kedes LH, et al. Evaluation of the effects of intramyocardial injection of DNA expressing vascular endothelial growth factor (VEGF) in a myocardial infarction model in the ratangiogenesis and angioma formation. J Am Coll Cardiol. 2000;35:1323-30.
97. Shintani S, Murohara T, Ikeda H, Ueno T, Honma T, Katoh A, et al. Mobilization of endothelial progenitor cells in patients with acute myocardial infarction. Circulation. 2001;103:2776-9.
98. Shi Q, Rafii S, Wu MH, Wijelath ES, Yu C, Ishida A, et al. Evidence for circulating bone marrow-derived endothelial cells. Blood. 1998;92:362-7.
99. Shujia J, Haider HK, Idris NM, Lu G, Ashraf M. Stable therapeutic effects of mesenchymal stem cell-based multiple gene delivery for cardiac repair. Cardiovasc Res. 2008;77:525-33.
100. Sim EK, Haider HK, Aziz S, Ooi OC, Law PK. Myoblast transplantation on the beating heart. Int Surg. 2005;90:148-50.
101. Sim EK, Zhang L, Shim WS, Lim YL, Ge R. Therapeutic angiogenesis for coronary artery disease. J Card Surg. 2002;17:350-4.
102. Siminiak T, Kalawski R, Fiszer D, Jerzykowska O, Rzezniczak J, Rozwadowska N, et al. Autologous skeletal myoblast transplantation for the treatment of postinfarction myocardial injury: phase I clinical study with 12 months of follow-up. Am Heart J. 2004;148:531-7.
103. Singla DK, Hacker TA, Ma L, Douglas PS, Sullivan R, Lyons GE, et al. Transplantation of embryonic stem cells into the infarcted mouse heart: Formation of multiple cell types. J Mol Cell Cardiol. 2006;40:195-200.

104. Smart N, Risebro CA, Melville AA, Moses K, Schwartz RJ, Chien KR, et al. Thymosin beta4 induces adult epicardial progenitor mobilization and neovascularization. Nature. 2007;445:177-82.

105. Smits PC, van Geuns RJ, Poldermans D, Bountioukos M, Onderwater EE, Lee CH, et al. Catheter-based intramyocardial injection of autologous skeletal myoblasts as a primary treatment of ischemic heart failure: clinical experience with six-month follow-up. J Am Coll Cardiol. 2003;42:2063-9.

106. Song MB, Yu XJ, Zhu GX, Chen JF, Zhao G, Huang L. Transfection of HGF gene enhances endothelial progenitor cell (EPC) function and improves EPC transplant efficiency for balloon-induced arterial injury in hypercholesterolemic rats. Vascul Pharmacol. 2009;51:205-13.

107. Springer ML, Hortelano G, Bouley DM, Wong J, Kraft PE, Blau HM. Induction of angiogenesis by implantation of encapsulated primary myoblasts expressing vascular endothelial growth factor. J Gene Med. 2000;2:279-88.

108. Stadtfeld M, Nagaya M, Utikal J, Weir G, Hochedlinger K. Induced pluripotent stem cells generated without viral integration. Science. 2008;322:945-9.

109. Stamm C, Kleine HD, Choi YH, Dunkelmann S, Lauffs JA, Lorenzen B, et al. Intramyocardial delivery of CD133+ bone marrow cells and coronary artery bypass grafting for chronic ischemic heart disease: safety and efficacy studies. J Thorac Cardiovasc Surg. 2007;133:717-25.

110. Suzuki K, Brand NJ, Allen S, Khan MA, Farrell AO, Murtuza B, et al. Overexpression of connexin 43 in skeletal myoblasts: Relevance to cell transplantation to the heart. J Thorac Cardiovasc Surg. 2001;122:759-66.

111. Takahashi K, Ito Y, Morikawa M, Kobune M, Huang J, Tsukamoto M, et al. Adenoviral-delivered angiopoietin-1 reduces the infarction and attenuates the progression of cardiac dysfunction in the rat model of acute myocardial infarction. Mol Ther. 2003;8:584-92.

112. Takahashi K, Tanabe K, Ohnuki M, Narita M, Ichisaka T, Tomoda K, et al. Induction of pluripotent stem cells from adult human fibroblasts by defined factors. Cell. 2007;131:861-72.

113. Takahashi K, Yamanaka S. Induction of pluripotent stem cells from mouse embryonic and adult fibroblast cultures by defined factors. Cell. 2006;126:663-76.

114. Takahashi T, Kalka C, Masuda H, Chen D, Silver M, Kearney M, et al. Ischemia- and cytokine-induced mobilization of bone marrow-derived endothelial progenitor cells for neovascularization. Nat Med. 1999;5:434-8.

115. Tambara K, Sakakibara Y, Sakaguchi G, Lu F, Premaratne GU, Lin X, et al. Transplanted skeletal myoblasts can fully replace the infarcted myocardium when they survive in the host in large numbers. Circulation. 2003;108 Suppl 1:II259-63.

116. Tang J, Wang J, Yang J, Kong X, Zheng F, Guo L, et al. Mesenchymal stem cells over-expressing SDF-1 promote angiogenesis and improve heart function in experimental myocardial infarction in rats. Eur J Cardiothorac Surg. 2009;36:644-50.

117. Templin C, Grote K, Schledzewski K, Ghadri JR, Schnabel S, Napp LC, et al. Ex vivo expanded haematopoietic progenitor cells improve dermal wound healing by paracrine mechanisms. Exp Dermatol. 2009;18:445-53.

118. Tomita S, Ishida M, Nakatani T, Fukuhara S, Hisashi Y, Ohtsu Y, et al. Bone marrow is a source of regenerated cardiomyocytes in doxorubicin-induced cardiomyopathy and granulocyte colony-stimulating factor enhances migration of bone marrow cells and attenuates cardiotoxicity of doxorubicin under electron microscopy. J Heart Lung Transplant. 2004;23:577-84.

119. Tomita S, Li RK, Weisel RD, Mickle DA, Kim EJ, Sakai T, et al. Autologous transplantation of bone marrow cells improves damaged heart function. Circulation. 1999;100:II247-56.

120. Uemura R, Xu M, Ahmad N, Ashraf M. Bone marrow stem cells prevent left ventricular remodeling of ischemic heart through paracrine signaling. Circ Res. 2006;98:1414-21.

121. Unger EF, Banai S, Shou M, Lazarous DF, Jaklitsch MT, Scheinowitz M, et al. Basic fibroblast growth factor enhances myocardial collateral flow in a canine model. Am J Physiol. 1994;266:H1588-95.
122. van Laake LW, Passier R, den Ouden K, Schreurs C, Monshouwer-Kloots J, Ward-van Oostwaard D, et al. Improvement of mouse cardiac function by hESC-derived cardiomyocytes correlates with vascularity but not graft size. Stem Cell Res. 2009;3:106-12.
123. van Laake LW, Passier R, Monshouwer-Kloots J, Verkleij AJ, Lips DJ, Freund C, et al. Human embryonic stem cell-derived cardiomyocytes survive and mature in the mouse heart and transiently improve function after myocardial infarction. Stem Cell Res. 2007;1:9-24.
124. Wang JS, Shum-Tim D, Chedrawy E, Chiu RC. The coronary delivery of marrow stromal cells for myocardial regeneration: Pathophysiologic and therapeutic implications. J Thorac Cardiovasc Surg. 2001;122:699-705.
125. Westenbrink BD, Lipsic E, van der Meer P, van der Harst P, Oeseburg H, Du Marchie Sarvaas GJ, et al. Erythropoietin improves cardiac function through endothelial progenitor cell and vascular endothelial growth factor mediated neovascularization. Eur Heart. J 2007;28:2018-27.
126. Yamakawa M, Liu LX, Date T, Belanger AJ, Vincent KA, Akita GY, et al. Hypoxia-inducible factor-1 mediates activation of cultured vascular endothelial cells by inducing multiple angiogenic factors. Circ Res. 2003;93:664-73.
127. Yau TM, Kim C, Li G, Zhang Y, Fazel S, Spiegelstein D, et al. Enhanced angiogenesis with multimodal cell-based gene therapy. Ann Thorac Surg. 2007;83:1110-9.
128. Yau TM, Kim C, Li G, Zhang Y, Weisel RD, Li RK. Maximizing ventricular function with multimodal cell-based gene therapy. Circulation. 2005;112:I123-8.
129. Yau TM, Kim C, Ng D, Li G, Zhang Y, Weisel RD, et al. Increasing transplanted cell survival with cell-based angiogenic gene therapy. Ann Thorac Surg. 2005;80:1779-86.
130. Ye L, Haider H, Jiang S, Tan RS, Ge R, Law PK, et al. Improved angiogenic response in pig heart following ischaemic injury using human skeletal myoblast simultaneously expressing VEGF165 and angiopoietin-1. Eur J Heart Fail. 2007;9:15-22.
131. Ye L, Haider H, Jiang S, Tan RS, Toh WC, Ge R, et al. Angiopoietin-1 for myocardial angiogenesis: a comparison between delivery strategies. Eur J Heart Fail. 2007;9:458-65.
132. Ye L, Haider H, Tan R, Toh W, Law PK, Tan W, et al. Transplantation of nanoparticle transfected skeletal myoblasts overexpressing vascular endothelial growth factor-165 for cardiac repair. Circulation. 2007;116:I113-20.
133. Yerebakan C, Sandica E, Prietz S, Klopsch C, Ugurlucan M, Kaminski A, et al. Autologous umbilical cord blood mononuclear cell transplantation preserves right ventricular function in a novel model of chronic right ventricular volume overload. Cell Transplant. 2009;18:855-68.
134. Yoon YS, Park JS, Tkebuchava T, Luedeman C, Losordo DW. Unexpected severe calcification after transplantation of bone marrow cells in acute myocardial infarction. Circulation. 2004;109:3154-7.
135. Young LS, Searle PF, Onion D, Mautner V. Viral gene therapy strategies: From basic science to clinical application. J Pathol. 2006;208:299-318.
136. Zhang F, Pasumarthi KB. Embryonic stem cell transplantation: Promise and progress in the treatment of heart disease. BioDrugs. 2008;22:361-74.
137. Zhou Y, Wang S, Yu Z, Hoyt RF Jr, Sachdev V, Vincent P, et al. Direct injection of autologous mesenchymal stromal cells improves myocardial function. Biochem Biophys Res Commun. 2009;390:902-7.
138. Zhu XY, Zhang XZ, Xu L, Zhong XY, Ding Q, Chen YX. Transplantation of adipose-derived stem cells overexpressing hHGF into cardiac tissue. Biochem Biophys Res Commun. 2009;379:1084-90.
139. Zisa D, Shabbir A, Suzuki G, Lee T. Vascular endothelial growth factor (VEGF) as a key therapeutic trophic factor in bone marrow mesenchymal stem cell-mediated cardiac repair. Biochem Biophys Res Commun. 2009;390:834-8.

Chapter

10

Cardiac Dysfunction and Therapies (Part 1): Pathophysiology, Diagnosis and Medical Management

Vamsee Yaganti, Snigdha Ancha, Catalin Boiangiu, Marc Cohen

Abstract. Heart failure is a complex clinical syndrome of epidemic proportion that affects approximately 23 million people worldwide. It is defined as the inability of the heart to maintain an adequate cardiac output to meet the metabolic demands of the body. The pathogenesis of HF involves the activation of neurohormonal system which includes the activation of sympathetic nervous system and renin-angiotensin-aldosterone system and the release of oxidative radicals, inflammatory cytokines and peripheral vasoconstrictors. The diagnosis of HF is based on detailed history, physical examination and diagnostic tests. The goal of pharmacological therapy in HF is to improve clinical symptoms, reduce hospitalization, prevent left ventricular remodeling and reduce mortality. Medications that are primarily used to improve symptoms in HF patients include diuretics, digoxin and intravenous inotropic agents. Medications that improve symptoms, prevent remodeling and reduce mortality include beta blockers, angiotensin converting enzyme (ACE) inhibitors, angiotensin receptor blockers, aldosterone receptor blockers and the hydralazine/nitrate combination.

Keywords. Heart failure, left ventricular remodeling, renin-angiotensin-aldosterone system, sympathetic nervous system, NYHA classification, pharmacological therapy.

INTRODUCTION

Heart failure (HF) is a complex clinical syndrome that is defined as the inability of the heart to maintain an adequate cardiac output to meet the metabolic demands of the body. HF affects approximately 23 million people worldwide. The prevalence of HF in the United States and the European population ranges from 0.4% to 2% (Kannel 2000, Swedberg et al 2005). In the United States, there are 5.7 million people with HF and approximately 550,000 new cases are diagnosed annually (Kannel 2000). The prevalence of heart failure increases exponentially with age. In the Rotterdam Heart Study, the prevalence of HF increased from 0.9% in subjects aged 55-64 years to 17.4% in subjects aged 85 years or older. (Bleumink et al 2004) Similarly the incidence of HF increased from 1.4% per 1000 patient years in subjects aged 55-64 years to 41.9% per 1000 patient years in subjects aged 85 years or older (Bleumink et al 2004). The incidence of HF in women is lower compared to men, however, because of their longer life expectancy women account for atleast 50% of patients diagnosed with HF (Levy et al 2002). The epidemiological data on HF in developing countries is unclear because of paucity of population based studies.

HF has an enormous impact on the socioeconomic well being of a country because of high mortality and rehospitalization rates seen in these patients. In 2006, HF was the underlying cause of death in 60,337 patients and was associated with another 282,754 deaths. The any mention mortality rate for HF was 89.2 per 100,000. The mortality rate was highest in men, older persons and blacks. Patients with HF also have a high rate hospitalization and rehospitalization which increases the health care costs exponentially. In 2006, 1.1 million patients were treated in hospitals for decompensated HF and another 3.4 million were treated on an outpatient basis. Approximately 50% of patients hospitalized for HF management were rehospitalized within 6 months of discharge. It is estimated that in the year 2010, the United States will spend $39.2 billion for management of HF patients (Lloyd-Jones et al 2009).

HF is a clinical diagnosis but should be classified into 2 groups based on the presence or absence of left ventricular systolic dysfunction; systolic heart failure or HF with reduced left ventricular ejection fraction (LVEF) and diastolic heart failure or HF with normal ejection fraction (HFnlEF). Approximately 50-55% of patients presenting with HF have HFnlEF (Owan et al 2006). The prevalence of HFnlEF increases more precipitously with age (compared to systolic heart failure) and is higher in women compared to men (Ceia et al 2002). The mortality rates in patients with HFnlEF are similar to ones seen in patients with systolic heart failure (Bhatia et al 2006, Owan et al 2006). Although mortality rates in patients with systolic heart failure have decreased over time, the survival rate for patients with HFnlEF hasn't improved (Owan et al 2006). In this chapter, we will focus primarily on the pathophysiology, clinical presentation, diagnosis and management of patients with systolic heart failure.

PATHOPHYSIOLOGY

Several models have been proposed to explain the pathogenesis of heart failure, however none have been completely successful in explaining the pathophysiology and progression of heart failure. One of the earliest proposed models postulated that abnormalities in the renal flow lead to excessive salt and water retention and ultimately caused heart failure ("Cardiorenal model") (Packer 1992). However, with a better understanding of cardiovascular hemodynamics it became apparent that increased peripheral vasoconstriction resulting from a decreased cardiac output, also contributed to the pathogenesis of heart failure ("Cardiocirculatory model") (Packer 1992). Although both these models could explain the excessive salt and water retention and the rationale for use of diuretics, inotropes and vasodilators in heart failure patients, they failed to explain the progressively worsening clinical course seen in this syndrome. The more recently proposed "Neurohormonal" model has been most successful in explaining the pathophysiology and progression of heart failure and hence has gained the most acceptance (Figure 10.1) (Mann and Bristow 2005).

According to the neurohormonal model, heart failure is a progressive syndrome which is initiated by an index event like myocardial infarction (acute onset) or hypertension (insidious onset). Irrespective of the nature of inciting event, HF ensues if there is a substantial decrease in the number of functional myocytes or an increase in the number of dysfunctional myocytes. Either of these mechanisms will ultimately cause a loss of myocardial contractility and a decrease in the cardiac output. Decrease in cardiac output activates the neurohormonal adaptations which try to increase myocardial contractility, maintain systemic pressure and increase intravascular volume. These hemodynamic changes increase the depressed cardiac output and restore (as much as is possible), perfusion to vital organs. However, sustained activation of these compensatory mechanisms leads to maladaptive changes in the structure of heart and cardiac myocytes called "Left ventricular (LV) remodeling". With the onset of LV remodeling, HF becomes a progressive disease. Apart from LV remodeling, neurohormonal activation also causes a number of maladaptive hemodynamic changes which ultimately leads to worsening of HF; including increase in cardiac filling pressures; increase in afterload, increase in myocardial wall stress and oxygen consumption causing myocardial ischemia (Mann and Bristow 2005).

The different components of the neurohormonal system involved in the pathogenesis and progression of HF include (a) Sympathetic nervous system, (b) Renin-Angiotensin-Aldosterone system, (c) Natriuretic peptides, (d) Arginine Vasopressin, (e) Reactive oxygen species, (f) Peripheral vasoconstrictors, (g) Nitric oxide, and (h) Cytokines (Figure 10.1)

Sympathetic Nervous System

Sympathetic nervous system (SNS) activation is one of the earliest compensatory mechanisms in heart failure patients. Under normal physiological conditions, SNS is primarily controlled by inhibitory impulses from the carotid sinus, aortic arch and cardiopulmonary mechanical and baroreceptors. Hence, a healthy individual under resting conditions displays very low SNS activity. Decrease in cardiac out and blood pressure in HF causes decrease in the stretch of the baroreceptors located in the carotid sinus and aortic arch. This leads to withdrawal of the inhibitory impulses from baroreceptors and activation of SNS. Increase in excitatory impulses from the metaboreceptors located in the muscles and the peripheral chemoreceptors also triggers SNS activity (Floras 2003). Activation of SNS leads to increased release and decreased reuptake of norepinephrine at the adrenergic nerve ending.

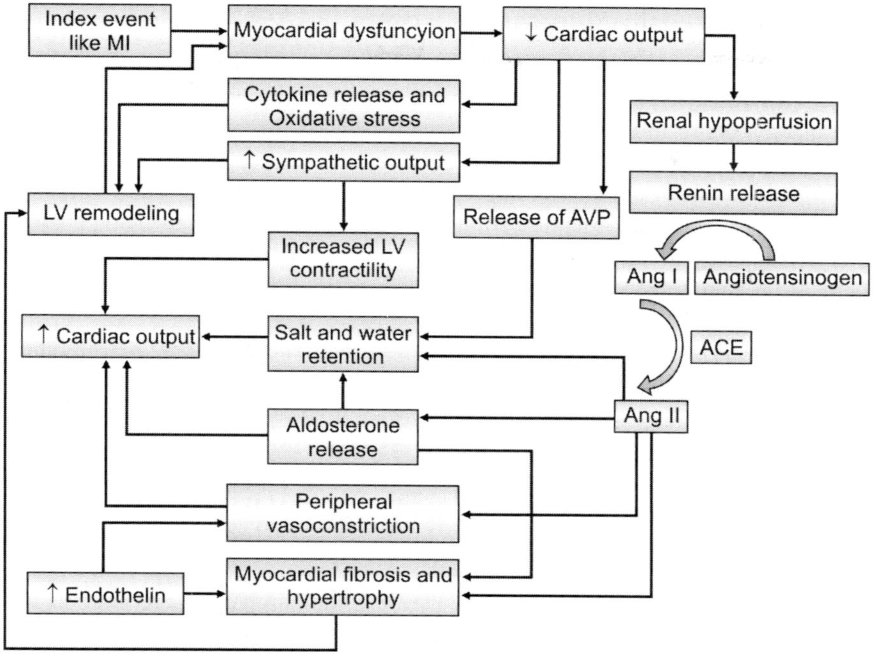

Figure 10.1: Pathophysiology of heart, failure. MI—myocardial infarction, Ang I—angiotensin I Ang II—angiotensin II

Downregulation of α-2 receptor function which normally inhibit NE release may contribute to increased release of NE in the nerve endings (Aggarwal et al 2001). There is also an increase in the systemic levels of norepinephrine in HF patients. In patients with HF, the level of NE is two to three times higher than the level found in normal subjects and reliable correlates directly with the severity of LV dysfunction and mortality (Anand et al 2003).

Activation of myocardial β-1 adrenergic receptors by SNS results in increased heart rate and contractility with a resultant increase in cardiac output. Similarly, activation of myocardial α-1 adrenergic receptors by heightened adrenergic activity exerts a positive inotropic effect on the heart. Action of increased adrenergic output on systemic and pulmonary vasculature results in an increase in peripheral vascular resistance (increased afterload) and an increase in venous tone (increased preload). Increased NE activity in the kidneys causes an activation of RAAS and increase in sodium reabsorption in the proximal tubule which leads to expansion of intravascular volume (increased preload). These lead to an increase in cardiac out and blood pressure resulting in restoration of organ perfusion. However, sustained SNS overactivity causes downregulation of cardiac β adrenergic receptors, expression of dysfunctional fetal protein isoforms in myocytes, desensitization of intracellular signaling cascades involved in myocardial contractility, increased myocyte apoptosis, myocardial ischemia and volume overload. These latter "maladaptations" all lead to progressive LV dysfunction and remodeling (Communal et al 1998, Nozawa et al 1998).

Renin-Angiotensin-Aldosterone System (RAAS)

Decreased cardiac output in HF patients causes renal hypoperfusion which activates the RAAS. Renal hypoperfusion results in a decreased amount of sodium reaching the macula densa in the distal tubule which triggers the release of a proteolytic enzyme 'Renin' from the granular cells of juxtaglomerular apparatus. Renin cleaves 4 amino acids from circulating angiotensinogen (formed in the liver) to form a biologically inactive decapeptide 'Angiotensin I'. Angiotensin-converting enzyme (ACE), found predominantly in the lung and endothelial surfaces, cleaves 2 amino acids from angiotensin I to form a biologically active octapeptide 'Angiotensin II' (AT- II) (Figure 10.1).

AT-II acts on two G protein coupled cell surface receptors: Angiotensin type 1 (AT1) and Angiotensin type 2 (AT2). AT1 receptors are present predominantly in the vasculature and on the nerves innervating the myocardium. Stimulation of AT1 receptors causes vasoconstriction, vascular smooth muscle cell proliferation, renal renin inhibition, sodium reabsorption in the proximal tubule, release of aldosterone and epinephrine from the adrenal gland, stimulation of thirst center and release of vasopressin, myocyte hypertrophy and increase in central sympathetic outflow (Goodfriend et al 1996). AT2 receptors are present in the myocardium (interstitium and fibroblasts), kidneys, brain and vasculature. Stimulation of AT2 receptor causes natriuresis, nitric oxide and bradykinin production promoting vasodilatation, inhibition of atherosclerosis, cardiac hypertrophy and apoptosis (Siragy 2009). In the short term, the octapeptide AT-II causes volume expansion, improves cardiac contractility and increases peripheral vascular resistance; all of which increase cardiac output and improve perfusion to vital organs. However, sustained release of AT-II causes myocardial hypertrophy, interstitial fibrosis, excessive fluid retention and increase in afterload resulting in elevated myocardial wall stress, increased in myocardial oxygen demand and progressive LV remodeling.

Additionally, AT-II stimulates the release of aldosterone from the zona glomerulosa region of the adrenal gland. It also induces aldosterone synthase (CYP11B2) enzyme in the failing myocardium which contributes to an increase in the local production of aldosterone (Silvestre et al 1999). Aldosterone causes the resorption of sodium chloride and secretion of potassium in the connecting segment and cortical collecting tubules of the kidney. Resorption of sodium causes water retention and an increase in the intravascular volume. However, sustained aldosterone secretion causes ventricular hypertrophy and fibrosis, volume overload, reduced vascular compliance secondary to fibrosis, endothelial dysfunction and increased norepinephrine (NE) levels. Cumulatively and over time, these effects undermine the adaptive response and cause progressive negative LV remodeling and worsening heart failure (Weber 2001).

Natriuretic Peptides

Natriuretic peptides are important counter-regulatory hormones secreted in increased levels in patients with HF. Volume expansion and increased wall stress seen in HF stimulates the release of natriuretic peptides from the myocardium

(Kinnunen et al 1993). Atrial natriuretic peptide (ANP) is a 28-amino acid peptide that is released from the atrial myocytes early in the course of HF. With progression of HF, the ventricular myocytes are recruited to release ANP and another analogous 32-amino acid peptide named brain natriuretic peptide (BNP). Apart from increased wall tension, other neurohormonal systems like angiotensin II and endothelin-1 also stimulate the release of these natriuretic peptides. The natriuretic peptides act on natriuretic peptide receptor A (NPR-A) and mediate the following actions: Natriuresis, diuresis, peripheral vasodilatation, inhibition of RAAS and inhibition of endothelin secretion. These actions collectively lead to a decrease in afterload and preload, suppression of neurohormonal activation, improvement in cardiac hemodynamics and reduction in myocardial wall stress. In addition to the aforementioned actions, BNP also inhibits cardiac fibrosis and prevents against LV remodeling (Tamura et al 2000).

Arginine Vasopressin

Arginine Vasopressin (AVP) or antidiuretic hormone (ADH) is a posterior pituitary hormone which is released in response to increased plasma osmolality and regulates free water clearance. AVP exerts its physiological actions by acting on 3 different receptors (1) V1a located on vascular smooth muscle cells and mediates vasoconstriction (2) V1b located in central nervous system and regulates ACTH secretion and (3) V2 located on epithelial cells in ascending loop of Henle and renal collecting ducts. Activation of V2 receptors causes insertion of preformed water channels 'aquaporins' on the luminal side of epithelial cells which increases free water retention. Hypotension in HF activates baroreceptors in the carotid sinus and aortic arch which trigger release of AVP from the posterior pituitary gland. Additionally, AT-II results in stimulation of the thirst center and release of AVP. Increase in AVP levels causes vasoconstriction and increase in free water retention. This resultant increase in systemic blood pressure and intravascular volume helps to restore organ perfusion. Continued release of AVP causes hyponatremia; which can cause neurological deficits (attention deficits and impaired gait) and is a poor prognostic indicator of HF. (Lee and Packer 1986, Renneboog et al 2006) Although AVP antagonists have been used in the management of HF patients, they haven't shown a decrease in mortality and heart failure related morbidity (Konstam et al 2007).

Oxidative Stress

Reactive oxygen species (ROS) like hydrogen peroxide and superoxide anion are produced as a normal byproduct of aerobic metabolism. Under normal physiological conditions, these ROS are scavenged by antioxidant mechanisms like superoxide dismutase, glutathione peroxidase, and catalase. In experimental models of HF, there is increased oxidative stress as evident by increased activity of xanthine oxidase and NADPH oxidase which increases the production of ROS in myocytes (Grieve and Shah 2003). The various factors that result in increased activity of these enzymes in HF include mechanical stretch of the myocardium, increases neurohormonal activation (AT-II, aldosterone, endothelin-1) and increased inflammatory cytokines (tumor necrosis factor, interleukin 1)

(Sawyer et al 2002). Evidence from animal studies also suggests that decrease in antioxidant mechanisms could contribute to onset and progression of HF. Transgenic mice deficient in mitochondrial superoxide dismutase developed dilated cardiomyopathy and died at a younger age whereas overexpression of glutathione peroxidase protected against ventricular dilatation and dysfunction (Lebovitz et al 1996, Shiomi et al 2004). ROS cause myocardial dysfunction by various mechanisms. These include myocardial hypertrophy, apoptosis, expression of dysfunctional fetal isoforms, increase in interstitial fibrosis and decreased bioavailability of nitrous oxide (NO) (Sawyer et al 2002). However, multiple clinical trials involving antioxidants like vitamin E, xanthine oxidase inhibitor and coenzyme Q10 did not show any improvement in clinical outcomes in HF patients (Khatta et al 2000, Keith et al 2001, Hare et al 2008).

Vasoconstrictor Peptides

A number of vasoconstrictor peptides like endothelin (ET), Urotensin II (U-II) and Neuropeptide Y (NPY) are released in heart failure patients for maintenance of systemic blood pressure. Endothelin is a 21 amino acid vasoconstrictor peptide; which is synthesized predominantly in the endothelial cells and also by other cell types like cardiac myocytes and fibroblasts. ET-1 is the predominant isoform found in the human vasculature and myocardium. ET acts on two different receptors: ET-A receptors found on vascular smooth muscle cells (VSMC) and cardiac myocytes and ET-B receptors found on VSMC, vascular endothelial cells and cardiac fibroblasts. In normal subjects ET-1 causes vasoconstriction, increased myocardial contractility and vascular smooth muscle proliferation. In patients with HF, the level of ET-1 is two to three times higher than the level found in normal subjects (Parker and Thiessen, 2004). The plasma level of ET-1 correlates positively with NYHA class and negatively with LV dysfunction (Wei et al 1994). Chronic activation of ET receptors in HF patients causes myocardial hypertrophy, fibroblast proliferation, sodium retention, release of NE, AT-II and inflammatory mediators; which cause worsening of HF and LV remodeling (Ito et al 1991, Fujisaki et al 1995, Ding et al 2002). However, clinical trials testing the use of endothelin antagonists did not show any benefit in ambulatory patients with HF (Teerlink 2002, Anand et al 2004).

Nitric Oxide

Nitric oxide (NO) is a vasodilatory peptide synthesized in the endothelial and myocardial cells by the action of NO synthase (NOS) enzyme on the amino acid L-Arginine. There are 3 different isoforms of NOS present in the heart: (1) NOS1 (neuronal NOS) expressed in the sarcoplasmic reticulum (SR), neurons and conduction tissue (2) NOS2 (cytokine inducible NOS) which is induced by the inflammatory cytokines and (3) NOS3 (endothelial NOS) which is expressed in the endothelium, endocardium and cell membrane of cardiac myocyte. Dysfunctional NO metabolism seen in HF can contribute to progression of HF and LV remodeling by different mechanisms. In HF patients, there is a decrease in the NOS3 expression and activity which leads to a blunting of NO mediated peripheral vasodilatation (Katz et al 1999). Also, increased levels of reactive oxygen species found in HF can bind and inactive NO. These result in an increase in after load and worsening of myocardial wall stress. Secondly, there is abnormal subcellular localization of NOS 1 from SR to the cell membrane in HF resulting in abnormal excitation-contraction coupling and decrease in cardiac contractility (Damy et al 2004). It has been shown in animal studies that cytokine induced production of NO inhibits mitochondrial energy production and results in impaired myocardial contractility (Tatsumi et al 2000). Finally, it has been observed that NO inhibits the positive inotropic effect of beta adrenergic stimulation on dysfunctional myocardium (Hare et al 1995).

Cytokines

Injury to cardiac myocytes due to any cause promotes the release of various pro-inflammatory cytokines like tumor necrosis factor α-(TNFa), IL-1, IL-2 and IL-6 in an attempt to initiate the repair of injured myocytes. Also, elevated levels of AT-II seen in HF result in further increase in the level of these cytokines. However sustained release of inflammatory cytokines causes increased oxidative stress, myocardial hypertrophy, myocardial fibrosis, expression of dysfunctional fetal protein isoforms in cardiac myocytes, myocyte apoptosis and necrosis (Mann 2002). This leads to deterioration of ventricular function, cardiac remodeling and progression of HF. The magnitude of cytokine elevation in HF patients correlates with the severity of heart failure and poor patient outcomes (Testa et al 1996, Deswal et al 2001).

CAUSES OF HEART FAILURE

The causes of HF vary according to the geographic location, race and socioeconomic status. In developing countries, the scant data available indicates that; rheumatic heart disease, systemic hypertension, idiopathic cardiomyopathy and postpartum cardiomyopathy are the major causes of heart failure (Sliwa et al 2005, Stewart et al 2008). In South and Central America, Chagas' disease caused by Trypanosoma Cruzi is the leading cause of dilated cardiomyopathy. In the United States and other western countries, coronary artery disease is the most common cause of HF accounting for 50-75% of all HF patients. The epidemiology of HF has changed over time. Over the past 4 decades in the Framingham Heart Study, the frequency of coronary artery disease and diabetes mellitus as the underlying cause of HF has progressively increased, while hypertension and valve abnormalities have become less common (Kannel et al 1994). In a substantial number of cases, the etiology of HF cannot be identified. Felker et al analyzed 1,230 patients with initially unexplained cardiomyopathy (Felker et al 2000). An underlying cause of HF couldn't be determined in 50% of the cohort (idiopathic cardiomyopathy). A detailed list of the causes of HF in the remaining 50% is outlined in Table. 10.1.

Table 10.1: Causes of heart failure

Causes of Heart Failure
1. **Coronary artery disease**
2. **Hypertension**
3. **Metabolic/endocrine causes** Diabetes mellitus Hyper and hypothyroidism Pheochromocytoma Hyper and hypoadrenalism Uremia
4. **Infectious causes** Virus (Coxsackie virus, HIV, Cytomegalovirus, Parvovirus, Echovirus, Epstein-Barr virus) Protozoa (Toxoplasmosis, Chagas' disease, shistosomiasis, Trichinosis) Bacteria (Streptococci, Salmonella, Rickettsia, Brucella, Borellia, Mycobacteria) Fungal (Histoplasma, Cryptococcus)
5. **Connective tissue/autoimmune Causes** Systemic lupus erythematosus Scleroderma Giant cell arteritis Celiac disease
6. **Infiltrative diseases** Amyloidosis Hemachromatosis Sarcoidosis
7. **Substance abuse** Chronic excessive alcohol use Cocaine Methamphetamine
8. **Valvular abnormalities** Aortic stenosis Mitral regurgitation Aortic insufficiency
9. **High output states** Hyperthyroidism AV fistulas Beriberi Paget's disease of the bone Anemia Albright's disease
10. **Tachyarrhythmia** Atrial fibrillation AV nodal reentrant tachycardia Atrioventricular reentrant tachycardia Atrial tachycardia
11. **Nutritional deficiency** Thiamine Selenium Zinc Phosphorous Carnitine Calcium
12. **Genetic causes** Duchenne dystrophy Emery-Dreifuss dystrophy Myotonic dystrophy Friedreich's ataxia Hypertrophic cardiomyopathy
13. **Drugs/toxins** Chemotherapeutic agents (Anthracyclines, Herceptin, Cyclophosphamide). Heavy metals (Cobalt, Mercury, Lead, Beryllium, Arsenic) Antiretroviral agents Antipsychotic medication Chloroquine
14. **Miscellaneous sepsis** Peripartum cardiomyopathy Sepsis LV Noncompaction syndrome Obstructive sleep apnea Takotsubo cardiomyopathy Congenital heart disease

CLINICAL PRESENTATION

Heart failure is principally a clinical diagnosis; hence, a thorough history and physical examination remains the cornerstone in the diagnosis of heart failure. It is extremely important to consider several noncardiac diseases such as pulmonary asthma, fluid overload from progressive renal insufficiency or acute exacerbation of systemic hypertension that can present just like true HF. The clinical signs and symptoms seen in HF patient can be attributed to 3 mechanisms: (1) Hypoperfusion secondary to decreased cardiac output, (2) Excessive fluid accumulation and (3) Neurohormonal activation in end stage heart failure. The clinical features seen in HF are summarized in Table 10.2. Although history and physical examination are pivotal in making a diagnosis of HF, the sensitivity and specificity of signs and symptoms used to diagnose HF are poor (Davie et al 1997) (Table 10.3). A number of diagnostic criteria have been developed for the diagnosis of heart failure. The

Table 10.2: Clinical characteristics of patients presenting with heart failure

Clinical Presentation		Physical Examination	
Hypoperfusion	**Fluid Overload**	**Hypoperfusion**	**Fluid Overload**
Dizziness	Dyspnea on exertion or at rest	Tachycardia	Jugular venous distention
Syncope	Orthopnea	Cool extremities	Pulmonary rales
Exercise intolerance	Paroxysmal nocturnal dyspnea	Hypotension	Tachypnea
Fatigue	Ankle edema	Narrow pulse pressure	S3/S4 gallop
Palpitations	Nocturia	Altered mentation	Positive hepatojugular reflex
Abdominal pain	Early satiety/ Anorexia		Edema (Legs, Sacral)
Peripheral cyanosis	Abdominal pain and bloating		Ascites/Pleural effusion
Confusion/ drowsiness	Nausea/vomiting		Splenomegaly/ hepatomegaly
Sleep disturbances	Wheezing		Cardiac murmurs
	Cough		Weight gain
End Stage Heart Failure		**End Stage Heart Failure**	
Weight loss/Cachexia		Muscle wasting/ Weight loss	Pulsus Alternans

Table 10.3: Predictive values of clinical signs and symptoms used to diagnose heart failure [Modified from Davie AP, Francis CM, Caruana L et al. 1997. Assessing diagnosis in heart failure: which features are any use? QJM 90:335-339 by permission of Oxford University Press. Proportional pulse pressure = (Systolic – diastolic)/Systolic blood pressure].

Feature	Sensitivity	Specificity	PPV	NPV
	Symptoms			
Dyspnea on exertion	100%	17%	18%	100%
Orthopnea	22%	74%	14%	83%
PND	39%	80%	27%	87%
Edema	49%	47%	15%	83%
	Signs			
Tachycardia	22%	92%	33%	86%
Jugular venous distension	17%	98%	64%	86%
Gallop	24%	99%	77%	87%
Murmur	49%	67%	22%	87%
Crackles	29%	77%	19%	85%
Wheezing	12%	82%	11%	83%
Edema	20%	86%	21%	85%
Displaced apex	66%	96%	75%	94%
Proportional pulse pressure <25%	0%	100%	–	84%

modified Framingham criteria require the presence of 2 major criteria or 1 major criterion in conjunction with 2 minor criteria to make the diagnosis of heart failure (Table 10.4). The minor criteria can be used only if they cannot be attributed to any concurrent medical condition like pulmonary hypertension, obstructive or restrictive lung disease, nephrotic syndrome, cirrhosis, and gastroesophageal reflux disease (Senni et al 1998). In National Health and Nutrition Survey (NHANES) criteria, points are assigned to patient reported symptoms, physical examination and chest radiography features. A score of $\geq$ 3 points is diagnostic of heart failure (Schocken et al 1992).

Heart failure can be classified based on the severity of heart failure symptoms (NYHA classification) and risk factors (ACC/AHA classification). The New York Heart Classification (NYHA) divides patients into 4 classes depending on the severity of heart failure symptoms (Table 10.5). Patients in NYHA class I are asymptomatic at rest and with exertion, NYHA class II patients develop dyspnea with ordinary exertion, NYHA class III patients develop dyspnea with less than ordinary exertion and NYHA class IV patients have dyspnea at rest. Although over a period of time patient with HF deteriorate symptomatically from class I to class IV; with adequate medical therapy, diet control and exercise patients can also move from a higher class to a lower one. Besides being a functional classification, NYHA

Table 10.4: Modified Framingham criteria for diagnosis of heart failure

Modified Framingham Criteria	
Major criteria	**Minor criteria**
Paroxysmal nocturnal dyspnea	Peripheral edema
Orthopnea	Night cough
Abnormal jugular venous pressure	Dyspnea on exertion
Pulmonary rales	Hepatomegaly
Cardiomegaly on chest X-ray	Pleural effusion
Pulmonary edema on chest X-ray	Heart rate >120/minute
S3 gallop	Weight loss of $\geq$ 4.5 kg in 5 days
Central venous pressure >16 cm of H2O	
Weight loss of > 4.5 kg in 5 days in response to therapeutic intervention for presumed HF	

Table 10.5: New York Heart association functional classification. Reprinted from "1994 Revisions to classification of functional capacity and objective assessment of patients with diseases of the heart" with permission from american heart association

New York Heart Classification of Cardiac Disease	
Class	**Symptoms**
Class I	Patients with cardiac disease but without resulting limitations of physical activity. Ordinary physical activity does not cause undue fatigue, palpitation, dyspnea, or anginal pain.
Class II	Patients with cardiac disease resulting in slight limitation of physical activity. They are comfortable at rest. Ordinary physical activity results in fatigue, palpitation, dyspnea, or anginal pain.
Class III	Patients with cardiac disease resulting in marked limitation of physical activity. They are comfortable at rest. Less than ordinary physical activity causes fatigue, palpitation, dyspnea, or anginal pain.
Class IV	Patient with cardiac disease resulting in inability to carry on any physical activity without discomfort. Symptoms of cardiac insufficiency or of the anginal syndrome may be present even at rest. If any physical activity is undertaken, discomfort is increased.

classification is used to guide medical and device therapy in HF patients and carries a prognostic significance. For example, patients in NYHA class III-IV with LVEF $\leq$ 35% benefit from initiation of aldosterone receptor blockers or hydralazine/nitrate combination along with beta blocker, ACE inhibitor and diuretics. The mortality of HF patients increases with increase in NYHA class. Patients in NYHA class II HF have an annual mortality rate of 5-15% which increases to 30-70% in class IV patients (Uretsky and Sheahan 1997). The mode of death in HF also varies with the NYHA functional class.

The majority of patients in NYHA class II-III die from sudden cardiac death whereas patients in NYHA class IV die from pump failure.

In contrast, the ACC/AHA heart failure classification scheme is based on risk factors not just prognosis. In addition to patients with established HF, the ACC/AHA heart failure classification includes patients who are at risk of developing heart failure. Patients are divided into 4 stages (Figure 10.2). Stage A includes patients who have risk factors for development of HF like hypertension, diabetes mellitus, or metabolic syndrome, but have no overt structural heart disease or clinical features of HF. Stage B includes patients who have structural heart disease like previous myocardial infarction, low ejection fraction, left ventricular hypertrophy, and valvular abnormalities but are asymptomatic. Stage C includes patients who have structural heart disease and clinical features of heart failure. Stage D includes patients with end stage heart failure who require specialized interventions like chronic intravenous inotropic support, left ventricular assist device (LVAD) and heart transplantation. While the NYHA classification focuses of clinical progression of HF, the ACC/AHA classification puts emphasis on both the development and progression of HF. The ACC/AHA classification encourages the physicians to identity patients at risk of developing HF and initiate preventive measures like management of hypertension, lipid disorders, metabolic syndrome and encourage smoking and alcohol cessation.

DIAGNOSTIC TESTS

As discussed above the sensitivity and specificity of signs and symptoms used to diagnose HF are poor. Hence, detailed history and physical examination must be complimented by diagnostic tests to support a diagnosis of HF.

Routine Laboratory Tests

Routine blood testing is essential for all patients presenting with signs and symptoms suggestive of HF, because they can provide valuable information about cause and severity of HF, identify exacerbating factors, and adverse effects of heart failure medications. Complete blood count can reveal anemia or infection which could exacerbate HF. Basic metabolic panel can reveal acute or chronic renal failure which could cause fluid retention and HF exacerbation. Alternatively, worsening prerenal failure could be the consequence of worsening HF. Serum electrolyte measurement can reveal hyponatremia, hypokalemia, hyperkalemia and hypomagnesemia. The degree of hyponatremia is directly related to the severity of HF and is an indicator of poor prognosis (Lee and Packer 1986). Hyperkalemia (ACE inhibitor therapy) or hypokalemia (diuretic therapy) could be secondary to medications used in HF management. Also, hypokalemia can predispose to nonsustained ventricular tachycardia or atrial arrhythmias which could cause HF exacerbation. High serum digoxin levels can cause atrial or ventricular arrhythmias. Hepatic congestion secondary to right heart failure can cause elevation in liver enzymes like alkaline phosphatase, aspartate aminotransferase and alanine aminotransferase. Hypomagnesemia can cause frequent ventricular ectopics or

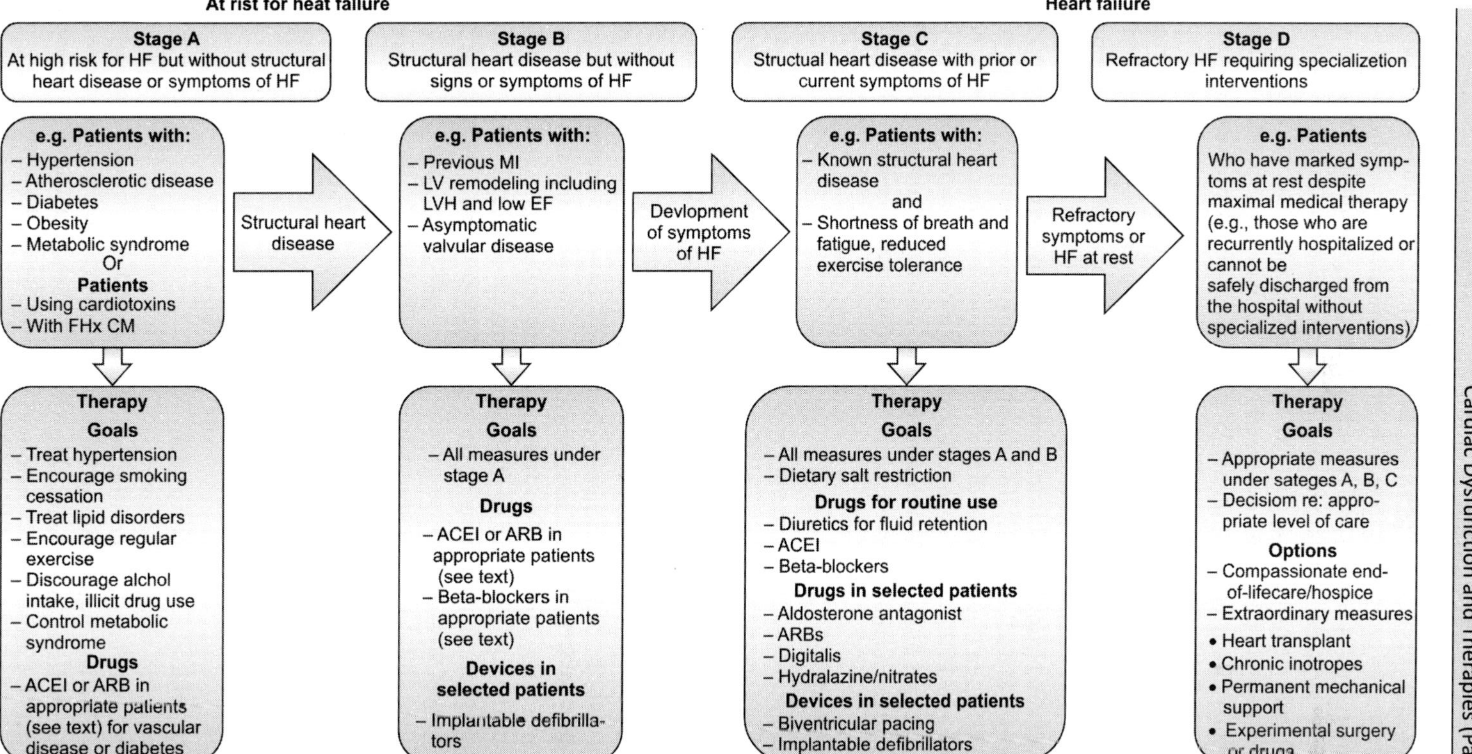

Figure 10.2: ACC/AHA classification of Heart Failure. Reprinted from J Am Coll Cardiol, 53, Hunt SA, Abraham WT, Chin MH, et al: Focused update incorporated into the ACC/AHA 2005 Guidelines for the Diagnosis and Management of Heart Failure in Adults A Report of the American College of Cardiology Foundation/American Heart Association Task Force on Practice Guidelines Developed in Collaboration With the International Society for Heart and Lung Transplantation, e1-e90; 2009, with permission from Elsevier

NSVT which can cause HF exacerbation. Urine analysis should be performed in all HF patients as it can reveal infection, microalbuminuria or microhematuria.

Measurement of cardiac specific biomarkers can provide information on cause and severity of HF. Increase in cardiac enzymes like troponin and creatine kinase (MB) indicate myocardial necrosis or infarction which could cause HF or exacerbate preexisting HF. As discussed earlier, BNP, a natriuretic peptide released from ventricular myocytes in response to volume expansion and pressure overload, can help identify HF patients. Most patients with shortness of breath secondary to HF have BNP levels above 400 pg/ml. BNP levels below 100 pg/ml have a strong negative predictive value. BNP levels between 100-400 pg/ml have low sensitivity and specificity in diagnosis of HF (Maisel 2002). In a multinational study Breathing Not Properly (BNP) study, BNP level was more accurate (83%) than Framingham criteria (73%) and National Health and Nutrition Examination Score (67%) in the diagnosis of HF (Maisel et al 2002). Increased BNP in patients with LV dysfunction and clinical HF is an important predictor of death and cardiovascular events. For every increase in BNP by 100 pg/ml, the relative risk of death increased by 35 percent (Doust et al 2005). BNP levels can be nondiagnostic in patients with certain conditions like renal failure, chronic heart failure, obesity and sepsis.

Electrocardiogram

Electrocardiogram (EKG) can provide vital information regarding the presence of systolic dysfunction, causes of HF and exacerbating factors. Most patients with HF have abnormalities on EKG. These include pathological Q waves, wide QRS secondary to interventricular conduction delay or bundle branch blocks, AV nodal blocks and left ventricular hypertrophy. A normal EKG makes the presence of systolic dysfunction very unlikely (98% negative predictive value). (Davie et al 1996) Evidence of ischemic changes (ST elevation/depression and T wave inversion) or arrhythmias (atrial fibrillation, supraventricular tachycardia, frequent ventricular ectopics or nonsustained ventricular tachycardia) on EKG could indicate the etiology of HF or the exacerbating cause. Certain EKG changes can have therapeutic implications in HF patients. Presence of wide QRS complex ($\geq$ 120 milliseconds) in patients with NYHA class III/IV and LVEF $\leq$ 35% on optimal medical therapy should be considered for biventricular pacer implantation.

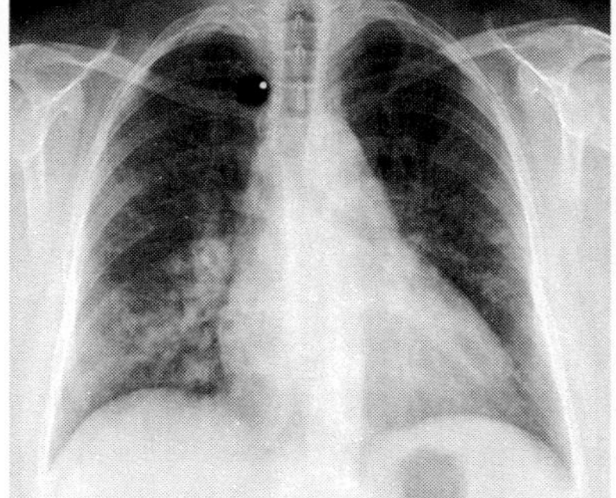

Figure 10.3: Chest X-ray of a patient diagnosed with HF showing cardiomegaly, cephalization, Kerley B lines and pulmonary edema

Chest X-ray

Chest X-ray provides valuable information about the size and shape of the heart, pulmonary vasculature, lead position of implantable devices, parenchymal and pleural abnormalities in patients with HF (Figure 10.3). Cardiothoracic ratio is defined as the ratio of the transverse cardiac diameter to the chest diameter and is usually ≤0.5. In patients in dilated cardiomyopathy the CT ratio is >0.5. The shape of heart on chest X-ray provides information about the etiology of HF (pressure-overload vs volume-overload of the ventricles), left atrial enlargement, right atrial enlargement and right ventricular enlargement.

Evaluation of pulmonary vasculature provides information about the left ventricular end diastolic pressure (LVEDP) and/or left atrial pressure. In patients with normal LVEDP (<8 mm of Hg), the pulmonary vascular pattern is normal. With an increase in LVEDP to 12 mm of Hg, there is prominence of pulmonary vasculature in the upper lobes called 'Cephalization'. Further increase in LVEDP to 18 mm of Hg causes extravasation of fluid into the interstitial space. This causes the presence of horizontal linear densities adjacent to the pleura called 'Kerley B lines'. Finally, elevation of LVEDP above 20 mm of Hg causes pulmonary edema along with substantial interstitial edema (perihilar bat wing appearance). The presence of interstitial edema, pulmonary edema and cephalization on chest X-ray has a specificity of 90% for HF (Knudsen et al 2004). However, in patients with chronic heart failure, there may be paucity of interstitial/pulmonary edema due to the increased capacity of lymphatics to clear interstitial fluid. Patients with high output states like anemia or left to right shunts also show prominent pulmonary vasculature in the peripheral lung fields. This pulmonary arterial hyperemia manifests as blood vessels with clear margins in contrast to the blurred margins seen in interstitial edema. Failure of dual chamber or biventricular pacing can lead to HF exacerbation. Evidence of lead dislodgement on chest X-ray can explain the malfunctioning of these devices. Evidence of parenchymal or pleural diseases like emphysema (honey comb appearance), COPD (hyperinflated lung fields), pulmonary fibrosis, pneumonia (pulmonary infiltrates), pleural effusion or pleural calcification can provide evidence of causes exacerbating HF or provide alternative diagnosis for shortness of breath.

Echocardiogram

2D Echocardiography is one of the most valuable noninvasive tools used in the evaluation of patients presenting with HF symptoms. Echocardiogram (2D Echo) is helpful in confirming the diagnosis of heart failure, determining the cause of heart failure, guiding management, providing prognostic information and monitoring response to medical management. In patients with new onset HF 2D echo is indispensable. 2D Echo can show wall motion abnormalities (indicating ischemic heart disease), valvular stenosis and/or regurgitation, papillary muscle dysfunction, right and left ventricular hypertrophy, chamber dilation, pericardial effusion and calcification which can help in determining the etiology of heart failure (Figure 10.4). Echocardiographic assessment of LVEF can guide pharmacological, device or surgical therapy in HF patients. Patients with NYHA class III/IV HF and LVEF ≤ 35% benefit from the initiation of aldosterone blockers and hydralazine/nitrate combination. Patients with NYHA class II/III HF and LVEF ≤ 35% should undergo implantable Cardioverter-defibrillator (ICD) implantation for primary prophylaxis against sudden cardiac death. Patients with NYHA class III/IV HF,

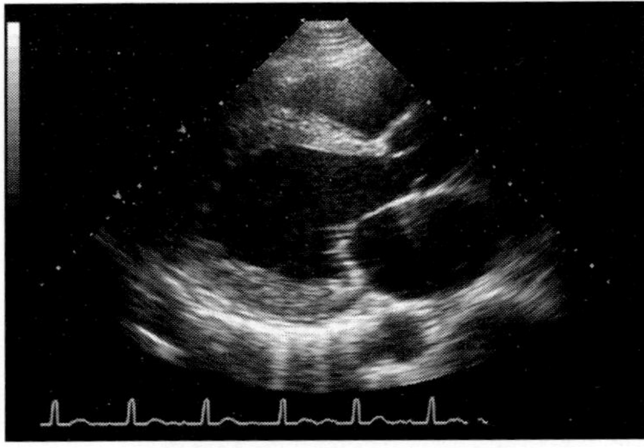

Figure 10.4: 2D Echocardiography of patient diagnosed with HF showing left ventricular hypertrophy, dilated left ventricle and left atrium. The left ventricular ejection fraction was 20%

LVEF $\leq$ 35% and QRS width $\geq$ 120 ms on EKG should undergo implantation of biventricular pacemaker. Echocardiography is also helpful in identifying patients who will benefit from biventricular pacing but with QRS < 120ms. Patients with echocardiographic evidence of mechanical dyssynchrony on tissue doppler imaging benefit from biventricular pacing as evident by increase in LVEF, decrease in mitral regurgitation and decrease in LV volume. Serial echocardiographic evaluation in HF patients can help in assessing the success of medical and device therapy and help in determining further management. Presence of certain valvular abnormalities like aortic stenosis, aortic regurgitation and mitral regurgitation in the setting of decreased LVEF and dilated left ventricle (for e.g. LV end systolic diameter $\geq$ 4.5 cm in mitral regurgitation) warrants surgical intervention. Echocardiogram is helpful in determining the severity of valvular abnormalities, LV function and LV dimensions in these patients. Certain echocardiographic parameters have prognostic significance in patients with heart failure. In patients with HF and LVEF < 35%, LV end-diastolic volume, severity of mitral regurgitation and deceleration time of mitral E velocity are the strongest predictor of survival (Grayburn et al 2005). Echocardiography also provides a noninvasive assessment of cardiac hemodynamics. It can be used to indirectly gauge cardiac output, pulmonary artery pressure, right ventricular pressure and left ventricular end diastolic pressure.

Stress Testing

Stress testing is used in HF patients to determine the cause of heart failure, assessment of functional status and prognostic stratification. Stress testing includes 2 components (1) Inducing myocardial stress by exercise, dobutamine, adenosine or dipyridamole infusion, and (2) Imaging by echocardiography and radionuclide imaging. Exercise stress testing is preferred over other stressing modalities as it also provides information about the functional status of the patient. A normal maximal exercise stress test makes the diagnosis of heart failure unlikely. Radionuclide imaging (RNI) is primarily used to exclude coronary artery disease (CAD) as an underlying cause of HF. RNI also provides information about the left ventricular function at rest and stress as well as viability of stunned or hibernating myocardium. Presence of wall motion abnormalities on stress echocardiography (SE) in HF patients indicates presence of CAD. Failure of LVEF to improve on SE indicate low myocardial contractive reserve and is a poor prognostic sign in HF patients.

Worsening of valvular regurgitation or increase in gradient across stenotic valves with symptom limitation implicates valvular abnormality as a cause of HF and would justify surgical intervention. Exercise testing to assess exertional capacity without imaging is used for prognostic stratification of patient with known HF, and for serial assessments after intervention. Patients with peak oxygen uptake (V02) less than 10 ml/kg/minute are classified as high-risk and should be considered for heart transplantation evaluation. Patients with Peak V02 above 18 ml/kg/minute are considered to be at low-risk.

Cardiovascular Magnetic Resonance (CMR)

CMR has been used in the assessment of HF patients to determine the cause of HF, evaluate LVEF, measure ventricular volumes and myocardial viability. Late enhancement after gadolinium injection (>10 minutes) can be used to distinguish-myocardial scar from viable tissue on CMR. The part of myocardium that hyperenhances >10 minutes after contrast injection is considered scar tissue, whereas; the nonenhancing part is considered to be viable myocardium. This data can be very helpful in guiding revascularization procedures in patients with ischemic cardiomyopathy. Also, the location of myocardial scar can help in distinguishing nonischemic cardiomyopathy (mid wall/epicardial) from ischemic cardiomyopathy (subendocardial/ transmural). CMR can help identify etiology of HFnlEF such as amyloidosis. More recently, coronary MR angiography (MRA) has been used for the assessment of coronary artery disease. This modality is helpful in the evaluation of proximal and middle coronary segments and bypass grafts. In one study, coronary MRA had a sensitivity and specificity of 82 % and 90% respectively in detecting coronary artery disease (Sakuma et al 2006). However, poor spatial resolution compared to cardiac CT angiogram, irregular heart rate and diaphragmatic movement provide diagnostic challenges in use of cardiac MRA for assessing coronary artery disease. Pharmacologic Stress CMR uses CMR along with pharmacological stressors like dobutamine; adenosine or dipyridamole for assessment of coronary artery disease. In one study, pharmacologic stress CMR was found to be more sensitive and specific than dobutamine stress echocardiography in detecting ischemic heart disease (Nagel et al 1999). CMR can detect myocyte injury and myocardial edema in myocarditis which can be the underlying cause of HF. Contrast enhanced CMR in patients with Chagas' cardiomyopathy reveals the presence of myocardial fibrosis in asymptomatic individuals which increases with advancing clinical stage of the disease (Rochitte et al 2005). Finally, Cine CMR can be used in the assessment of regurgitant and stenotic valvular lesions which can be the underlying cause of HF (Yoshida et al 1991, John et al 2003).

Invasive Catheterization

Invasive catheterization procedures like right heart catheterization, coronary angiography and myocardial biopsy are helpful in determining the cause of heart failure, assessing cardiac hemodynamics and guiding therapy. Right heart catheterization using a pulmonary artery catheter (PAC) provides information on cardiac hemodynamics including central venous pressure, right ventricular pressure, pulmonary artery pressure, pulmonary capillary wedge pressure and cardiac output. PAC is used in patients with severe hemodynamic compromise or cardiogenic shock, patients with prerenal failure with anuria or oliguria secondary to hypoperfusion and in patients with inadequate response to conventional HF therapy. However, use of PAC to guide therapy in HF hasn't shown to be beneficial. In the ESCAPE (The Evaluation Study of Congestive Heart Failure and Pulmonary Artery Catheterization Effectiveness) trial, 433 HF patients were randomized to either PAC guided therapy or clinical assessment guided therapy. There was no difference in reduction of volume overload, mortality or hospitalization in both groups. There was an increase in incidence of anticipated adverse events in the PAC group (Binanay et al 2005). Coronary angiography is used to identify coronary artery disease in (1) Patients with known HF presenting with angina, (2) Patients presenting with unexplained HF, (3) Patients presenting with HF symptoms who have positive stress test and (4) Patients with known HF who have severely dyskinetic myocardium. Left ventriculography performed during left heart catheterization provides assessment of LVEF, wall motion abnormalities and severity of valvular regurgitation. Myocardial biopsy is performed in patients with unexplained heart failure to determine underlying causes like infiltrative heart disease, storage disorders, myocarditis and anthracycline toxicity.

MANAGEMENT OF HEART FAILURE

The management of newly diagnosed HF involves (a) Management of acute exacerbation (b) Preventive Measures (c) Pharmacological Therapy (Figure 10.5):

Management of Acute Exacerbation

Acute management of HF begins with a determination of what could have destabilized the patient (sometimes not more complicated than the patient being noncompliant). Therapy for HF begins with maintaining adequate oxygenation, stabilization of blood pressure, management of fluid overload and treatment of exacerbating features. Patients with acute HF who are hypoxic ($SaO2 < 95\%$) on presentation should receive supplemental oxygenation. Patients with persistent respiratory distress and hypoxia should receive noninvasive positive pressure ventilation (NIPPV) like continuous positive airway pressure (CPAP) or bilevel positive pressure support (BiPAP). NIPPV reduces the in-hospital mortality by 45% and the intubation rate by 50%. (Masip et al 2005) Patient with acute HF can be hypertensive or hypotensive on presentation. Hypertension leads to increase in afterload and increases the myocardial oxygen demand. Vasodilators like nitroprusside, nitroglycerin and hydralazine can be used for the management of elevated blood pressure. Patients presenting with hypotension should be treated with positive inotropic medications like dobutamine, milrinone, dopamine or vasoconstrictors like high dose dopamine, vasopressin, norepinephrine and epinephrine. The use of vasoconstrictors can be detrimental in patients with HF as they increase the afterload. Volume overload is treated by administration of intravenous diuretics, nesiritide, ultrafiltration (diuretic resistance or renal failure)

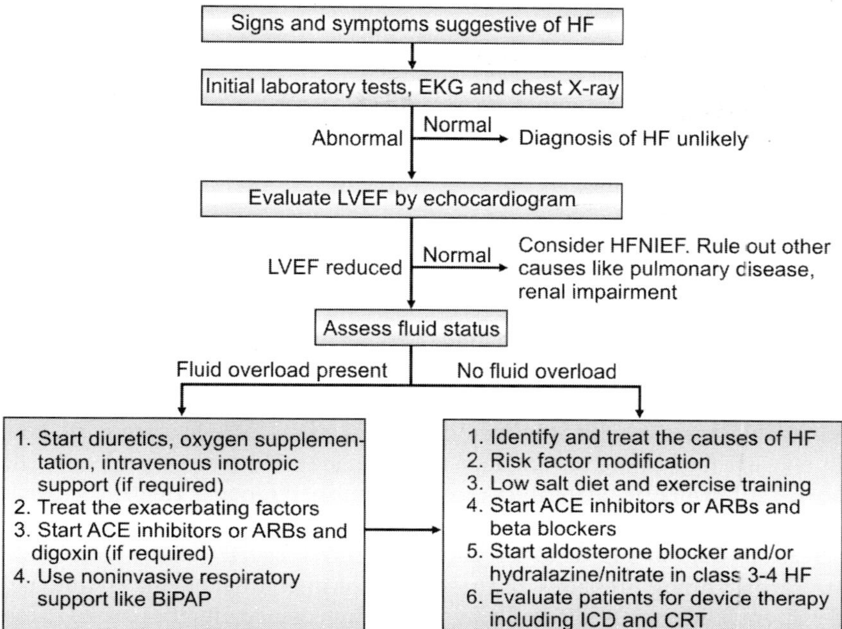

Figure 10.5: Approach to diagnosis and management of heart failure. HFNIEF—heart failure with normal ejection fraction; ICD—Implantable Defibrillator-Cardioverter, CRT—cardiac resynchronization therapy

or hemodialysis (in end stage renal failure patients). Exacerbating causes like myocardial ischemia, arrhythmias (atrial fibrillation, frequent ventricular ectopics or non sustained ventricular tachycardia), worsening of preexisting pulmonary diseases like COPD exacerbation, hypertensive emergency, infections and acute renal failure should be appropriately treated.

Preventive Measures

After the management of acute exacerbation of HF, emphasis should be placed on identification of reversible causes of HF, exacerbating factors and patient education. Patients should be advised to stop smoking, avoid excessive alcohol and salt consumption and avoid medications that worsen HF (NSAIDs, calcium channel blockers, thiazolidinediones and class I antiarrhythmic agents). One of the most common causes of HF exacerbation is noncompliance with medications. The importance of HF medications like ACE inhibitors and beta blockers in cardiac remodeling, preventing HF progression, and reducing hospitalizations should be reemphasized. Patients should be advised to perform routine and modest isotonic exercises like walking or riding a stationary bicycle. However, heavy physical exertion should be discouraged. Patients should be encouraged to check their weight regularly and report any weight gain to their physician or increase their diuretic dose.

Pharmacological Therapy

Medications used in heart failure can be divided into 2 broad categories (a) Medication that improve survival: Beta blockers, ACE inhibitors, angiotensin receptor blockers (ARBs), aldosterone antagonists, hydralazine/nitrate combination. (b) Medication that cause only symptomatic relief: Diuretics, digoxin and intravenous inotropes.

a. Diuretics

The 2009 focused update of 2005 ACC/AHA guidelines for the management and diagnosis of heart failure in adults recommend the use of diuretics along with salt restriction for the management of fluid overload in patients with prior or current symptoms of HF and reduced LVEF (Class I recommendation) (Hunt et al 2009). The diuretics used in HF include loop diuretics, thiazide diuretics, aldosterone receptor blockers, carbonic anhydrase inhibitors and vasopressin antagonists. Loop diuretics like furosemide, torsemide and bumetanide act by reversibly inhibiting the Na^+-K^+-$2Cl^-$ symporter in the thick ascending limb of the loop of Henle. This results in 20-25% increase in the excretion of filtered sodium and free water clearance. Increase in fluid loss leads to a reduction in intravascular volume, decrease in intracardiac filling pressures and resolution of interstitial edema (pulmonary edema, ankle edema). Additionally, administration of loop diuretics causes release of vasodilatory prostaglandins which leads to venodilatation and a decrease in right atrial pressure and pulmonary capillary wedge pressure. However, administration of intravenous loop diuretics causes transient activation of RAAS and increase in norepinephrine levels which causes vasoconstriction, increase in LV afterload and increase in pulmonary capillary wedge pressure. Hence vasodilators should be administered along with loop diuretics in patients with decompensated HF. The efficacy of loop diuretics is dependent on the renal blood flow and bioavailability. Loop diuretics are secreted actively in the proximal tubule by the organic acid transport system. There is a decrease in renal blood flow in HF patients which leads to a decrease in the secretion of loop diuretics into the tubular lumen. Hence, these patients may need higher doses of loop diuretics to achieve adequate response. Torsemide and bumetanide have a high oral bioavailability (80%); however, oral bioavailability of furosemide in only 50%. Presence of intestinal edema in HF can further decrease the absorption of furosemide. Hence patients with acute HF who are resistant to oral furosemide should be switched to either intravenous furosemide or oral bumetanide or torsemide. Use of loop diuretics is associated with adverse effects like electrolyte abnormalities (hypokalemia, hypocalcaemia, and hypomagnesemia), azotemia, hypotension, hyperuricemia and ototoxicity.

Thiazide diuretics like hydrochlorothiazide inhibit the Na^+-K^+ symporter in the distal convoluted tubule and result in increased sodium (5-10%) and free water excretion. Because of their weaker diuretic action compared to loop diuretics and loss of efficacy in patients with renal impairment, thiazide diuretics are primarily used as adjunctive therapy in heart failure patients. Administration of thiazide diuretics like chlorthiazide or metalazone along with loop diuretics results in sequential blockade of sodium absorption in loop of Henle and distal tubule and increases natriuretic response. Carbonic anhydrase inhibitors like acetazolamide cause complete loss of sodium bicarbonate resorption in the proximal tubule. Acetazolamide is a weak diuretic and is primarily used for the management of contraction metabolic acidosis that develops in response to administration of other diuretics. Although, short term use of diuretics in decompensated HF patients results in symptomatic improvement, it is unclear if long-term use of these agents results in a decrease in mortality and morbidity in these patients. In the DIG (Digitalis Investigation Group) trial, use of nonpotassium sparing diuretics was associated with increase in all-cause mortality, cardiovascular mortality, sudden cardiac death, progressive HF death and HF hospitalizations (Domanski et al 2006). Faris et al performed a metanalysis of double blinded randomized controlled trials comparing diuretic therapy to placebo or another active agent (digoxin, ACE inhibitor). The metanalysis showed that patients in the diuretic arm showed a significant reduction in mortality and rates of hospitalization for HF exacerbation compared to the placebo arm. There was also a significant improvement in the exercise capacity in patients receiving diuretic therapy (Faris et al 2006). Hence, long term studies evaluating the effect of diuretic therapy on mortality and morbidity are required.

b. Beta Blockers

The 2009 focused update of 2005 ACC/AHA guidelines for the management and diagnosis of heart failure in adults recommend the use of beta blockers in all stable patients with current or prior symptoms of HF and reduced LVEF (Class I recommendation) (Hunt et al 2009). Beta blockers are also recommended in patients who have asymptomatic LV dysfunction irrespective of the underlying etiology (Class I recommendation) (Hunt et al 2009). As discussed in pathophysiology, there is an overactivation of sympathetic nervous system in HF patients. Beta blockers antagonize the harmful actions of sympathetic overactivation by blocking beta 1, beta 2 and/or alpha1 receptors in myocardium and systemic vasculature. Beta blockers have been shown to improve symptoms, reduce hospitalization rates, prevent LV remodeling and reduce mortality in multiple placebo controlled randomized trials (Table 10.6). Three beta blockers have been approved for use in heart failure patients: sustained release Metoprolol succinate (β-1 antagonist), Bisoprolol (β-1 antagonist) and Carvedilol (β-1, β-2 and α-1 antagonist).

In the MERIT-HF (Metoprolol CR/XL Randomized Intervention Trial in Congestive Heart Failure) trial, 3991 patients with NYHA class II-IV HF, LVEF $\leq$ 40% and on optimum medical therapy which included digoxin, diuretics and ACE inhibitors were randomized to receive placebo or sustained release metoprolol succinate. At the end of 12 month follow-up, there was a 34% relative risk reduction in all-cause mortality, 49% relative risk reduction in deaths from worsening heart failure, 41% relative risk reduction in sudden cardiac deaths and decrease in the number of hospitalization due to HF exacerbation in the metoprolol arm. (317 vs 451; $p < 0.001$) (1999b) In the United States Carvedilol Heart Failure Study Group trial; 1094 patients with NYHA class II-III HF, LVEF $\leq$ 35% and on medical therapy which included digoxin, diuretics and ACE inhibitors were randomized to receive placebo or carvedilol. The study was prematurely terminated because

Table 10.6: Randomized placebo control trials reporting effect of beta blockers on mortality in HF patients (Waagstein et al., 1993; 1994; Packer et al., 1996; 1999b; 1999a; 2001; Packer et al. 2002)

Beta Blocker Trials				
Trial	**Medication**	**NYHA Class**	**No. of Patients**	**Mortality Reduction**
MERIT-HF	Metoprolol	II-IV	3391	7.2 vs 11.0%, p = 0.006
MDC	Metoprolol	II/III	383	12.0 vs 10.0%, P = NS
U.S-Carvedilol	Carvedilol	II/III	1094	3.2 vs 7.8%, p < 0.001
COPERNICUS	Carvedilol	III/IV	2289	10.7 vs 12.8%, P = 0.00013
CIBIS I	Bisoprolol	III/IV	641	20.9 vs 16.6 % , p = 0.22
CIBIS II	Bisoprolol	III/IV	2647	11.8 vs 17.3 % , p < 0.0001
BEST	Bucindolol	III/IV	2708	30.0 vs 33.0%, p = NS

of 65% reduction in mortality seen in the carvedilol arm. There was also 27% reduction in the risk of hospitalization for cardiovascular cause and 38% increase in event free survival (Packer et al 1996). In the CIBIS II (The Cardiac Insufficiency Bisoprolol Study II) trial, 2647 patients with NYHA class III/IV HF and LVEF ≤ 35% were randomized to receive placebo or bisoprolol. The study was prematurely terminated after 16 month average follow-up because patients in the bisoprolol group showed a 32 % reduction in all-cause mortality and 30% reduction in hospitalizations for HF (1999a). Certain β-blockers like bucindolol have not shown a mortality benefit in clinical trials. Hence the beneficial effects of β-blockers in HF cannot be considered a class effect. In the BEST (The β-blocker stroke) trial, 2708 patients with NYHA class III/IV HF and LVEF ≤ 35% were randomized to receive placebo or bucindolol. At 2 year follow up; there was no difference in all-cause mortality amongst the study groups but patients in the bucindolol arm showed a 14% reduction in cardiovascular mortality (2001). Interestingly, subgroup analysis showed that only nonblack patients in the bucindolol arm had a significant reduction in mortality (19%) whereas black patients had a nonsignificant trend towards increase in mortality (17%). The preferential mortality benefit seen in white patients is attributed to beta 1 receptor polymorphism (Arginine 389) (Liggett et al 2006).

Although the current guidelines don't recommend preferential selection of any one β-blocker, carvedilol has shown to be superior to metoprolol and bisoprolol in clinical trials. In the COMET (Carvedilol or Metoprolol European Trial) trial involving 3029 patients with NYHA class II-IV HF and LVEF < 35%, patients randomized to the carvedilol arm had a significant reduction in mortality (34%) compared to the metoprolol arm (40%). However, patients in the carvedilol arm had significantly lower heart rates and blood pressure which could have accounted for this difference (Poole-Wilson et al 2003).

Beta blockers should be initiated at a low dose in patients with stable HF. The dose of β-blockers should be increased gradually at atleast 2 week intervals as rapid up-titration can lead to fluid retention and decompensated HF. Gradual up-titration of β-blockers can also lead to fluid retention within 3-5 days of initiation of therapy which can be managed by increasing the diuretic dose. Treatment with β-blockers can also cause fatigue, bradycardia, hypotension, worsening claudication in patients with peripheral vascular disease and bronchospasm. Attempts should be made to initiate β-blockers prior to discharge from hospitalization. In the IMPACT-HF (The Initiation Management Predischarge: Process for Assessment of Carvedilol Therapy in Heart Failure) trial, initiation of carvedilol predischarge was associated with increased use at 60 day follow-up compared to post-discharge initiation of the medication. (91.2% vs 73.4%, $p < 0.0001$) The incidence of adverse reaction was same in both groups (Gattis et al 2004).

c. ACE Inhibitors

The 2009 focused update of 2005 ACC/AHA guidelines for the management and diagnosis of heart failure in adults recommend the use of ACE inhibitors in patients with current or prior symptoms of HF and reduced LVEF (Class I recommendation) (Hunt et al 2009). ACE inhibitors are also recommended in patients who have asymptomatic LV dysfunction (LVEF $\leq$ 40%) irrespective of the underlying etiology (Class I recommendation) (Hunt et al 2009). ACE inhibitors act primarily by inhibiting the production of angiotensin II and aldosterone and preventing their deleterious effects on preload, afterload and myocardial structure. Angiotensin converting enzyme also has kininase activity; hence, ACE inhibitors cause an increase in the levels of kinins like bradykinin. Bradykinin causes release of endothelium derived nitric oxide and vasodilatation which is beneficial in HF patients. However, increase in bradykinin is responsible for adverse reaction like angioedema and cough seen after the administration of ACE inhibitors. Other mechanisms by which ACE inhibitors are beneficial effects in HF include inhibition of cytokines, inhibition of intracardiac renin-angiotensin system, reduction of sympathetic activity and improvement in arterial compliance.

The benefit of ACE inhibitors in patients with symptomatic HF and asymptomatic LV dysfunction has been demonstrated in multiple randomized placebo controlled trials (Table 10.7). In the SOLVD-Treatment (Studies of Left Ventricular Dysfunction-Treatment) trial, 2569 patient with NYHA class II/III HF and LVEF $\leq$ 35% were randomized to receive enalapril or placebo. At an average follow-up of 41 months, there was a significant reduction in the all-cause mortality (35% vs 40%, $p = 0.0036$), deaths due to pump failure and hospitalizations for HF exacerbation in the enalapril arm. (1991) In the AIRE (Acute Infarction Ramipril Efficacy Study) trial, 2006 patients who developed overt heart failure symptoms after myocardial infarction were randomized to receive ramipril or placebo. After an average follow-up of 15 months, there was a significant reduction in all-cause mortality (17% vs 23%, $p = 0.002$), incidence of resistant HF and sudden death in the ramipril arm.(1993) In the SOLVD-Prevention (Studies of Left Ventricular Dysfunction-Prevention) trial, 4228 patients with asymptomatic LV dysfunction with LVEF < 35% were randomized to receive enalapril or placebo. After a median follow-up approximately 3 years, there was no significant difference in the mortality

Table 10.7: Randomized placebo control trials reporting effect of ACE inhibitors and Angiotensin receptor blockers on mortality in HF patients. (1987, 1991, 1992, 1993, Pitt et al 2000, Cohn and Tognoni 2001, Granger et al 2003, McMurray et al 2003)

Trial	Medication	NYHA Class	No. of Patients	Mortality Reduction
Angiotensin Converting Enzyme Inhibitors Trials				
CONSENSUS	Enalapril	IV	253	39.0 vs 54.0%, p = 0.003
SOLVD-Treatment	Enalapril	II/III	2569	35.2 vs 39.7%, p = 0.0036
SOLVD-Prevention	Enalapril	I	4228	14.8 vs 15.7 %, P = 0.30
AIRE	Ramipril	Clinical HF	2006	17.0 vs 23.0%, p = 0.002
Angiotensin Receptor Blockers Trials				
Val-HeFT	Valsartan	II-IV	5010	17.0 vs 27.0%, p = 0.017
CHARM-Alternate	Candesartan	II-IV	2028	21.6 vs 24.8%, p = 0.02
CHARM-Added	Candesartan	II-IV	2548	23.7 vs 27.3%, p = 0.021
ELITE II	Losartan	II-IV	3152	17.5 VS 16.0%, P = NS

rate among both groups. (14.8 vs 15.7 %, P = 0.30) However, there was a significant decrease in the combined end point of death and new onset heart failure (30% vs 39%, p < 0.001) and hospitalization or death secondary for HF. (20.5% vs 24.5%, p < 0.001). Use of ACE inhibitors is associated with following side effects: symptomatic hypotension, acute renal failure, hyperkalemia, cough (10-15% of patients) and rarely angioedema (1% of patients).

Angiotensin converting enzyme is encoded by ACE gene which is located on chromosome 17. There are 3 different genotypes of ACE gene based on insertion (I) or deletion (D) of 287 base pair within intron 16 of the ACE gene: DD, ID and II. Patients with DD genotype have the highest tissue and plasma ACE levels, ID genotype have intermediate levels and II genotype have the lowest levels. Patients with DD genotype have higher incidence of myocardial infarction, coronary artery disease, left ventricular hypertrophy, cardiomyopathy, mortality and reduced transplant free survival. (Danser et al 1995) The ACE gene polymorphism affects the response to pharmacological therapy in HF patients. Patients with DD genotype require higher doses of ACE inhibitors to achieve ACE inhibition compared to ID and II genotypes. Also, addition of beta blockers to ACE inhibitor therapy in patients with DD genotype improves mortality and transplant free survival in these patients comparable to ID and II genotype patients (McNamara et al 2001).

d. Angiotensin Receptor Blockers (ARBs)

The 2009 focused update of 2005 ACC/AHA guidelines for the management and diagnosis of heart failure in adults recommend the use of ARBs as a substitute to ACE inhibitors in patients with current or prior symptoms of HF, reduced LVEF and intolerance of ACE inhibitors (Class I recommendation) (Hunt et al 2009). Guidelines also recommend the use of ARBs in patients with reduced LVEF who are persistently symptomatic on conventional therapy (beta blocker, ACE inhibitor and diuretics) (Class IIb recommendation) (Hunt et al 2009). ARBs act primarily by blocking the action of AT-II on AT 1 receptor. Additionally, they also reduce the activation of SNS in HF, decrease cytokine levels and prevent remodeling after myocardial infarction. Unlike the ACE inhibitors, ARBs don't not block the degradation of kinins like bradykinin. Hence, they don't cause angioedema or cough like ACE inhibitors. Among patients with systolic heart failure, ARBs have been evaluated in patients with ACE inhibitor intolerance, as an additive therapy for patients symptomatic on conventional therapy and as a primary therapy in HF patients in place of ACE inhibitors (Table 10.7). In the ELITE-II (Losartan Heart Failure Survival Study) trial, 3152 patients with NYHA class II-IV HF were randomized to receive losartan or captopril. After a median follow-up of 555 days, there was no difference in the all-cause mortality, sudden death, progression of HF and resuscitated cardiac arrest between both arms. Compared to the captopril arm, significantly fewer patients discontinued losartan because of adverse reactions. (Pitt et al 2000) In the CHARM-Alternate (Candesartan in Heart Failure -- Assessment of Mortality and Morbidity- Alternate) trial, 2028 patients with NYHA class II-IV HF, LVEF $\leq$ 40% and intolerance to ACE inhibitors (cough, hypotension and renal failure) were randomized to receive candesartan or placebo. After a median follow-up of 34 months, there was a significant reduction in the primary end point of cardiovascular death or hospitalization for HF (33 versus 40 percent; adjusted hazard ratio 0.70; 95% CI 0.60-0.81), sudden cardiac death and death due to heart failure (Granger et al 2003).

Angiotensin II is primarily produced by the activation of circulating renin angiotensin system in the kidney and lungs. However, AT II can also be produced by renin-independent and ACE independent pathways in the myocardium, vasculature and brain. Angiotensinogen can be enzymatically converted to angiotensin I in the tissue by kallikrein and cathespin G. The action of proteases like myocardial chymases on angiotensin I leads to the local production of AT II. These pathways are not blocked by ACE inhibitors. Hence, combination of ACE inhibitors and ARBs may provide additive benefit by blocking both pathways. This hypothesis was tested in CHARM-Added (Candesartan in Heart Failure — Assessment of Mortality and Morbidity- Added) trial in which 2548 patients with NYHA class II-IV HF, LVEF $\leq$ 40% and on ACE inhibitor therapy were randomized to receive Candesartan or placebo. At 41 month median follow-up, there was a small but_significant reduction in primary end point of cardiovascular death or hospitalization for HF (38 versus 42%; adjusted hazard ratio 0.85; 95% CI 0.75-0.96), sudden death and death due to progression of HF (McMurray et al 2003). The side effects associated with the use of ARBs includes hyperkalemia, azotemia, hypotension and infrequently anigoedema.

e. Digoxin

The 2009 focused update of 2005 ACC/AHA guidelines for the management and diagnosis of heart failure in adults recommend the use of digoxin in patients with current or prior symptoms of HF and reduced LVEF to reduce the hospitalization for HF exacerbation (Class IIa recommendation) (Hunt et al 2009). Digoxin is one of the oldest medications used in the management of heart failure. It is a cardiac glycoside which acts by inhibiting the Na^+-K^+ ATPase pump in the myocardial cells. Inhibition of Na^+-K^+ ATPase pump results in an increase in the intracellular sodium content which in turn promotes sodium-calcium exchange and results in a rise in intracellular calcium. This results in an increase in myocardial contractility and improvement in LV systolic function. (Smith 1988) Additionally, digoxin increases the sensitivity of Na^+-K^+ ATPase pump in the vagal afferent nerves which results in an increase in vagal output to the heart. This counteracts the increased adrenergic input to the heart seen in HF patients. Increase in vagal output secondary to digoxin use is particularly beneficial in HF patients with rapid atrial fibrillation. Digoxin relieves the HF symptoms by slowing the ventricular rate and increasing the LV contractility (Gheorghiade et al 2006). Digoxin favorably affects the neurohormonal system in HF patients by decreasing NE release, regulating pathologic baroreceptors reflexes, increasing the release of natriuretic peptides, decreasing cytokine release and by decreasing RAAS activation (Gheorghiade et al 2006).

Intravenous administration of digoxin results in an immediate increase in LVEF, left ventricular stroke work index, cardiac index and a decrease in pulmonary capillary wedge pressure (PCWP) (Gheorghiade et al 1987). Data to support the chronic use of digoxin in HF comes from the DIG (Digoxin Investigators' Group) trial. In this study 6800 patients with symptomatic HF, LVEF $\leq$ 45% and normal sinus rhythm were randomly to digitalis or placebo. At 3 year follow-up there was no difference in overall mortality between both groups; however, patients assigned to the digoxin arm had a reduction in mortality from worsening HF and also had fewer hospitalizations for cardiovascular causes. Similar results were seen in the two randomized trials (PROVED and RADIANCE) where withdrawal of digoxin resulted in worsening of HF, decrease in exercise tolerance, reduction in LVEF and increased weight gain (Packer et al 1993; Uretsky et al 1993). A post-hoc analysis of DIG trial involving men with LVEF $\leq$ 45% revealed a decrease in all cause mortality in patients with serum digoxin level between 0.5-0.8 ng/ml. However, there was an increase in the all cause mortality rate with increase in the serum digoxin level (Rathore et al 2003). This effect suggests a very narrow therapeutic window for digoxin. The major adverse effects seen with digoxin use are cardiac arrhythmias (atrial arrhythmias, heart blocks, accelerated junctional rhythm and bidirectional ventricular tachycardia), neurological deficits (visual disturbances and confusion) and gastrointestinal symptoms (nausea, vomiting and anorexia).

f. Inotropic Medications

The inotropic agents used in HF can be divided into 3 categories (1) Phosphodiesterase inhibitors: Milrinone, inamrinone and enoximone (2) Beta adrenergic receptor agonists: dobutamine, dopamine and xametrol (3) Calcium sensitizing agents: levosimendan and pimomendan.

f.1. Phosphodiesterase Inhibitors

Phosphodiesterase IIIa (PDE IIIa) is an intracellular enzyme located in cardiac myocytes and vascular smooth muscle cells which degrades cyclic AMP (cAMP) into AMP. Administration of PDE IIIa inhibitors like milrinone inhibits the degradation of cAMP which results in an increase in the level of intracellular cAMP. This results in an increase in the intracellular calcium in the cardiac myocytes and increase in myocardial contractility. Additionally, inhibition of PDE IIIa in vascular smooth cells results in arterial and venous dilatation in systemic and pulmonary vasculature. Hence, intravenous administration of PDE IIIa inhibitor results in a decrease in preload (systemic and pulmonary venous dilatation), decrease in after load (systemic arterial dilatation), increase in cardiac index and improvement in cardiac hemodynamics (Colucci et al 1986). However, short-term administration of milrinone in patients hospitalized for management of acute exacerbation of chronic HF did not show any clinical benefit in the OPTIME CHF (Outcomes of a Prospective Trial of Intravenous Milrinone for Exacerbations of Chronic Heart Failure) trial (Cuffe et al 2002). In this trial 951 patients were randomized to receive intravenous milrione or placebo infusion for 48 hours. There was no difference in in-hospital mortality, 60 day mortality and days of hospitalization secondary to cardiovascular causes. There was also increased incidence of sustained hypotension requiring intervention and new atrial arrhythmias in patients receiving milrinone. Similarly, chronic use of oral milrinone in NYHA class III/IV HF patients with advanced LV dysfunction did not any clinical benefit in the PROMISE (Prospective Randomized Milrinone Survival Evaluation) trial. In this trial patients who were randomized to the trial arm had a 28% increase in all cause mortality and 34% increase in cardiovascular mortality. Also the rate of hospitalization, adverse drug reactions (hypotension and syncope) and medication discontinuation rates were higher in patients receiving oral milrinone therapy (Packer et al 1991).

f.2. Beta adrenergic receptor agonist

Dobutamine is the most commonly used intravenous inotropic medication in United States. Activation of myocardial beta receptors by dobutamine increases intracellular cAMP and calcium which results in increased myocardial contractility and cardiac output. The activation of beta 1 and alpha receptors by low dose dobutamine infusion results in vasodilatation and decrease in systemic vascular resistance. This results in a decrease in after load and increase in cardiac output. At higher doses dobutamine causes vasoconstriction and increase in afterload. Dobutamine is preferred in hypotensive decompensated HF patients who have renal failure. Dobutamine is safer in patients with renal failure compared to milrinone which has renal elimination. Also, low dose dobutamine infusion results in improvement in renal perfusion. It has been suggested that brief infusion of dobutamine (72 hours) results in sustained improvement in cardiac hemodynamics lasting for more than 30 days in certain cases. This effect is called 'dobutamine holiday' (Liang et al 1984). However, dobutamine infusion can cause adverse reactions like sinus tachycardia, atrial and ventricular arrhythmias, worsening of myocardial ischemia, atrial fibrillation with rapid ventricular response and myocyte apoptosis. These adverse reactions could be responsible for increased mortality seen in HF patients receiving dobutamine infusion. In CASINO (Calcium Sensitizer or Inotrope or None in Low-Output Heart Failure) trial, 299 patients with NYHA class IV HF were randomized to receive levosimendan, dobutamine or placebo infusion. Patients receiving dobutamine infusion had higher mortality (39.6%) at 6 months compared to the placebo group (24.7%) (Coletta et al 2004).

f.3. Calcium sensitizing agents (CSAs)

All the above mentioned inotropic agents exert their action by increasing intracytosolic calcium; however, this predisposes patients to fatal cardiac arrhythmias. Calcium sensitizers like levosimendan exert a positive inotropic on the myocardium without increasing the intracytosolic calcium concentration. CSAs bind to N-terminal of troponin C and stabilize the troponin C-Ca^{2+} complex. This interaction prevents the inhibition of actin/myosin ATPase by troponin I and leads to increase in myocardial contractility (Kass and Solaro 2006). CSAs also activate the ATP sensitive potassium channels in the vascular smooth muscles which causes coronary and peripheral vasodilatation. Peripheral vasodilatation leads to decrease in afterload and increase in cardiac output. Hence, intravenous administration of CSAs causes increase in stroke volume, cardiac output, cardiac index and decrease in intracardiac filling pressures, systemic vascular resistance and mean arterial pressure. The short and long term safety and efficacy of administration of CSAs have been studied in randomized trials. In the LIDO (Levosimendan Infusion Versus Dobutamine) trial, 203 patients with severe low output HF were randomized to receive 24 hour infusion of levosimendan or dobutamine. At the end of 24 hours, more patients in levosimendan group had hemodynamic improvement than dobutamine group (28% vs 15%, p=0.022). Also, 6 month mortality was lower in levosimendan group (26% vs 38%, p=0.029). (Follath et al 2002) In the SURVIVE (Survival of Patients With Acute Heart Failure in Need of Intravenous Inotropic Support) trial, 1237 patients with acute decompensated HF requiring inotropic support were randomized to levosimendan and dobutamine infusions. There was a greater decrease in the level of BNP and incidence of HF in the levosimendan arm. However, there was no difference in all cause mortality (at 180 days), cardiovascular mortality, subjective dyspnea at 24 hours and out of hospital days (Mebazaa et al 2007). In the REVIVE-II (Randomized Evaluations of Levosimendan) trial, patients in the levosimendan arm had increased incidence of hypotension, headache, atrial fibrillation, ventricular arrhythmias and non-significant trend towards increased mortality at 90 days (Cleland et al 2006). In conclusion, CSAs like levosimendan cause short-term improvement in cardiac hemodynamics but there is no reduction in long-term mortality and in some cases there may be increased mortality.

HYDRALAZINE/NITRATE COMBINATION

The 2009 focused update of 2005 ACC/AHA guidelines for the management and diagnosis of heart failure in adults recommend the use of hydralazine/nitrate combination in self described African-American patients with NYHA class III/IV symptoms on optimal medical therapy including beta blockers, ACE inhibitors and diuretics (Class I recommendation) (Hunt et al 2009). Hydralazine is an arterial dilator and isosorbide dinitrate (ISD) is a venous dilator. The use of hydralazine/ISD combination results in reduction of cardiac preload and afterload resulting in improved cardiac filling pressures. It is also postulated that hydralazine/ISD combination increases the bioavailability of NO as antioxidant property of hydralazine reduces nitric oxide consumption and ISD acts as NO donor. The use of this combination in HF patients results in symptomatic improvement and improved survival. The initial evidence of benefit from the use of hydralazine/ISD came from the V-HeFT 1 (Vasodilator-Heart Failure Trial) study. In this trial, 642 men with NYHA class II/III HF and LV systolic dysfunction were randomized to placebo, prazosin or hydralazine/ISD. At the end of 2.3 year follow-up, there was a trend towards mortality benefit in the hydralazine/ISD arm (Cohn et al 1986). A post hoc analysis of V-HeFT I trial showed that only black patients receiving this combination showed a significant reduction in mortality (Carson et al 1999). This observation was further substantiated in A-HeFT (African-American Heart Failure Trial) study (Taylor et al 2004). In this trial 1050 self identified black patients with NYHA class III/IV HF were randomly assigned to placebo or fixed dose hydralazine/ISD. All patients were receiving the standard HF therapy, including ACE inhibitors, ARBs, beta blockers and spironolactone. The trial was stopped prematurely at 10 months as there was significant reduction in mortality in the trial arm (6.2 vs 10.2%). There was also a significant reduction in the rate of hospitalizations for HF and an improvement in quality of life in the trial arm.

ALDOSTERONE ANTAGONISTS

The 2009 focused update of 2005 ACC/AHA guidelines for the management and diagnosis of heart failure in adults recommend the use of aldosterone antagonists in patients with NYHA class III/IV symptoms on optimal medical therapy including β-blockers, ACE inhibitors and diuretics (Class I recommendation) (Hunt et al 2009). The data supporting the use of aldosterone antagonists like spironolactone and eplerenone in patients with moderate to severe HF comes primarily from two randomized double blind placebo controlled clinical trials: RALES trial and EPHESUS trial. In the RALES (Randomized Aldactone Evaluation Study) trial, 1663 patients with NYHA class III (with class IV symptoms in last 6 months) and NYHA class IV HF and LVEF $\leq$ 35% were randomized to receive spironolactone or placebo. Majority of patients in this study received the standard HF therapy; including ACE inhibitors, diuretics and digoxin. However, only 10-11% of patients were on beta blockers. The study was prematurely terminated at a mean follow-up of 24 months as there was a significant reduction (30%) in the all-cause mortality in the spironolactone arm compared to placebo arm. (0.6 to 0.82; $p< 0.001$) This reduction was attributed to reduction in sudden death and deaths from HF. Additionally, there was a significant reduction in the rate of hospitalization for HF exacerbation (35%; 0.54.54 to 0.77; $P<0.001$) and improvement in the NYHA class in the spironolactone arm (Pitt et al 1999). In the EPHESUS (Eplerenone Post-AMI Heart Failure Efficacy and Survival Study) trial, 6642 patients who experienced myocardial infarction 3-14 days prior to initiation of study drug and also had clinical evidence of HF and/or diabetes mellitus were randomized to eplerenone arm or placebo arm. Unlike the RALES trial, majority of patients in this trial were on all HF medications including β-blockers (75%). At 16 month follow-up, there was a significant reduction in the all-cause mortality (0.75-0.96; $p = 0.008$), cardiovascular mortality (0.72-0.94; $p = 0.005$), rate of hospitalization for HF and sudden death (Pitt et al 2003).

The use of aldosterone antagonists in HF appears to be beneficial by 2 different mechanisms (1) Raising serum potassium concentration: In the SOLVD trial, HF patients receiving nonpotassium sparing diuretics had higher incidence of arrhythmic deaths compared to patients receiving potassium sparing diuretics (relative risk 1.37; $p=0.007$) (Cooper et al 1999). Hence, increase in serum potassium by aldosterone antagonists in hypokalemic HF patients ($K < 4.0$ mEq/L) may reduce the incidence of arrhythmic deaths. (2) Blocking the direct deleterious effects of systemic and locally produced aldosterone on the heart (Refer to pathophysiology section). Blockage of mineralocorticoid receptors in the heart may benefit by preventing cardiac hypertrophy and fibrosis, decreasing tissue angiotensin II production, decreasing oxidative stress and inflammation, preventing myocyte apoptosis and blocking proarrhythmic effect of mineralocorticoid receptor activation.

Aldosterone antagonists should be used cautiously in patients with underlying renal insufficiency as they can cause life-threatening arrhythmias. Patient receiving these agents should get their basic metabolic panel checked in 3 days and 1 week after initiation of the medication and then monthly for at least the first 3 months to monitor their serum potassium level and renal function. Use of these agents is not recommended in patients with serum creatinine > 2.5 mg/dl, creatinine clearance < 30 ml/min and baseline serum potassium > 5.0 mEq/L. As spironolactone binds nonspecifically to androgen and progesterone receptors, painful gynecomastia, impotence, menstrual irregularities and decreased libido are seen in 5-10% of patients receiving this medication (Pitt et al 1999). In these patients, spironolactone should be substituted with eplerenone as it has higher specificity to mineralocorticoid receptors and hence causes lesser endocrine side effects.

BIBLIOGRAPHY

1. Aggarwal A, Esler MD, Socratous F, Kaye DM. Evidence for functional presynaptic alpha-2 adrenoceptors and their down-regulation in human heart failure. J Am Coll Cardiol. 2001;37:1246-51.
2. Anand I, McMurray J, Cohn JN, Konstam MA, Notter T, Quitzau K, et al. Long-term effects of darusentan on left-ventricular remodelling and clinical outcomes in the EndothelinA Receptor Antagonist Trial in Heart Failure (EARTH): Randomised, double-blind, placebo-controlled trial. Lancet. 2004;364:347-54.
3. Anand IS, Fisher LD, Chiang YT, Latini R, Masson S, Maggioni AP, et al. Changes in brain natriuretic peptide and norepinephrine over time and mortality and morbidity in the Valsartan Heart Failure Trial (Val-HeFT). Circulation. 2003;107:1278-83.
4. A trial of the beta-blocker bucindolol in patients with advanced chronic heart failure. N Engl J Med. 2001;344:1659-67.
5. Bhatia RS, Tu JV, Lee DS, Austin PC, Fang J, Haouzi A, et al. Outcome of heart failure with preserved ejection fraction in a population-based study. N Engl J Med. 2006;355:260-9.

6. Binanay C, Califf RM, Hasselblad V, O'Connor CM, Shah MR, Sopko G, et al. Evaluation study of congestive heart failure and pulmonary artery catheterization effectiveness: the ESCAPE trial. JAMA. 2005;294:1625-33.
7. Bleumink GS, Knetsch AM, Sturkenboom MC, Straus SM, Hofman A, Deckers JW, et al. Quantifying the heart failure epidemic: Prevalence, incidence rate, lifetime risk and prognosis of heart failure The Rotterdam Study. Eur Heart J. 2004;25:1614-9.
8. Carson P, Ziesche S, Johnson G, Cohn JN. Racial differences in response to therapy for heart failure: Analysis of the vasodilator-heart failure trials. Vasodilator-Heart Failure Trial Study Group. J Card Fail. 1999;5:178-87.
9. Ceia F, Fonseca C, Mota T, Morais H, Matias F, de Sousa A, et al. Prevalence of chronic heart failure in Southwestern Europe: The EPICA study. Eur J Heart Fail. 2002;4:531-9.
10. Cleland JG, Freemantle N, Coletta AP, Clark AL. Clinical trials update from the American Heart Association: REPAIR-AMI, ASTAMI, JELIS, MEGA, REVIVE-II, SURVIVE, and PROACTIVE. Eur J Heart Fail. 2006;8:105-10.
11. Cohn JN, Archibald DG, Ziesche S, Franciosa JA, Harston WE, Tristani FE, et al. Effect of vasodilator therapy on mortality in chronic congestive heart failure. Results of a Veterans Administration Cooperative Study. N Engl J Med. 1986;314:1547-52.
12. Cohn JN, Tognoni G. A randomized trial of the angiotensin-receptor blocker valsartan in chronic heart failure. N Engl J Med. 2001;345:1667-75.
13. Coletta AP, Cleland JG, Freemantle N, Clark AL. Clinical trials update from the European Society of Cardiology Heart Failure meeting: SHAPE, BRING-UP 2 VAS, COLA II, FOSIDIAL, BETACAR, CASINO and meta-analysis of cardiac resynchronisation therapy. Eur J Heart Fail. 2004;6:673-6.
14. Colucci WS, Wright RF, Jaski BE, Fifer MA, Braunwald E. Milrinone and dobutamine in severe heart failure: Differing hemodynamic effects and individual patient responsiveness. Circulation. 1986;73:III175-83.
15. Communal C, Singh K, Pimentel DR, Colucci WS. Norepinephrine stimulates apoptosis in adult rat ventricular myocytes by activation of the beta-adrenergic pathway. Circulation. 1998;98:1329-34.
16. Cooper HA, Dries DL, Davis CE, Shen YL, Domanski MJ. Diuretics and risk of arrhythmic death in patients with left ventricular dysfunction. Circulation. 1999;100:1311-5.
17. Cuffe MS, Califf RM, Adams KF Jr, Benza R, Bourge R, Colucci WS, et al. Short-term intravenous milrinone for acute exacerbation of chronic heart failure: A randomized controlled trial. JAMA. 2002;287:1541-7.
18. Damy T, Ratajczak P, Shah AM, Camors E, Marty I, Hasenfuss G, et al. Increased neuronal nitric oxide synthase-derived NO production in the failing human heart. Lancet. 2004;363:1365-7.
19. Danser AH, Schalekamp MA, Bax WA, van den Brink AM, Saxena PR, Riegger GA, et al. Angiotensin-converting enzyme in the human heart. Effect of the deletion/insertion polymorphism. Circulation. 1995;92:1387-8.
20. Davie AP, Francis CM, Caruana L, Sutherland GR, McMurray JJ. Assessing diagnosis in heart failure: Which features are any use? QJM. 1997;90:335-9.
21. Davie AP, Love MP, McMurray JJ. Value of ECGs in identifying heart failure due to left ventricular systolic dysfunction. BMJ. 1996;313:300-1.
22. Deswal A, Petersen NJ, Feldman AM, Young JB, White BG, Mann DL. Cytokines and cytokine receptors in advanced heart failure: an analysis of the cytokine database from the Vesnarinone trial (VEST). Circulation. 2001;103:2055-9.
23. Ding SS, Qiu C, Hess P, Xi JF, Clozel JP, Clozel M. Chronic endothelin receptor blockade prevents renal vasoconstriction and sodium retention in rats with chronic heart failure. Cardiovasc Res. 2002;53:963-70.
24. Domanski M, Tian X, Haigney M, Pitt B. Diuretic use, progressive heart failure, and death in patients in the DIG study. J Card Fail. 2006;12:327-32.

25. Doust JA, Pietrzak E, Dobson A, Glasziou P. How well does B-type natriuretic peptide predict death and cardiac events in patients with heart failure: Systematic review. BMJ. 2005;330:625.
26. Effect of enalapril on survival in patients with reduced left ventricular ejection fractions and congestive heart failure. The SOLVD Investigators. N Engl J Med. 1991;325:293-302.
27. Effect of metoprolol CR/XL in chronic heart failure: Metoprolol CR/XL Randomised Intervention Trial in Congestive Heart Failure (MERIT-HF). Lancet. 1999b;353:2001-7.
28. Effect of ramipril on mortality and morbidity of survivors of acute myocardial infarction with clinical evidence of heart failure. The Acute Infarction Ramipril Efficacy (AIRE) Study Investigators. Lancet. 1993;342:821-8.
29. Effects of enalapril on mortality in severe congestive heart failure. Results of the Cooperative North Scandinavian Enalapril Survival Study (CONSENSUS). The CONSENSUS Trial Study Group. N Engl J Med. 1987;316:1429-35.
30. Faris R, Flather MD, Purcell H, Poole-Wilson PA, Coats AJ. Diuretics for heart failure. Cochrane Database Syst Rev. 2006;CD003838.
31. Felker GM, Thompson RE, Hare JM, Hruban RH, Clemetson DE, Howard DL, et al. Underlying causes and long-term survival in patients with initially unexplained cardiomyopathy. N Engl J Med. 2000;342:1077-84.
32. Floras JS. Sympathetic activation in human heart failure: Diverse mechanisms, therapeutic opportunities. Acta Physiol Scand. 2003;177:391-8.
33. Follath F, Cleland JG, Just H, Papp JG, Scholz H, Peuhkurinen K, et al. Efficacy and safety of intravenous levosimendan compared with dobutamine in severe low-output heart failure (the LIDO study): A randomised double-blind trial. Lancet. 2002;360:196-202.
34. Fujisaki H, Ito H, Hirata Y, Tanaka M, Hata M, Lin M, et al. Natriuretic peptides inhibit angiotensin II-induced proliferation of rat cardiac fibroblasts by blocking endothelin-1 gene expression. J Clin Invest 1995;96:1059-65.
35. Gattis WA, O'Connor CM, Gallup DS, Hasselblad V, Gheorghiade M. Predischarge initiation of carvedilol in patients hospitalized for decompensated heart failure: Results of the Initiation Management Predischarge: Process for Assessment of Carvedilol Therapy in Heart Failure (IMPACT-HF) trial. J Am Coll Cardiol. 2004;43:1534-41.
36. Gheorghiade M, St Clair J, St Clair C, Beller GA. Hemodynamic effects of intravenous digoxin in patients with severe heart failure initially treated with diuretics and vasodilators. J Am Coll Cardiol. 1987;9:849-57.
37. Gheorghiade M, van Veldhuisen DJ, Colucci WS. Contemporary use of digoxin in the management of cardiovascular disorders. Circulation. 2006;113:2556-64.
38. Goodfriend TL, Elliott ME, Catt KJ. Angiotensin receptors and their antagonists. N Engl J Med. 1996;334:1649-54.
39. Granger CB, McMurray JJ, Yusuf S, Held P, Michelson EL, Olofsson B, et al. Effects of candesartan in patients with chronic heart failure and reduced left-ventricular systolic function intolerant to angiotensin-converting-enzyme inhibitors: The CHARM-Alternative trial. Lancet. 2003;362:772-6.
40. Grayburn PA, Appleton CP, DeMaria AN, Greenberg B, Lowes B, Oh J, et al. Echocardiographic predictors of morbidity and mortality in patients with advanced heart failure: The Beta-blocker Evaluation of Survival Trial (BEST). J Am Coll Cardiol. 2005;45:1064-71.
41. Grieve DJ, Shah AM. Oxidative stress in heart failure. More than just damage. Eur Heart J. 2003;24:2161-3.
42. Hare JM, Loh E, Creager MA, Colucci WS. Nitric oxide inhibits the positive inotropic response to beta-adrenergic stimulation in humans with left ventricular dysfunction. Circulation. 1995;92:2198-203.
43. Hare JM, Mangal B, Brown J, Fisher C Jr, Freudenberger R, Colucci WS, et al. Impact of oxypurinol in patients with symptomatic heart failure. Results of the OPT-CHF study. J Am Coll Cardiol. 2008;51:2301-9.

44. Hunt SA, Abraham WT, Chin MH, Feldman AM, Francis GS, Ganiats TG, et al. 2009 Focused update incorporated into the ACC/AHA 2005 Guidelines for the Diagnosis and Management of Heart Failure in Adults A Report of the American College of Cardiology Foundation/American Heart Association Task Force on Practice Guidelines Developed in Collaboration With the International Society for Heart and Lung Transplantation. J Am Coll Cardiol. 2009;53:e1-e90.
45. Ito H, Hirata Y, Hiroe M, Tsujino M, Adachi S, Takamoto T, et al. Endothelin-1 induces hypertrophy with enhanced expression of muscle-specific genes in cultured neonatal rat cardiomyocytes. Circ Res. 1991;69:209-15.
46. John AS, Dill T, Brandt RR, Rau M, Ricken W, Bachmann G, et al. Magnetic resonance to assess the aortic valve area in aortic stenosis: how does it compare to current diagnostic standards? J Am Coll Cardiol. 2003;42:519-26.
47. Kannel WB, Ho K, Thom T. Changing epidemiological features of cardiac failure. Br Heart. J 1994;72:S3-9.
48. Kannel WB. Incidence and epidemiology of heart failure. Heart Fail Rev. 2000;5:167-73.
49. Kass DA, Solaro RJ. Mechanisms and use of calcium-sensitizing agents in the failing heart. Circulation. 2006;113:305-15.
50. Katz SD, Khan T, Zeballos GA, Mathew L, Potharlanka P, Knecht M, et al. Decreased activity of the L-arginine-nitric oxide metabolic pathway in patients with congestive heart failure. Circulation. 1999;99:2113-7.
51. Keith ME, Jeejeebhoy KN, Langer A, Kurian R, Barr A, O'Kelly B, et al. A controlled clinical trial of vitamin E supplementation in patients with congestive heart failure. Am J Clin Nutr. 2001;73:219-24.
52. Khatta M, Alexander BS, Krichten CM, Fisher ML, Freudenberger R, Robinson SW, et al. The effect of coenzyme Q10 in patients with congestive heart failure. Ann Intern Med. 2000;132:636-40.
53. Kinnunen P, Vuolteenaho O, Ruskoaho H. Mechanisms of atrial and brain natriuretic peptide release from rat ventricular myocardium: Effect of stretching. Endocrinology. 1993;132:1961-70.
54. Knudsen CW, Omland T, Clopton P, Westheim A, Abraham WT, Storrow AB, et al. Diagnostic value of B-Type natriuretic peptide and chest radiographic findings in patients with acute dyspnea. Am J Med. 2004;116:363-8.
55. Konstam MA, Gheorghiade M, Burnett JC Jr, Grinfeld L, Maggioni AP, Swedberg K, et al. Effects of oral tolvaptan in patients hospitalized for worsening heart failure: the EVEREST Outcome Trial. JAMA. 2007;297:1319-31.
56. Lebovitz RM, Zhang H, Vogel H, Cartwright J Jr, Dionne L, Lu N, et al. Neurodegeneration, myocardial injury, and perinatal death in mitochondrial superoxide dismutase-deficient mice. Proc Natl Acad Sci USA. 1996;93:9782-7.
57. Lee WH, Packer M. Prognostic importance of serum sodium concentration and its modification by converting-enzyme inhibition in patients with severe chronic heart failure. Circulation. 1986;73:257-67.
58. Levy D, Kenchaiah S, Larson MG, Benjamin EJ, Kupka MJ, Ho KK, et al. Long-term trends in the incidence of and survival with heart failure. N Engl J Med. 2002;347:1397-402.
59. Liang CS, Sherman LG, Doherty JU, Wellington K, Lee VW, Hood WB Jr. Sustained improvement of cardiac function in patients with congestive heart failure after short-term infusion of dobutamine. Circulation. 1984;69:113-9.
60. Liggett SB, Mialet-Perez J, Thaneemit-Chen S, Weber SA, Greene SM, Hodne D, et al. A polymorphism within a conserved beta(1)-adrenergic receptor motif alters cardiac function and β-blocker response in human heart failure. Proc Natl Acad Sci USA. 2006;103:11288-93.
61. Lloyd-Jones D, Adams RJ, Brown TM, Carnethon M, Dai S, De Simone G, et al. Heart Disease and Stroke Statistics--2010 Update. A Report From the American Heart Association. Circulation. 2009.

62. Maisel A. B-type natriuretic peptide levels: Diagnostic and prognostic in congestive heart failure: What's next? Circulation. 2002;105:2328-31.
63. Maisel AS, Krishnaswamy P, Nowak RM, McCord J, Hollander JE, Duc P, et al. Rapid measurement of B-type natriuretic peptide in the emergency diagnosis of heart failure. N Engl J Med. 2002;347:161-7.
64. Mann DL, Bristow MR. Mechanisms and models in heart failure: The biomechanical model and beyond. Circulation. 2005;111:2837-49.
65. Mann DL. Inflammatory mediators and the failing heart: Past, present, and the foreseeable future. Circ Res. 2002;91:988-98.
66. Masip J, Roque M, Sanchez B, Fernandez R, Subirana M, Exposito JA. Noninvasive ventilation in acute cardiogenic pulmonary edema: Systematic review and meta-analysis. JAMA. 2005;294:3124-30.
67. McMurray JJ, Ostergren J, Swedberg K, Granger CB, Held P, Michelson EL, et al. Effects of candesartan in patients with chronic heart failure and reduced left-ventricular systolic function taking angiotensin-converting-enzyme inhibitors: The CHARM-Added trial. Lancet. 2003;362:767-71.
68. Mebazaa A, Nieminen MS, Packer M, Cohen-Solal A, Kleber FX, Pocock SJ, et al. Levosimendan vs dobutamine for patients with acute decompensated heart failure: The SURVIVE Randomized Trial. JAMA. 2007;297:1883-91.
69. Nagel E, Lehmkuhl HB, Bocksch W, Klein C, Vogel U, Frantz E, et al. Noninvasive diagnosis of ischemia-induced wall motion abnormalities with the use of high-dose dobutamine stress MRI: Comparison with dobutamine stress echocardiography. Circulation. 1999;99:763-70.
70. Nozawa T, Igawa A, Yoshida N, Maeda M, Inoue M, Yamamura Y, et al. Dual-tracer assessment of coupling between cardiac sympathetic neuronal function and downregulation of beta-receptors during development of hypertensive heart failure of rats. Circulation. 1998;97:2359-67.
71. Owan TE, Hodge DO, Herges RM, Jacobsen SJ, Roger VL, Redfield MM. Trends in prevalence and outcome of heart failure with preserved ejection fraction. N Engl J Med. 2006;355:251-59.
72. Packer M, Bristow MR, Cohn JN, Colucci WS, Fowler MB, Gilbert EM, et al. The effect of carvedilol on morbidity and mortality in patients with chronic heart failure. US Carvedilol Heart Failure Study Group. N Engl J Med. 1996;334:1349-55.
73. Packer M, Carver JR, Rodeheffer RJ, Ivanhoe RJ, DiBianco R, Zeldis SM, et al. Effect of oral milrinone on mortality in severe chronic heart failure. The PROMISE Study Research Group. N Engl J Med. 1991;325:1468-75.
74. Packer M, Gheorghiade M, Young JB, Costantini PJ, Adams KF, Cody RJ, et al. Withdrawal of digoxin from patients with chronic heart failure treated with angiotensin-converting-enzyme inhibitors. RADIANCE Study. N Engl J Med. 1993;329:1-7.
75. Packer M. The neurohormonal hypothesis: A theory to explain the mechanism of disease progression in heart failure. J Am Coll Cardiol. 1992;20:248-54.
76. Parker JD, Thiessen JJ. Increased endothelin-1 production in patients with chronic heart failure. Am J Physiol Heart Circ Physiol. 2004;286:H1141-5.
77. Pitt B, Poole-Wilson PA, Segal R, Martinez FA, Dickstein K, Camm AJ, et al. Effect of losartan compared with captopril on mortality in patients with symptomatic heart failure: Randomised trial—the Losartan Heart Failure Survival Study ELITE II. Lancet. 2000;355:1582-7.
78. Pitt B, Remme W, Zannad F, Neaton J, Martinez F, Roniker B, et al. Eplerenone, a selective aldosterone blocker, in patients with left ventricular dysfunction after myocardial infarction. N Engl J Med. 2003;348:1309-21.
79. Pitt B, Zannad F, Remme WJ, Cody R, Castaigne A, Perez A, et al. The effect of spironolactone on morbidity and mortality in patients with severe heart failure. Randomized Aldactone Evaluation Study Investigators. N Engl J Med. 1999;341:709-17.

80. Poole-Wilson PA, Swedberg K, Cleland JG, Di Lenarda A, Hanrath P, Komajda M, et al. Comparison of carvedilol and metoprolol on clinical outcomes in patients with chronic heart failure in the Carvedilol Or Metoprolol European Trial (COMET): Randomised controlled trial. Lancet. 2003;362:7-13.
81. Rathore SS, Curtis JP, Wang Y, Bristow MR, Krumholz HM. Association of serum digoxin concentration and outcomes in patients with heart failure. JAMA. 2003;289:871-8.
82. Renneboog B, Musch W, Vandemergel X, Manto MU, Decaux G. Mild chronic hyponatremia is associated with falls, unsteadiness, and attention deficits. Am J Med. 2006;119:71 e71-8.
83. Rochitte CE, Oliveira PF, Andrade JM, Ianni BM, Parga JR, Avila LF, et al. Myocardial delayed enhancement by magnetic resonance imaging in patients with Chagas' disease: A marker of disease severity. J Am Coll Cardiol. 2005;46:1553-8.
84. Sakuma H, Ichikawa Y, Chino S, Hirano T, Makino K, Takeda K. Detection of coronary artery stenosis with whole-heart coronary magnetic resonance angiography. J Am Coll Cardiol. 2006;48:1946-50.
85. Sawyer DB, Siwik DA, Xiao L, Pimentel DR, Singh K, Colucci WS. Role of oxidative stress in myocardial hypertrophy and failure. J Mol Cell Cardiol. 2002;34:379-88.
86. Schocken DD, Arrieta MI, Leaverton PE, Ross EA. Prevalence and mortality rate of congestive heart failure in the United States. J Am Coll Cardiol. 1992;20:301-6.
87. Senni M, Tribouilloy CM, Rodeheffer RJ, Jacobsen SJ, Evans JM, Bailey KR, et al. Congestive heart failure in the community: A study of all incident cases in Olmsted County, Minnesota, in 1991. Circulation. 1998;98:2282-9.
88. Shiomi T, Tsutsui H, Matsusaka H, Murakami K, Hayashidani S, Ikeuchi M, et al. Overexpression of glutathione peroxidase prevents left ventricular remodeling and failure after myocardial infarction in mice. Circulation. 2004;109:544-9.
89. Silvestre JS, Heymes C, Oubenaissa A, Robert V, Aupetit-Faisant B, Carayon A, et al. Activation of cardiac aldosterone production in rat myocardial infarction: effect of angiotensin II receptor blockade and role in cardiac fibrosis. Circulation. 1999;99:2694-701.
90. Siragy HM. The potential role of the angiotensin subtype 2 receptor in cardiovascular protection. Curr Hypertens Rep. 2009;11:260-2.
91. Sliwa K, Damasceno A, Mayosi BM. pidemiology and etiology of cardiomyopathy in Africa. Circulation. 2005;112:3577-83.
92. Smith TW. Digitalis. Mechanisms of action and clinical use. N Engl J Med. 1988;318:358-65.
93. Stewart S, Wilkinson D, Hansen C, Vaghela V, Mvungi R, McMurray J, et al. Predominance of heart failure in the Heart of Soweto Study cohort: Emerging challenges for urban African communities. Circulation. 2008;118:2360-7.
94. Swedberg K, Cleland J, Dargie H, Drexler H, Follath F, Komajda M, et al. [Guidelines for the Diagnosis and Treatment of Chronic Heart Failure: Executive summary (update 2005)]. Rev Esp Cardiol. 2005;58:1062-92.
95. Tamura N, Ogawa Y, Chusho H, Nakamura K, Nakao K, Suda M, et al. Cardiac fibrosis in mice lacking brain natriuretic peptide. Proc Natl Acad Sci USA. 2000;97:4239-44.
96. Tatsumi T, Matoba S, Kawahara A, Keira N, Shiraishi J, Akashi K, et al. Cytokine-induced nitric oxide production inhibits mitochondrial energy production and impairs contractile function in rat cardiac myocytes. J Am Coll Cardiol. 2000;35:1338-46.
97. Taylor AL, Ziesche S, Yancy C, Carson P, D'Agostino R Jr, Ferdinand K, et al. Combination of isosorbide dinitrate and hydralazine in blacks with heart failure. N Engl J Med. 2004;351:2049-57.
98. Teerlink JR. Recent heart failure trials of neurohormonal modulation (OVERTURE and ENABLE): Approaching the asymptote of efficacy? J Card Fail. 2002;8:124-7.
99. Testa M, Yeh M, Lee P, Fanelli R, Loperfido F, Berman JW, et al. Circulating levels of cytokines and their endogenous modulators in patients with mild to severe congestive heart failure due to coronary artery disease or hypertension. J Am Coll Cardiol. 1996;28:964-71.

100. The Cardiac Insufficiency Bisoprolol Study II (CIBIS-II): A randomised trial. Lancet. 1999a;353:9-13.
101. Uretsky BF, Sheahan RG. Primary prevention of sudden cardiac death in heart failure: Will the solution be shocking? J Am Coll Cardiol. 1997;30:1589-97.
102. Uretsky BF, Young JB, Shahidi FE, Yellen LG, Harrison MC, Jolly MK. Randomized study assessing the effect of digoxin withdrawal in patients with mild to moderate chronic congestive heart failure: Results of the PROVED trial. PROVED Investigative Group. J Am Coll Cardiol. 1993;22:955-62.
103. Weber KT. Aldosterone in congestive heart failure. N Engl J Med. 2001;345:1689-97.
104. Wei CM, Lerman A, Rodeheffer RJ, McGregor CG, Brandt RR, Wright S, et al. Endothelin in human congestive heart failure. Circulation. 1994;89:1580-6.
105. Yoshida K, Yoshikawa J, Hozumi T, Akasaka T, Yamaura Y, Minagoe S, et al. Assessment of aortic regurgitation by the acceleration flow signal void proximal to the leaking orifice in cinemagnetic resonance imaging. Circulation. 1991;83:1951-5.

Chapter

11

Cardiac Dysfunction and Therapies (Part 2): Nonpharmacological Management and Future Directions

Vamsee Yaganti, Catalin Boiangiu, Snigdha Ancha, Marc Cohen

Abstract. Recent advances in pharmacological therapy have lead to an improvement in survival and quality of life in patients with heart failure. Despite the reductions in morbidity and mortality with pharmacotherapy; the prognosis of these patients remains poor. Use of various nonpharmacological interventions including device based therapies, coronary artery and valvular surgeries, ventricular assist devices and heart transplantation have lead to further reductions in morbidity and mortality in these patients. The major cause of mortality in patients with HF is either sudden cardiac death due to fatal arrhythmias or progressive pump failure. Implantable cardioverter-defibrillators reduce the incidence of sudden cardiac death and hence are used for primary and secondary prevention in patients with ischemic and nonischemic cardiomyopathy. Cardiac resynchronization therapy prevents and reverses left ventricular remodeling and results in improved ventricular function, functional status and survival. Development of implantable devices that are capable of monitoring fluid status and cardiac hemodynamics can help in preclinical detection of HF exacerbation and prevent hospitalizations. Surgical or percutaneous coronary revascularization of hibernating myocardium in patients with ischemic cardiomyopathy and repair of valvular regurgitant lesions improves left ventricular function, functional status and survival. Use of passive cardiac restraining devices limits ventricular dilatation, improves cardiac dimensions, prevents LV remodeling and improves functional status of HF patients.

For patients with end stage heart failure, refractory to medical therapy, ventricular assist devices and cardiac transplantation are the only therapeutic alternatives available. Ventricular assist devices have been used as destination therapy, bridge-to-transplantation and bridge-to-recovery. Increasing surgical experience with device implantation and advances in device designs have lead to a decrease in the surgical complication rates and device failures. Orthotopic heart transplantation is the definitive therapy in patients with end-stage heart failure. Approximately 2200 patients undergo heart transplantation annually in the United States. Implementation of stringent donor and recipient selection criteria and use of potent antirejection therapy has resulted in excellent outcomes after heart transplantation with survival rates exceeding 80% at 10 years in selected patients. The use of stem cell therapy, gene therapy and new neurohormonal agents in the management of heart failure is currently being investigated.

Keywords. Sudden cardiac death, implantable cardioverter defibrillator, cardiac resynchronization therapy, cardiac surgery, ventricular assist device, heart transplantation, stem cell therapy, gene therapy.

INTRODUCTION

Recent advances in pharmacological therapy have improved survival and quality of life in patients with heart failure. Despite reduction in morbidity and mortality rates with pharmacotherapy including β-blockers, angiotensin converting enzyme inhibitors, angiotensin receptor blockers, aldosterone receptor blocker and the hydralazine/nitrate combination, the prognosis of these patients remains poor. Analysis of a Medicare patient database revealed 1-year all-cause mortality rate between 32-37% and 1-year readmission rate of 66% in HF patients (Kosiborod et al 2006, Curtis et al 2008). The two major causes of mortality in HF patients are sudden cardiac death secondary to fatal arrhythmias and death due to progressive pump failure. The mode of death varies with the NYHA (New York Heart Association) functional class of the patient. The majority of patients in NYHA class II/III HF die secondary to sudden cardiac death and patients in NYHA class IV die predominantly from progressive pump failure (Table 11.1) (Uretsky and Sheahan 1997). In this chapter we will focus on nonpharmacological therapies that are being used to improve left ventricular function and functional status in HF patients and prevent sudden cardiac death and progressive pump failure. These include device-based therapies (implantable cardioverter-defibrillators and cardiac resynchronization therapy) nonreplacement surgical therapy (including coronary revascularization, valvular repair, reconstructive procedures or passive cardiac restraining devices) and cardiac replacement (total artificial heart or transplantation).

Table 11.1: Sudden cardiac death by severity of heart failure symptoms [Reprinted from J Am Coll Cardiol, 30, Uretsky BF and Sheahan RG: Primary prevention of sudden cardiac death in heart failure: Will the solution be shocking?, 1589-1597; 1997, with permission from Elsevier]

NYHA Functional Class	Annual Mortality (%)	Sudden Death (%)
II	5-15	50-80
III	20-50	30-50
IV	30-70	5-30

DEVICE-BASED THERAPY FOR HEART FAILURE

Implantable Cardioverter-Defibrillators (ICD)

In spite of many years of experience with antiarrhythmic drugs, ICD therapy has emerged as the only evidence-based therapy that reduces mortality in patients with cardiomyopathy (primary prevention) and in those surviving life-threatening arrhythmias (secondary prevention). ICDs have been compared to medical therapy in multiple randomized clinical trials for primary and secondary prevention of sudden cardiac death in patients with ischemic and nonischemic cardiomyopathy.

a. ICD for Secondary Prevention

Several randomized trials compared ICD with medical treatment for secondary prevention of SCD in heart failure patients (Table 11.2) (Can and Tholakanahalli 2009). The AVID trial enrolled patients who have been resuscitated from ventricular fibrillation (VF) or ventricular tachycardia (VT), had ventricular tachycardia (VT)

Table 11.2: Randomized placebo control trials reporting effect of implantable cardioverter defibrillators on mortality in HF patients

Trial	Patients (N)	LVEF (%)	Follow-up (Months)	Control Treatment	Relative Risk (95% CI)	p Value
Primary Prevention Trials						
MADIT I	196	26	27	Conventional	0.46 (0.26-0.82)	0.009
MADIT II	1232	23	20	Conventional	0.69 (0.51-0.93)	0.016
MUSST	704	30	32	Antiarrhythmic or Conventional	0.45 (0.32-0.63)	<0.001
CABG Patch	900	27	32	No ICD	1.07 (0.81-1.42)	0.63
DINAMIT	674	28	30	No ICD	1.08 (0.76-1.55)	0.66
DEFINITE	458	21	29	No ICD	0.65 (0.40-1.06)	0.08
SCD-HeFT	2521	25	45	No ICD	0.77 (0.62-0.96)	0.007
Secondary Prevention Trials						
AVID	1016	35	18	Amiodarone or sotolol	0.66 (0.51-0.85)	0.02
CIDS	659	34	35	Amiodarone	0.85 (0.67-1.10)	0.14
CASH	288	45	57	Amiodarone or Metoprolol	0.82 (0.60-1.11)	0.08

AVID—Arrhythmias Versus Implantable Defibrillators, CABG—Coronary Artery Bypass Graft, CABG Patch—Coronary Artery Bypass Graft Patch, CASH—Cardiac Arrest Study Hamburg, CIDS—Canadian Implantable Defibrillator Study, DEFINITE—Defibrillators in nonischemic cardiomyopathy treatment and evaluation, DINAMIT—Defibrillator in acute myocardial infarction and Trial, ICD—Implantable Cardioverter Defibrillator, MADIT-Multicenter Automatic Defibrillator Implantation Trial, MUSST—Multicenter Unsustained Tachycardia Trial, SCD-HeFT-Sudden Cardiac Death in Heart Failure Trial.

with syncope or had symptomatic VT in the presence of systolic dysfunction (LVEF ≤ 40%). The subjects were randomized to medical therapy (sotalol or amiodarone) or ICD implantation. The study was terminated early due to a significantly better survival in the ICD arm (89.3% versus 82.3% in the antiarrhythmic-drug group at 1 year, 81.6% versus 74.7% at 2 years, and 75.4% versus 64.1% at 3 years, $p < 0.02$), corresponding to reductions in mortality of 39 ± 20%, 27 ± 21% and 31 ± 21% at 1, 2, and 3 years respectively in the group receiving ICD therapy (1997).

b. ICD for Primary Prevention in Ischemic Cardiomyopathy

One of the earliest primary prevention trials, the MADIT-I (Multicenter Automatic Defibrillator Implantation Trial) trial, studied patients with prior myocardial infarction (MI), depressed systolic function (LVEF ≤ 35%) and inducible VT non-suppressible by procainamide during electrophysiological testing. The patients were assigned to ICD implantation or antiarrhythmic drugs. ICD therapy provided a 54% risk reduction in all-cause mortality during an average follow-up of more than 2 years (Moss et al 1996). The MUSST (Multicenter Unsustained Tachycardia Trial) study randomized patients with coronary artery disease (CAD), LVEF ≤ 40% and inducible VT to ICD therapy, antiarrhythmic medication or no therapy. After 5 years of follow-up, the all-cause mortality and SCD were reduced by 56% (24% versus 55%) and 76% (9% versus 37%) respectively by ICD implantation as compared to the other groups (Buxton et al 1999). The MADIT-II (Multicenter Automatic Defibrillator Implantation Trial) trial investigated the role of prophylactic ICD implantation in patients with ischemic cardiomyopathy. Patients with remote history of MI, LVEF ≤ 30% and on optimum medical therapy were randomized to receive an ICD or conventional therapy. After an average follow-up of 20 months, there was a 31% relative reduction in all-cause mortality (14.2% versus 19.8%) in the ICD group (Moss et al 2002). In contrast to the aforementioned trials which studied patients with remote ischemic events, DINAMIT (Hohnloser et al 2004) and CABG Patch (Bigger 1997) trials studied the role of ICD implantation in patients with a recent history of MI or at the time of coronary artery bypass graft surgery (CABG), respectively. The DINAMIT trial enrolled 332 patients with a recent history of MI (within preceding 6 to 40 days), LVEF ≥ 35% and either increased resting heart rate (≥ 80 beats/minute) or decreased heart rate variability. There was no significant difference in annual all-cause mortality between the ICD and control arm (6.9 vs 7.5%). In the CABG Patch trial, 900 patients undergoing CABG, with LVEF ≥ 35% and a positive signal averaged ECG were randomized to receive epicardial ICD or placebo. After an average follow-up of 32 months, there was no difference in all-cause mortality between both groups. Based on these two negative trials, the current guidelines do not recommend a prophylactic implantation of ICD within 40 days after an MI or within 3 months after CABG.

c. ICD for Primary Prevention in Nonischemic Cardiomyopathy

The efficacy of ICD implantation in preventing SCD in patients with nonischemic cardiomyopathy was addressed by the DEFINITE and SCD-HeFT trials. DEFINITE (Defibrillators in Nonischemic Cardiomyopathy Treatment Evaluation) trial randomized patients with NYHA Class I, II or III HF, LVEF ≤ 35% and history of nonsustained VT or frequent premature ventricular contractions (PVC) to receive standard medical therapy alone or in combination with an ICD. After a mean follow-up of 29 months, there was a 34% relative risk reduction in all-cause mortality in the ICD arm and the greatest benefit was seen in NYHA Class III patients (Kadish et al 2004). SCD-HeFT, the longest and largest trial on prophylactic use of ICD, enrolled patients with ischemic or nonischemic cardiomyopathy, LVEF ≤ 35% and NYHA Class II or III heart failure and randomized them to ICD, amiodarone therapy or placebo. ICD therapy significantly reduced mortality by 23% as compared to the other arms. Interestingly, the benefit was demonstrated exclusively for patients in Class II NYHA. Also importantly, therapy with amiodarone in this study increased the mortality risk by 44% in patients with Class III NYHA heart failure as compared to placebo (Bardy et al 2005).

The timing of ICD implantation for primary prophylaxis of SCD following the diagnosis of nonischemic cardiomyopathy remains a subject of debate. While an arbitrary 9 month wait period was recommended by the Centers for Medicare and Medicaid, there is no reliable evidence supporting this recommendation. In addition, a recent trial demonstrated that these patients experienced equivalent episodes of treated and potentially lethal arrhythmias irrespective of duration since diagnosis (< 9 months or > 9 months) (Makati et al 2006). The current ACC/AHA/HRS guidelines recommend ICD implantation therapy in patients with nonischemic cardiomyopathy if a potentially reversible cause of transient LV dysfunction has been excluded and the response to optimal medical therapy has been assessed (Epstein et al 2008).

Cardiac Resynchronization Therapy (CRT)

A significant number of patients with HF exhibit electromechanical dyssynchrony (atrioventricular (AV), intraventricular, interventricular or intramural delay) which leads to decrease in cardiac output and increase in mortality (Baldasseroni et al 2002). Approximately 30% of patients with LVEF ≤ 35% demonstrate ventricular conduction delay as evident by prolongation of QRS duration ≥ 120 ms. CRT involves simultaneous pacing of right ventricle (RV) and LV free wall which results in correction of inter/intraventricular conduction delays with subsequent increase in stroke volume and cardiac output. The RV is paced using a conventional pacing lead or an ICD lead implanted in RV apex or interventricular septum and the LV free wall is paced by placing a pacing lead via the coronary sinus into one of the branches of the great cardiac vein (Figure 11.1). CRT also reduces the AV mechanical asynchrony by optimizing the AV interval. Restoration of ventricular synchrony during systole improves LVEF, exercise capacity, quality of life and reduces hospitalization for worsening heart failure (Abraham et al 2002). CRT has also been shown to promote reversing of LV remodeling, reduce mitral regurgitation and heart size (Jessup and Brozena 2003).

Two major trials have assessed the morbidity and mortality benefits of CRT. In the COMPANION (Comparison of Medical Therapy, Pacing and Defibrillation in Heart Failure) trial, 1520 patients with Class III or IV NYHA heart failure, LVEF ≤ 35% and QRS duration ≥ 120 ms were randomized to 3 groups: Optimal medical therapy alone, medical therapy with CRT (CRT-P), and medical therapy with CRT

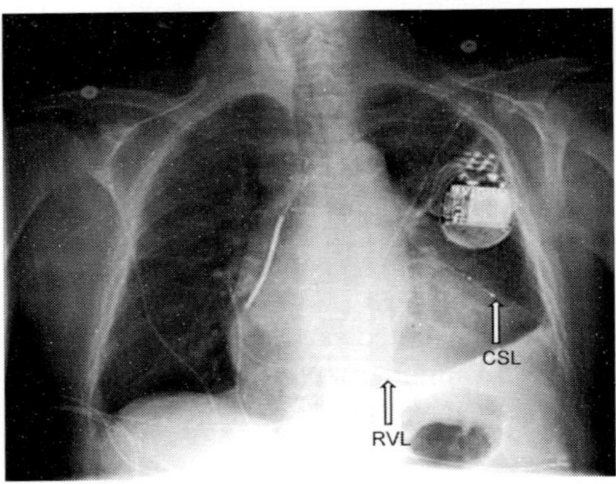

Figure 11.1: Chest X-ray of a HF patient with an implanted CRT-D device. RVL stands for right ventricular (ICD/Pacemaker) lead and CSL stands for coronary sinus lead (left ventricular lead). The right atrial lead is not clearly visible

and defibrillator (CRT-D) (Bristow et al 2004). At 1 year follow-up, there was a 19% reduction in primary composite end-point of all-cause mortality or all-cause hospitalization in the CRT-P arm ($p = 0.014$) and 20% reduction in the CRT-D arm ($p = 0.01$). Patients receiving CRT-D also enjoyed a significant 36% decrease in the secondary end-point of all-cause mortality vs medical therapy alone, ($p = 0.003$) in. There was no significant reduction in all-cause mortality in the CRT-P arm as the trial was not powered to show a mortality benefit in the CRT-P arm. Patients in both CRT arms also showed improvement in NYHA class, 6 minute walk distance, LVEF and systolic blood pressure. The CARE-HF (Cardiac Resynchronization in Heart Failure) trial randomized patients with Class III or IV NYHA heart failure, LVEF $\leq$ 35% and QRS duration $\geq$ 120 msec, to optimal medical therapy alone or with CRT (Cleland et al 2005). There was a 37% relative risk reduction in primary composite end-point of all-cause mortality or unplanned hospitalization for a cardiovascular event in the CRT group compared to the medical therapy alone arm (39% versus 55%, hazard ratio [HR] 0.63, 95% CI 0.51-0.77). The secondary end-point of all-cause mortality was also significantly reduced by 36% in CRT arm (20% versus 30%). The reduction in mortality was primarily due to a reduction in deaths due to worsening HF. (8.1% vs 13.9%) The mortality benefit in the CRT only arm in CARE-HF and COMPANION trials began approximately 8 months after the initiation of biventricular pacing whereas mortality benefit in CRT plus defibrillator arm was seen immediately after implantation. One possible explanation for this observation is that ICD benefits immediately by reducing SCD whereas CRT benefits from reverse remodeling which takes approximately 8 months. Very recently in the MADIT-CRT trial, 1820 patients with ischemic or nonischemic cardiomyopathy, NYHA Class I or II HF symptoms, LVEF $\leq$ 30% and QRS duration $\geq$ 130 msec were randomized to receive CRT plus ICD (CRT-ICD) or ICD alone (Moss et al 2009). During an average follow-up of 2.4 years, CRT-ICD therapy significantly reduced the occurrence of the primary composite end-point of death from any cause or nonfatal heart failure events in patients with ischemic or nonischemic cardiomyopathy (25.3% in the CRT-ICD group versus 17.2% in the ICD-only group, hazard ratio = 0.66, 95% confidence interval 0.52 to 0.84, $p = 0.001$). Interestingly, the superiority of CRT-ICD was driven by a 41% reduction in the risk of heart-failure events, without a significant difference in the overall risk of death between the two groups (3% annual mortality rate in each treatment arm).

It has been demonstrated in CRT trials that at least 85-90% biventricular capture is required for effective resynchronization therapy. This goal is difficult to achieve in patients with advanced HF and atrial fibrillation because the intrinsic ventricular rate can be faster than the programmed pacemaker rate which prevents resynchronization. A meta-analysis comparing the effectiveness of CRT in patients with atrial fibrillation and sinus rhythm demonstrated a lesser improvement in functional outcomes like 6 minute walk test and Minnesota scale in patients with atrial fibrillation (Upadhyay et al 2008). Hence, pharmacological and/or nonpharmacological (AV nodal ablation) methods should be used to control ventricular rate that will facilitate effective CRT therapy. Several CRT trials are currently investigating the efficacy of epicardial LV pacing, multisite LV pacing and the use of CRT in patients with narrow QRS complex. In conclusion, the findings of the major ICD and CRT trials suggest that patients with severely reduced LVEF, ventricular dyssynchrony and mildly symptomatic (NYHA Class I or II) HF benefit most from CRT secondary to reduction in heart failure related events with a lesser influence on mortality rate. However, patients with more advanced heart failure (NYHA Class II-IV) benefit from ICD/CRT therapy secondary to a significant reduction in all-cause mortality and reduction in rates of rehospitalizations for heart failure.

Implanted Device Based Invasive Hemodynamic Monitoring

Hospitalization for HF exacerbation is associated with increased mortality risk (4%) and predicts subsequent morbidity (Abraham 2009). The signs and symptoms of heart failure are a consequence of elevated cardiac filling pressures. It is known that an increase in ventricular filling pressure precedes symptom worsening by 7–14 days. Hence, continuous invasive cardiac pressure/fluid monitoring in an outpatient setting could potentially be beneficial in averting heart failure exacerbations and hospitalizations. One approach used for hemodynamic monitoring in the ambulatory setting consists of monitoring the intra-thoracic impedance which acts as a surrogate for fluid status. The OptiVol® Fluid Status Monitoring System (Medtronic, Minneapolis, MN) is a monitoring device which is embedded in selected CRT-D or ICD devices to measure the intrathoracic impedance. In a recent clinical trial, OptiVol® was more sensitive compared to weight monitoring in accurately predicting future heart failure events (76% vs 23%; $p<0.0001$) However, the specificity of impedance changes in predicting heart failure events was poor. Approximately 88% of impedance triggers were not followed by a clinical event. Hence, impedance monitoring can trigger inappropriate therapeutic decisions (diuretic dose increases, etc) with potential detrimental effects.

A second type of device-based hemodynamic monitoring is performed with implantable hemodynamic monitors (IHM). Chronicle® is an IHM system that monitors RV pressure along with heart rate, physical activity and body temperature. The device is implanted subcutaneously and has a transvenous pressure-sensing electrode placed in the RV outflow tract. The device can record RV systolic pressure (maximum pressure on RV pressure waveform) which corresponds to PA systolic pressure and RV diastolic pressure (measure at onset of R wave) which corresponds to RA pressure. The maximum rate of change in RV pressure over time (RV dp/dt $_{max}$) corresponds to the moment of opening of pulmonic valve. The right ventricular pressure at the time of RV dp/dt $_{max}$ provides an estimate of PA diastolic pressure. The PA diastolic pressure is reflective of LV filling pressure (LV end diastolic pressure) in the absence of significant lung disease. The COMPASS-HF study is a multicenter randomized clinical trial which accessed the safety and efficacy of continuous intracardiac pressure monitoring using the Chronicle® device in reducing HF related morbidity. Although the trial demonstrated a good safety profile of the implantable device, there was no significant reduction in all HF-related events (hospitalizations and emergency room or urgent care clinic visits requiring intravenous therapy) in the trial arm (Bourge et al 2008). A number of similar devices have been developed and evaluated for ambulatory intra-cardiac pressure monitoring. The HeartPOD® system (St. Jude Medical, St. Paul, MN) is a device for continuous monitoring of left atrial pressure. It is implanted through a transseptal puncture and anchored to the interatrial septum. The RemonCHF® device (Boston Scientific) is an implantable pulmonary artery pressure monitor delivered in a stent-like anchoring device using a percutaneous approach. The device provides on-demand pulmonary artery hemodynamics with the help of a handheld device and an acoustic transducer. CardioMEMS® (Atlanta, GA) manufactures a pulmonary pressure monitor that can be percutaneously delivered in the distal pulmonary artery and secured with a flexible wire structure. The device is currently being evaluated in a clinical study.

NONREPLACEMENT SURGICAL THERAPIES

Coronary Artery Bypass (CABG) Surgery

Hibernating myocardium is defined as dysfunctional myocardium which results from mismatch in the oxygen supply and demand at the cellular level secondary to reduced resting coronary blood flow. Restoration of coronary blood flow results in partial or complete recovery of function in the hibernating myocardium. Hence, presence of myocardial viability (hibernating myocardium) is an important determinant for the success of revascularization. In a metanalysis of 24 nonrandomized trials comparing revascularization to medical therapy in ischemic cardiomyopathy, patients with viable myocardium who underwent revascularization had an 80% reduction in annual mortality (3.2% versus 16%, $p<0.001$) compared to medical therapy. In contrast, in patients without myocardial viability there was no difference in mortality between revascularization vs medical therapy. (7.7% versus 6.2%, p = NS) The noninvasive tests that can be used to detect hibernating myocardium include dobutamine stress echocardiography (most specific test), thallium rest-redistribution single photon emission computed tomography (SPECT), thallium stress-redistribution-reinjection SPECT, fluorodeoxyglucose (FDG)-positron emission tomography (PET) scan (highest predictive value) and cardiac magnetic resonance (CMR) imaging with delayed gadolinium enhancement.

Multiple observation studies have shown that patients with ischemic cardiomyopathy and reduced LVEF who undergo surgical revascularization (CABG) have higher survival rates compared to medical therapy alone. In a retrospective trial by Bounous et al 710 patients with ischemic cardiomyopathy and LVEF $\leq$ 40% underwent CABG (284) or medical therapy (409). After a follow-up of 3 years, the survival in the surgical arm (86%) was better compared to medical therapy arm (68%) (Bounous et al 1988). In a prospective observation trial, 261 patients with ischemic cardiomyopathy, LVEF $\leq$ 40% and myocardial viability on FDG-PET scan underwent either surgical revascularization (94) or medical management (167). After a median follow-up of 2.1 years, the cardiac death rate was significantly lower in the revascularization arm (13% versus 24%, $p < 0.05$) and there was trend towards increased survival as well (85% versus 75%, p = NS) (Desideri et al 2005). However, there are no randomized clinical trials comparing the efficacy of surgical revascularization and medical therapy in ischemic cardiomyopathy patients with viable myocardium. The STICH trial (Coronary revascularization hypothesis) that is currently underway will address this issue. Patients with ischemic cardiomyopathy and severely reduced LVEF should be evaluated for myocardial viability and possible revascularization before they undergo transplant evaluation. Hausmann et al compared the efficacy of CABG and heart transplantation in 514 transplant eligible patients with ischemic cardiomyopathy (predominantly NYHA Class III-IV HF), low LVEF (10-30%), and viable myocardium. Patients who underwent CABG had an operative mortality of 7.1%, an actuarial survival rate of 78.9% at 6 years, improvement in NYHA functional class and improvement in LVEF. Patient who underwent heart transplantation had an operative mortality of 18.2%, an actuarial survival rate of 68.9 % at 6 years and improvement in NYHA functional class. It was also observed that presence of viable myocardium $\geq$ 20% of the total heart mass predicted favorable outcome after CABG (Hausmann et al 1997). Currently, identification of at least 4 viable myocardial segments representing >30% of left ventricular mass is considered to be associated with a significant improvement in LV function after revascularization.

Mitral Valve Repair

Majority of patients with dilated cardiomyopathy have varying degrees of mitral regurgitation (MR) irrespective of the cause of LV dysfunction. Mitral regurgitation results in progressive volume overload of the left ventricle leading to LV and mitral annular dilatation and further worsening of mitral regurgitation. Progressive LV dilatation causes a change in the LV geometry and leads to noncoaptation of mitral valve leaflets. Similarly, papillary muscle dysfunction secondary to ischemia and dyskinesis or aneurysm of left ventricular wall also contributes to this process. Mitral valve (MV) repair procedure is preferred over MV replacement for the management of mitral regurgitation because preservation of the native sub-valvular apparatus during MV repair results in better postoperative left ventricular function, avoids the complications associated with prosthetic mitral valves and results in improved survival. Repair of the MV can be accomplished by mitral ring annuloplasty with adjunctive artificial cord replacement and/or placement of 'Alfieri stitch'. Mitral valve annuloplasty involves insertion of an annuloplasty ring done via a percutaneous approach or through a conventional surgical approach. The percutaneous MV annuloplasty can be performed antegradely through the coronary sinus (e.g. Viacor percutaneous transvenous mitral valvuloplasty device Monarc system) or retrogradely via a transaortic approach (AccuCinch system or the Mitralign system). In addition to MV annuloplasty, placement of a figure-of-eight stitch (i.e. Alfieri stitch) across the mitral valve leaflets can be performed in selected patients to create a more competent, double-orifice valve. In patients with severe mitral regurgitation and high-surgical risk, a similar procedure can be performed by a percutaneous approach. The procedure involves percutaneous, transseptal delivery of a mitral clip device and placement of clip across the mitral valve leaflets resulting in better leaflet coaptation. (e.g. MitraClip system) In the EVEREST trial, 107 patients with 3-4+ MR underwent percutaneous mitral repair with MitralClip device. The survival rates at 1, 2 and 3 years were 95.9%, 94% and 90.1%, respectively with majority of patients having < 2+ MR. (Feldman et al 2009) Combined surgical revascularization and mitral valve repair in patients with ischemic cardiomyopathy and significant MR has been shown good survival rates. When used in patients with LVEF < 25%, 1-year survival was 87%, approaching that of cardiac transplantation (Gangemi et al 2000).

Surgical Ventricular Reconstruction (SVR)

Left ventricle undergoes negative remodeling after myocardial infarction which results in ventricular dilatation, increase in wall stress and change in ventricular geometry. Left ventricular reconstructive surgery involves exclusion of akinetic and/or dyskinetic myocardium and/or scar which decreases the LV volume and restores the LV geometry. This causes decrease in neurohormonal activation, decrease in end-systolic and end-diastolic wall stress, restoration of a normal ventricular anatomy (decrease in LV volume and a more ellipsoid shape) with subsequent improvement in LV function and prognosis. The partial left ventriculectomy or Batista procedure involves resection of ventricular myocardium between papillary muscles extending from apex to mitral annulus. Although the short and midterm studies showed promising results with improvement in LVEF and clinical functional status, long-term follow-up showed recurrence of heart failure, increased occurrence of fatal arrhythmias and poor survival rate (55% at 2 years). Dynamic cardiomyoplasty involves wrapping the latissimus dorsi muscle around the heart and synchronously pacing it during systole. Although there is an improvement in LVEF, stroke volume index and NYHA functional class in patients undergoing cardiomyoplasty, this technique has high procedural mortality and poor long-term survival. Hence, currently this procedure should be considered only as a destination therapy or a biological bridge to heart transplantation (Chachques et al 2009).

Endoventricular circular patch plasty (EVCPP) or Dor procedure was initially developed in the early 1980s for LV aneurysm repair. Subsequently, EVCPP has been used in the management of patients with symptomatic ischemic cardiomyopathy and large areas of LV akinesis or dyskinesis. The procedure involves partial exclusion of nonviable scarred myocardium using a purse string suture and closure of the residual defect with a pericardial or Dacron patch. The excluded aneurysmal scar is sutured to reinforce the repair. SAVER (Surgical Anterior Ventricular Endocardial Restoration) procedure is a modification of the Dor procedure which involves exclusion of noncontracting remodeled ventricular myocardium after an anterior myocardial infarction. Athanasuleas et al studied early and late outcomes in 1198 HF patients (67% in NYHA class III-IV HF) who underwent SAVER procedure. Majority of these patients also underwent concomitant surgeries including CABG (95%), mitral valve repair (22%) and mitral valve replacement (1%). Patients undergoing SAVER procedure showed improvement in LVEF (29% pre-versus 39% post-procedure), end-systolic volume index (80 ml pre-versus 57 ml post-procedure) and NYHA functional class. They also had an excellent 5-year survival (69%) and a low peri-operative mortality rate (5.3%) (Athanasuleas et al 2004). The routine use of SVR along with CABG in patients with ischemic cardiomyopathy and anteroapical LV dysfunction was investigated in the recently published STICH (LV reconstruction hypothesis) (Surgical Treatment of Ischemic Heart Failure) trial (Jones et al 2009). The STICH trial randomized 1000 patients with coronary artery disease amenable to CABG, anteroapical left ventricular dysfunction and LVEF $< 35\%$ to CABG alone or in conjunction with SVR (CABG + SVR). After a median follow-up of 4 years, there was no difference in the primary end-point of death and cardiac re-hospitalization (58% versus 59%, $p = 0.90$), NYHA functional class and quality of life between the groups despite a significant reduction in the end-systolic volume index in patients undergoing SVR. These findings do not support the routine use of SVR along with CABG in patients with ischemic cardiomyopathy who have dysfunctional myocardium. Hence appropriate patient selection (dyskinetic or aneurysmal myocardium) is critical for long-term success of SVR procedure.

Passive Cardiac Restraint Devices (PCRD)

Passive cardiac restraint devices (PCRDs) are helpful in restoring optimum ventricular geometry by limiting ventricular dilatation. Restoration of ventricular geometry leads to a decrease in myocardial wall stress and facilitates to reverse cardiac remodeling in patients with advanced HF. CorCap cardiac support device (CSD) or Acorn wrap consists of a thin polyester mesh which is surgically implanted around both ventricles. This device was prospectively evaluated in the Acorn trial. In this trial, 300 patients were randomized to receive 1 of 4 therapeutic options: Medical therapy only, mitral valve surgery only, CSD with medical therapy and CSD with mitral valve surgery. The use of CSD was associated with a significant reduction in LV dimensions (LV end-systolic and end-diastolic volume and sphericity index), improvement in NYHA functional class, reduction in the need for advanced cardiac surgery (LVAD placement, heart transplantation) and improvement in quality of life (Mann et al 2007). The beneficial effects on LV dimension were preserved at 3 year follow-up (Starling et al 2007). However, there was no survival benefit in patients receiving CSD. The Myocor Myosplint device is another PCRD which consists of a series of epicardial pads connected by tension bands from apex to base, drawing the LV walls inward and reducing the ventricular volumes. In a pilot clinical study, use of Myosplint device was associated with improvement in NYHA functional class, LV dimensions and LVEF. However, patients who underwent simultaneous Myosplint and mitral valve repair (for mitral regurgitation) did not show an improvement in LV function (Fukamachi and McCarthy 2005).

CIRCULATORY SUPPORT DEVICES (CSD)

Circulatory support devices are required in patients with severe, life-threatening hemodynamic deterioration on maximal pharmacological therapy and in whom survival is unlikely without heart transplantation. Hemodynamic instability can be defined as presence of persistent systemic hypotension (< 75-80 mm Hg), a cardiac index of <1.5-1.8 l/min/m^2 or pulmonary venous oxygen saturation < 50%. The different types of CSDs include intraaortic balloon pump (IABP), extracorporeal membrane oxygenation (ECMO), Impella circulatory assist device and ventricular assist device (uni or biventricular). CSDs are used in 5 clinical settings: "bridge-to-transplantation" (BTT), "bridge-to-recovery" (BTR), triage ("bridge to next step"), "bridge-to-bridge" (BTB, from short-term to long-term devices), or as destination therapy (DT) (Table 11.3). The choice of CSD depends on the anticipated duration of use, potential reversibility of hemodynamic instability, need for uni- or biventricular support, patient's size and availability. There are four major categories of patients who benefit from short-term circulatory support: Patients with cardiogenic shock after cardiac surgery, patients who develop cardiogenic shock as a consequence of acute myocardial infarction, patients with acute myocarditis and patients with acute, but reversible, myocardial dysfunction. Catheter-based devices like IABP, Impella and ECMO are usually used for short-term hemodynamic support. Insertion is rapid and does not require direct surgical access to the heart. These devices can be use in acute clinical situation and exchanged at a later time to a more permanent type of mechanical assistance ("bridge-to-bridge").

Intraaortic Balloon Counterpulsation

The most commonly used circulatory support device is an intraaortic balloon pump (IABP). The IABP is placed via the femoral artery into the descending thoracic aorta with its proximal tip lying just below the origin of the left subclavian artery. Inflation of IABP in early diastole augments the aortic diastolic pressure and augments coronary perfusion. Deflation of IABP just before the onset of ventricular ejection decreases the afterload which results in an increase in the effective stroke volume and cardiac output and a decrease in the work of the heart. Use of IABP in cardiogenic shock is associated with an increase in diastolic blood pressure by 30%, decrease in systolic blood pressure by 20%, increase in cardiac output by 20%, decrease in pulmonary capillary wedge pressure by 20% and reduction in heart rate by 20% (which decreases cardiac work load) (Scheidt et al 1973). Use of IABP is contraindicated in patients with significant aortic regurgitation, aortic dissection, abdominal aortic aneurysm, severe peripheral artery disease and with contraindication to anticoagulation. Complications associated with the use of IABP include hemorrhage, arterial dissection, vascular laceration, limb ischemia, cholesterol embolization, thrombocytopenia, hemolysis, sepsis and rarely stroke and balloon rupture. In the Benchmark Registry, the incidence of major IABP complications (severe bleeding, balloon rupture, major limb ischemia and death caused by balloon insertion or failure) was 2.6%, (Ferguson et al 2001). In the absence of large randomized trials, data regarding the benefit of using IABP comes from observational reports or registries. In the SHOCK trial, the use of IABP in the setting of cardiogenic shock due to myocardial infarction significantly improved in-hospital mortality (50% versus 72% without IABP, $p<0.0001$). (Hochman et al 2000) A recent meta-analysis including more than 10,000 patients with STEMI and cardiogenic shock showed that IABP use in patients treated with thrombolysis was associated with an 18% decrease in 30 day mortality, helped by a significantly higher revascularization rate compared to patients without support (Sjauw et al 2009). On the contrary, in patients treated with primary percutaneous coronary intervention, IABP was associated with a 6% increase in 30-day mortality. Overall, this analysis did not support the routine use of intraaortic balloon counterpulsation in patients developing cardiogenic shock in the setting of STEMI, challenging the current guidelines of therapy.

Extracorporeal Membrane Oxygenation (ECMO)

ECMO uses a mechanical pump to extract blood from the patient and circulate it through a membrane oxygenator system for oxygenation of blood and removal of carbon dioxide. The venous or outlet cannula is usually placed via the femoral vein and advanced to the junction of inferior vena cava and right atrium. The inlet or arterial cannula is placed in the aorta or femoral artery. The pump requires anticoagulation and can cause significant hemolysis. ECMO is used to provide cardiopulmonary support as a BTB (exchange to a long-term VAD system) or BTT.

Impella Circulatory Assist Device

The Impella system is microaxial flow device which consists of a rotary pump incorporated within a catheter. The device can be placed either percutaneously (via femoral artery) or surgically across the aortic valve. The pump draws blood via the inflow port placed in the left ventricle and delivers it into the ascending aorta via the outflow port. The system can also be used as a right ventricular assist device when the inflow port is placed in the right atrium and outflow port is placed in the pulmonary artery. This device can deliver a flow of 2.5 or 5 l/min, and is currently used for hemodynamic support in patients with cardiogenic shock secondary to myocardial infarction or acute myocarditis and also during high-risk percutaneous coronary interventions. In a retrospective study, use of Impella in acute surgical and nonsurgical heart failure as a BTR device was accompanied by 45% and 23% early mortality respectively (Granfeldt et al 2009).

Table 11.3: Classification and characteristics of ventricular assist devices

	Type	Placement	Support	Anticoagulation	Disadvantages	Ambulation
Short-term ventricular assist devices						
IABP	Pulsatile	Percutaneous	Uni (left) ventricular	Heparin	Vascular complication and Bleeding	No
Abiomed BVS 5000	Pulsatile	Surgical	Uni- or biventricular	Heparin	Bleeding Thromboembolism	Limited
Abiomed AB 5000				Heparin/ Warfarin		
ECMO	Nonpulsatile Centrifugal flow	Surgical	Uni- or biventricular	Heparin	Bleeding Hemolysis	No
Impella LP 2.5	Nonpulsatile Axial flow	Surgical/ Percutaneous	Univentricular	Heparin	Bleeding Thromboembolism	No
TandemHeart	Nonpulsatile Centrifugal flow	Percutaneous	Univentricular		Ventricular arrhythmia Hemolysis Catheter displacement	No
Levitronix CentriMag	Nonpulsatile	Surgical	Univentricular			No

Contd...

Contd...

	Type	Placement	Support	Anticoagulation	Disadvantages	Ambulation
Intermediate and long-term ventricular assist devices						
First generation						
Thoratec pVAD or IVAD	Pulsatile flow	Surgical	Uni- or biventricular	Heparin/ Warfarin	Bleeding Thromboembolic events	Yes
HeartMate IP1000, VE, XVE			Univentricular (left)	No, aspirin only	High incidence of device failure	Yes
Novacor				Heparin/Warfarin	Bleeding Thromboembolic events	Yes
LionHeart			Uni- or biventricular		Totally implantable; no percutaneous lead – less infection	Yes
Second generation						
HeartMate II Jarvik 2000 DeBakey	Rotary Axial flow	Surgical	Uni- or biventricular	Warfarin	Hemolysis Thromboembolic events Ventrilar suction	Yes
Third generation						
VentrAssist DuraHeart HVAD EVAHEART	Rotary Centrifugal flow	Surgical	Uni- or biventricular	Warfarin	Bleeding Hemolysis	Yes

Ventricular Assist Devices (VAD)

a. Short-term VADs

The TandemHeart is a percutaneously placed short-term circulatory support device which removes blood from the left atrium (via a catheter placed by transseptal puncture) and returns it the iliac artery (via a cannula placed in the femoral artery) TandemHeart was compared to IABP in patients with revascularized acute myocardial infarction complicated by cardiogenic shock. TandemHeart demonstrated better hemodynamic improvement compared to IABP, however, the mortality rate in both arms was similar at 30 days (45% versus 43%, $p = 0.86$) (Thiele et al 2005).

b. Intermediate and Long-term VADs

The intermediate and long-term VADs can be classified depending on the type of flow (pulsatile or nonpulsatile), placement (extracorporeal, intracorporeal or paracorporeal) or chronological development (Generation). Most of these devices require chronic anticoagulation; hence, there is a risk of bleeding or thrombotic events with their use. Based on their chronological development and engineering design, these devices can be divided into three generations (Table 11.3).

i. *First generation*: The first generations VADs include a pneumatically or electrically driven pulsatile volume displacement pump, a pumping chamber and two valves (inflow and outflow). These devices can achieve a stroke volume of 65-83 ml. Thoratec PVAD (pneumatic) can be used as a uni- or biventricular device and has been approved for use as BTT or BTR. The pump is extracorporeal; hence, it can be exchanged in cases of infection, thrombosis or malfunction and is suitable for use in smaller patients. If the duration of cardiac support is anticipated to be longer, Thoratec IVAD (implantable) can be used. HeartMate VAD (HeartMate I) is a long-term circulatory support device and has FDA approval for use as a BTT or DT device. This device is available in three versions: Rarely used implantable pneumatic version (IP), a vented electric version (VE) and an improved vented electric version (XVE). All three versions of HeartMate have porcine valves and a textured inner surface that becomes covered by nonthrombogenic "pseudoneointimal" layer overtime. Hence, these devices have a low incidence of thromboembolism and do not require chronic anticoagulation. The use of HeartMate XVE as a destination therapy was evaluated in the REMATCH (Randomized Evaluation of Mechanical Assistance in Treatment of Chronic Heart Failure) trial. In this trial, 129 NYHA class IV HF patients who were ineligible for heart transplantation were randomized to receive HeartMate XVE device or optimal medical therapy. Patients in the HeartMate XVE arm had a higher survival rate at 1 year (52% vs 25%, $p = 0.002$) and 2 year follow-up (23% vs 8%, $p = 0.09$) which represents a 48% reduction in all-cause mortality in HeartMate XVE arm compared to medical therapy arm (Rose et al 2001). A subgroup analysis of REMATCH trial showed that the survival benefit from use of HeartMate XVE was seen only in inotrope-dependent patients (Stevenson et al 2004).

These results lead to FDA approval of this device for use in inotrope-dependent HF patients who are ineligible for transplantation. One of the major limitations of these devices is their poor durability. The rate of device exchange or fatal failure was 17.9% at 1 year and 72.9% at 2 years. (Morgan et al 2004) The first generation devices were generally large because of the need for a reservoir for blood accumulation before ejection. Their size made them less suitable for use in smaller patients (women, children).

ii. *Second generation*: The second generations VADs are rotary pumps with axial flow and have several advantages compared to first generation VADs: Smaller size (hence simpler implantation and reduced risk of infection), fewer moving parts, absence of valves, smaller surfaces in contact with blood and reduced energy requirements. These devices also have better durability with an estimated device life between 5 and 10 years. The HeartMate II is the only FDA approved continuous flow LVAD and provides excellent hemodynamic support in the outpatient setting. In a prospective study evaluating the use of HeartMate II for BTT, 42% of transplant eligible candidates underwent cardiac transplantation within 6 months of support. The overall survival was 75% at 6 months and 68% at 1 year, which was significantly better when compared with historical controls. (Miller et al 2007) Recently, a similar study reported a survival rate of 86.9% at 6 months and a low device malfunction rate (3%). (John et al 2008) The HeartMate II device is approved for BTT use and is also a good device for DT. The Jarvik 2000 is a small axial flow pump which is placed within the left ventricle. This eliminates the need to create a device pocket and reduced the incidence of device-related infections. Jarvik 2000 did not have any internal component failures over an accumulated support period of 59 year and had only 5% external component failures at 1-4 years. This shows the reliability of this device and makes it a good device for BTT and DT (Siegenthaler et al 2006).

iii. *Third generation*: The third generation VADs are centrifugal continuous-flow pumps with an impeller (rotor) suspended in the blood flow path by means of a nonbearing, magnetic (DuraHeart) or hydrodynamic (VentrAssist LVAD) levitation. This feature promises longer durability and higher reliability. Indeed, in a prospective multicenter study using the VentrAssist as a BTT device, overall survival was 82% at 5 months (Esmore et al 2008). When DuraHeart was used as a BTT device, survival rate was 86% at 6 months and 77% at 1 year (Nojiri et al 2008). The incidence of thromboembolic events or hemolysis is greatly reduced with the third generation devices, but they still require anticoagulation putting the patient at risk of bleeding complications. The EVAHEART LVAD has a unique thromboresistant coating over its parts that are in contact with blood. This reduces the incidence of thromboembolic events and bleeding complications due to anticoagulation. In a small study, survival was 91% at 1 year and 78% at 2 years using this device as a BTT (Yamazaki et al 2008).

REPLACEMENT SURGICAL THERAPY

Total Artificial Heart (TAH)

Despite more than 4000 transplants being performed annually, the current waiting list for heart transplantation exceeds 15000. Total artificial hearts (TAH) were developed to meet this immense demand for cardiac replacement. The CardioWest Total Artificial Heart (TAH) system is a pulsatile biventricular device that replaces a patient's native ventricles and valves and pumps blood to both the pulmonary and systemic circulation. The device has a large external command console which restricts mobility and the presence of mechanical valves necessitates anticoagulation. The CardioWest TAH system has been implanted in over 715 patients at multiple centers worldwide as a bridge to transplantation since 1993. In a prospective trial, the survival rate with CardioWest TAH was 79% compared to 46% in control patients awaiting transplantation. Long-term survival of patients receiving CardioWest implantation was 86% at 1 year and 64% at 5 years (Copeland et al 2004).

Heart Transplantation

Cardiac transplantation is the definitive treatment modality for patients with end-stage heart failure which improves quality of life and survival. The survival rates of patients undergoing heart transplantation depends on the underlying etiology of cardiomyopathy. Patients with ischemic cardiomyopathy have a survival rate of 39% at 10 years and the ones with nonischemic cardiomyopathy have a survival rate of 80% at 10 years (Aziz et al 2001). Implementation of stringent selection criteria and improvement in immunosuppressive therapy has lead to increased survival rate in heart transplantation patients. Metabolic stress testing represents the definitive test in assessing the severity of functional capacity limitation and assesses the eligibility of patients for heart transplantation. Patients with compensated chronic heart failure and peak oxygen consumption of <14 ml/kg/min or <50% of predicted value are considered suitable for transplantation. Once patients are considered eligible for transplantation, they are entered into a national waiting list database maintained by the UNOS (United Network of Organ Sharing). The patients are assigned a specific UNOS status depending on their clinical condition (Table 11.4). Patients who are designated status IA are considered the sickest and are prioritized for organ allocation.

Prerequisites

a. Patients should be on optimal medical therapy for heart failure, including an angiotensin-converting enzyme inhibitor (or an angiotensin-receptor blocker, if intolerant to ACE Inhibitor), diuretic, a β-blocker and spironolactone.
b. Medically reversible causes of congestive heart failure have been excluded (hypothyroidism, tachycardia-mediated cardiomyopathy, alcohol abuse, etc).
c. Surgically reversible causes of congestive heart failure have been excluded (valvular heart disease, ischemic cardiomyopathy, hypertrophic obstructive cardiomyopathy, LV aneurysms).

Table 11.4: UNOS status of adult patients awaiting heart transplantation (Modified from http://www.unos.org/PoliciesandBylaws2/policies/pdfs/policy_9.pdf by permission of United Network of Organ Sharing).

UNOS Status	Definition
1A	1. Requires admission to listing transplant center hospital (Note exceptions). 2. Mechanical circulatory support for acute hemodynamic decompensation with right and/or left ventricular assist device (for any 30 days after implantation, hospital admission not required), total artificial heart, intraaortic balloon pump or ECMO. 3. Device-related complications like thromboembolism, device infection, mechanical failure and/or life-threatening ventricular arrhythmias (Hospital admission not required). 4. Continuous mechanical ventilation. 5. Continuous infusion of single high-dose intravenous inotrope (dobutamine > 7.5 mcg/kg/min or milrinone 0.5 > mcg/kg/min) or multiple intravenous inotropes. Continuous hemodynamic monitoring of left ventricular pressures is required.
1B	1. Continuous infusion of intravenous inotropes. 2. Implantation of right and/or left ventricular assist device.
2	Candidates not meeting Status 1A or 1B definition.
7	Inactive on the list (Improved clinical status or short-term contraindication to transplantation like infection).

d. Patients with suboptimal response to cardiac resynchronization therapy (CRT) or with life expectancy less than 1 year.

Indications

1. Cardiogenic shock requiring mechanical support (VAD, IABP).
2. Cardiogenic shock requiring continuous intravenous inotropic support.
3. NYHA Class III or IV symptoms, especially if worsening.
4. Recurrent life-threatening arrhythmias refractory to pharmacological therapy or catheter-based ablation.
5. End-stage complex congenital heart disease without pulmonary hypertension.
6. Refractory angina without potential medical or surgical therapeutic options.

Exclusion criteria

1. Irreversible pulmonary parenchymal disease.
2. Irreversible pulmonary hypertension (PVR > 4 Wood units after vasodilators).
3. Renal dysfunction (Cr > 2.0-2.5 mg/dl or CrCl < 30-50 ml/min) (unless combined heart-kidney transplant is performed).

4. Irreversible hepatic dysfunction (unless combined heart-liver transplant is performed).
5. Severe peripheral or cerebrovascular atherosclerotic obstructive disease.
6. Insulin-dependent diabetes with end-organ damage.
7. Acute pulmonary embolism.
8. History of malignancy with probability of recurrence.
9. Advanced age (>70 years).
10. Severe obesity.
11. Active infection.
12. Severe osteoporosis.
13. Psychosocial instability or substance abuse.

Orthotopic cardiac transplantation is performed via a median sternotomy. After the recipient heart is explantated, the donor heart is anastomosed in sequence, to the left atrial cuff, right atrium (at atrial level or bicaval level), aorta and pulmonary artery. The most common perioperative complication after heart transplantation is pericardial effusion with or without cardiac tamponade. Early systolic left ventricular dysfunction is common after transplantation and often requires short-term inotropic support. Diastolic LV dysfunction is also common immediately posttransplantation but usually resolves in several days or weeks. After transplantation, patients should be closely monitored for right ventricular dysfunction because 20% of postoperative deaths after transplantation occur due to RV failure. RV failure usually manifests as RV dilatation and severe tricuspid regurgitation. Inotropic agents are commonly needed to overcome the right ventricular pump failure, with most severe cases requiring inhaled nitric oxide, temporary right VAD or even ECMO support.

The immunosuppressive agents represent the mainstay of therapy after cardiac transplantation. Traditionally, posttransplant immunosuppressive regimen includes three medications: A corticosteroid (dexamethasone and prednisone), a calcineurin-inhibitor (cyclosporine or tacrolimus) and an antiproliferative agent (Mycophenolate mofetil—MMF or azathioprine). Newer immunosuppressive regimens have been tried with substantial success. One approach involves rapid weaning of corticosteroids between 8 and 12 weeks posttransplant which reduces complications related to steroid use. Another approach involves monotherapy with tacrolimus. In a prospective study, transplant patients were randomized to monotherapy with tacrolimus (MMF was discontinued after 14 days post-transplant) or dual therapy with tacrolimus and MMF. The freedom from rejection grade of 2R or higher (moderate or severe) at 6 and 12 months was 93.3% with tacrolimus alone and 92.9% in the dual therapy arm and the primary end-point of mean 6-month International Society of Heart and Lung Transplantation (ISHLT) biopsy score was 0.44 +/- 0.04 in the monotherapy group and 0.60 +/- 0.05 in the combined therapy group ($p = 0.013$) (Baran et al 2007). The survival after cardiac transplantation continues to improve on a yearly basis. By mid-2009, the 1-year survival rate was 88% in men and 77.2% in women, the 3-year survival rate was 79.3% in men and 77.2% women and the five-year survival rate was 73.1% in men and 67.4% in women. However, the 10-year survival in these patients is only

Table 11.5: Causes of death after heart transplantation

Mortality after Heart Transplantation			
Time After Transplantation	**Cause of Death**		
	I	**II**	**II**
0-30 days	Graft failure (40%)	Multiple organ failure (14%)	Non-CMV infection (13%)
31-365 days	Non-CMV infection (33%)	Graft failure (18%)	Acute Rejection (12%)
1-5 years	Graft failure & TV (37%)	Malignancy (19%)	Non-CMV infection (11%)
> 5 years	Graft failure & TV (30%)	Malignancy (22%)	Non-CMV infection (10%)

CMV—cytomegalovirus TV—transplant vasculopathy.

50% because of long-term complications like ischemic heart disease secondary to transplant vasculopathy, malignancy or liver failure.

The complications seen in patients undergoing heart transplantation include graft failure, allograft rejection, transplant vasculopathy, infections and increased risk of malignancy (Table 11.5).

i. *Allograft rejection*: Allograft rejection can be classified as cellular rejection or antibody-mediated (humoral) rejection. Cellular rejection is characterized by lymphocyte infiltration of the myocardium accompanied by myocyte necrosis. In the absence of hemodynamic compromise, patients are usually treated with oral corticosteroids as outpatients. Therapy with intravenous corticosteroids, thymoglobulin, OKT3, plasmapheresis and total lymphocyte irradiation are reserved for cases with hemodynamic compromise or recurrent severe episodes of rejection. Antibody mediated (humoral) rejection is characterized by the interaction of preformed or denovo generated antibodies with donor HLA I and II antigens and complement activation which results in myocardial capillary injury. Patients diagnosed with humoral rejection may require high doses of corticosteroids, plasmapheresis or immunoadsorption. Allograft rejection can also be classified as hyperacute rejection (occurs within hours of transplantation), acute rejection (weeks to months after transplantation) and chronic rejection (years after transplantation). Hyperacute rejection is usually secondary to ABO incompatibility and is often fatal. However, because of comprehensive pretransplant work-up, hyperacute rejection is rare in modern era. Majority of patients who are detected to have acute allograft rejection on surveillance endomyocardial biopsy are asymptomatic. Symptoms due to acute rejection can be attributed to LV dysfunction which include dyspnea on exertion and at rest, orthopnea, palpitation, dizziness and syncope. Acute cellular rejection contributes significantly to mortality and morbidity after cardiac transplantation. It is responsible for 6.4% mortality during the first month and for 9.3% mortality during the first year after transplantation (Taylor et al 2007). Hence, surveillance endomyocardial biopsies are performed routinely to monitor for allograft rejection. The 2004-updated grading scale for endomyocardial biopsies classifies rejection as 1R, 2R or 3R (mild, moderate or severe, respectively) (Stewart et al 2005). A typical surveillance schedule involves biopsies performed every week for 1 month after transplant, then every 2 weeks up to 12 weeks and monthly thereafter up to 6 months. After 6 months, biopsies are performed every other month for the remainder of the first year after transplant, every 3-4 months during the second year and biannually during the 3rd and 4th year. After 4 years, biopsies are performed only when clinically indicated. Rejection monitoring can also be achieved using the gene expression profiling (GEP), known as the AlloMap test. This test uses real-time polymerase chain reaction (PCR) to measure the expression of 20 genes (11 informative plus 9 control and normalization) and generates a score from 0 to 40. Score less than 34 have more than 99% negative predictive value in ruling out moderate to severe (grade≥ 2R) rejection (Deng et al 2006).

ii. *Transplant vasculopathy*: Transplant vasculopathy (TV) (transplant coronary artery disease) along with graft failure is the leading cause of death in patients after the 1st year of transplantation (30-37%) (Table 11.5). TV only affects the allograft and is characterized by diffuse concentric intimal hyperplasia involving the mid to distal segments of epicardial coronary arteries and concentric medial disease involving microvasculature causing stenotic microvasculopathy. The pathogenesis of TV is multifactorial. The factors involved in pathogenesis of TV include vascular injury secondary to multiple episodes of rejection (cellular and humoral), HLA mismatch, CMV infection, hyperlipidemia, insulin resistance and production of inflammatory cytokines. TV is a slowly progressive disease, however, in some patients it can progress rapidly causing diffuse occlusive coronary artery disease. The prevalence of TV is 7% at 1 year, 32% at 5 years and 53% at 10 years after transplantation. Ischemia secondary to transplant vasculopathy is clinically silent. Patients with TV usually present with silent myocardial infarction, heart failure or sudden cardiac death. Hence routine screening is vital to make an early diagnosis of TV. Because of its diffuse nature, TV can be missed on routine coronary angiography. Hence, annual coronary angiography along with adjunctive intravascular ultrasound (IVUS) is the screening modality of choice in a majority of institutions including ours. Increase in maximal intimal thickness (MIT) by ≥ 0.5 mm at 1 year posttransplantation on IVUS is associated with increased mortality, graft loss, non-fatal major adverse cardiac events (Kobashigawa et al 2005). Other adjunctive modalities that have been used along with coronary angiography include TIMI frame count and measurement of coronary flow reserve. Treatment of TV includes augmentation of immunosuppression, percutaneous or surgical revascularization or retransplantation. However, once the TV manifests through an ischemic event, the survival is very poor with only 20% of patients alive at 1 year. Hence, effective prevention of TV seems to be a more reasonable approach. Medications that have shown to prevent TV include statins, sirolimus, everolimus, mycophenolate mofetil and diltiazem.

iii. *Infections*: Immunosuppressive medications used to prevent allograft rejection increase the susceptibility of the transplant recipients to community acquired bacterial infections, viral infections and opportunistic infections. Lack of inflammatory reaction to microbial agents, failure of seroconversion and antibiotic resistance makes the diagnosis and treatment of infections challenging and leads to high mortality. NonCMV infections are the most common cause of mortality between 30-365 days of transplantation. The epidemiology of infections in transplant recipients depends on the time from transplantation. In the first month after transplantation, patients are predisposed to donor or recipient derived infections, procedure related or nosocomial infections. Between 1 and 6 months posttransplantation, opportunistic infections like Pneumocystis jiroveci pneumonia, toxoplasmosis, herpes viruses, mycobacterial infections, cryptosporidiosis etc are the most common cause of infection in transplant recipients. 6 months after transplantation, community acquired pathogens (e.g. bacterial and viral pneumonias) are the predominant cause of infection. Because of high morbidity and mortality in infected transplanted patients, prophylaxis with vaccination and medications is of paramount importance to improve survival. American Society of Transplantation recommends pretransplantation prophylaxis against Hepatitis B, Influenza, *Streptococcus pneumoniae*, Hepatitis A, Poliovirus, *Clostridium tetani*, Varicella zoster and Neisseria meningitidis (only in selected patients). Posttransplant antibiotic prophylaxis includes the use of gancyclovir, valgancyclovir or valacylovir against Cytomegalovirus (CMV), Herpes simplex and Varicella zoster, trimethoprim-sulfamethoxazole against *Pneumocystis jiroveci* and *Toxoplasma gondii* and fluconazole or liposomal amphotericin B against fungal pathogens (in selected population).

iv. *Malignancy*: Posttransplant malignancy is the second most common cause of mortality after 1st year of transplantation. The use of immunosuppressive medications in transplanted patients increases the incidence of certain malignancies compared to the general population. The incidence of malignancies in heart transplant recipients is 2-4 times higher than the renal transplant patients because of higher level of immunosuppression required in these patients. The malignancies that occur with increased frequency in this population include skin cancers (sqamous cell carcinoma, melanoma, basal cell carcinoma and Merkel cell carcinoma), posttransplantation lymphoproliferative disorder (PTLD) (Non-Hodgkin's lymphoma, multiple myeloma, lymphoid leukemia and Hodgkin's lymphoma), Kaposi's carcinoma, lung cancers and anogenital cancers. The risk of developing posttransplant malignancy also depends on the type of immunosuppressive medication used. Patients treated with cyclosporine and azathioprine or anti-lymphocyte antibodies are at higher risk of developing certain malignancies like PTLD and skin cancers. Use of target-of-rapamycin inhibitors (sirolimus and everolimus) and in some cases MMF has been associated with decreased incidence of posttransplant malignancies (Kauffman et al 2005; Robson et al 2005). PTLD develops due to malignant transformation and proliferation of

B lymphocytes due to Epstein-Barr infection. Majority of patients manifest extra nodal masses involving gastrointestinal tract, lungs, heart, skin, liver or central nervous system. The management of PTLD involves reduction in the dose of immunosuppressive therapy (atleast by 50% in certain cases) and stopping certain immunosuppressive medications like azathioprine. In selected patients, antiviral therapy, chemotherapy, radiation therapy, surgical resection and immunoglobulin therapy may be necessary. Preventive measures like avoidance of sun exposure, use of sunscreens, regular physical examination, avoidance of azathioprine (if possible) and treatment of premalignant lesions should be employed to reduce the occurrence of posttransplant skin cancers. Besides reduction in the doses of immunosuppressive medications, the management of skin cancers in transplanted patients is similar to the one in nontransplanted patients. Change in immunosuppressive medications can be curative for certain skin cancers. For example, discontinuation of cyclosporine and initiation of sirolimus has been associated with complete regression of Kaposi's carcinoma. The management of other posttransplant visceral malignancies involves reduction in immunosuppressive regimen, surgical therapy, chemotherapy and radiation therapy.

FUTURE DIRECTIONS

Stem Cell Therapy

As reviewed in Part 1, HF develops as a consequence myocardial cell death or dysfunction; hence, replacement of dead or dysfunctional myocardium with stem cells appears to be a logical and promising therapy for management of HF. Data from animal studies and human blood and heart transplantation provides supportive evidence towards the possible use of this novel therapy in future. Transplantation of hematopoietic stem cells, mesenchymal stem cells, stromal cells or neonatal cardiomyocytes into myocardium has lead to the formation of cardiac tissue, improvement in ventricular function and reversal of LV remodeling (Murry et al 2005).

The stem cells that have been investigated for potential therapeutic use can be divided into two major categories depending on their embryological origin: (a) Embryonic stem cell (b) Adult stem cells.

a. Embryonic Stem Cells

Embryonic stem cells (ESC) are derived from the inner cell layer of trophoblast and have the capability to differentiate into any cell type depending on cultivation conditions. Under appropriate conditions, functionally active cardiomyocytes have been cultivated from mouse and human ESC. These cardiomyocytes show anatomic integration with the surrounding cells, propagation of electrical activity, spontaneous pacemaker activity and sarcomeric organization. Unfortunately, animal studies have shown that there is a dose-dependent incidence of teratocarcinoma in mice models after transplantation of ESC (Kehat et al 2001).

b. Adult Stem Cells

Adult stem cells (ASC) have been cultivated from 3 different sources: Bone marrow, blood and tissues (myocardium and adipose tissue).

i. The bone marrow derived stem cells that have been used in clinical trials include hematopoietic stem cells (HSC), stromal cells and mesenchymal stem cells (MSC). Injection of bone marrow derived mononuclear cells into viable dysfunctional myocardium in HF patients has shown a reduction in the area of reversible ischemia, improvement in the mechanical contractility of the injected areas and an increase in LV ejection fraction (Perin et al 2003).
ii. The circulating blood derived progenitor cells include the endothelial progenitor cells (EPC) and mesoangioblasts. The EPC were initially thought be responsible for postinfarction neovascularisation by differentiating into endothelial cells but it is now evident that they also have clonal potential and can form cardiac myocytes (Urbich and Dimmeler 2004).
iii. The tissue based stem cells have been found in the myocardium and in the adipose tissue. Although different population of stem cells have been found in the human myocardium, the cardiac side population cells (SP) which express Sca-1 have the most potential for cardiomyogenic differentiation (Mouquet et al 2005). The adipose tissue contains MSC and EPC which have shown therapeutic potential in experimental studies (Fraser et al 2006). Implantation of autologous skeletal myoblasts isolated from skeletal muscle satellite cells into the human myocardium have shown to improve contractility and increase LV ejection fraction (Murry et al 2005).

The exact mechanism of benefit of stem cell therapy is unclear. Although it is intuitive to assume that stem cell therapy benefits by transdifferentiation of pleuripotent cells into cardiac myocytes, the data from animal studies suggests additional mechanisms. The MSC and ESC cells have the capability to differentiate into cardiomyocytes; however, studies have shown that the HSC and skeletal myoblasts do not transdifferentiate into cardiac myocytes. It has been proposed that these cells release growth factors, cytokines and other signaling molecules which act in a paracrine fashion in the myocardium. These signaling molecules may cause differentiation of cardiac stem cells into myocytes, promote angiogenesis and increase the longevity of cardiac myocytes, all of which lead to better myocardial perfusion and improved contractility (Murry et al 2005). In addition to carcinogenic potential of stem cells discussed above, there are other complications associated with stem cell therapy. It has been noted that patients who underwent myoblast injections experienced multiple episodes of ventricular tachycardia. Although the exact mechanism of these arrhythmias is unknown, it is postulated that electrical inhomogeneity between the trans-differentiated and native cells facilitates reentrant arrhythmias (Murry et al 2005). Differentiation of the bone marrow derived stem cells into myofibroblasts can lead to perivascular fibrosis and LV remodeling (Endo et al 2007). It has also been noted that patients with stem cell therapy have increased incidence of in-stent restenosis leading to increase risk or coronary ischemia and acute coronary syndrome (Kang et al 2004). In conclusion, stem cell therapy appears to be a promising therapeutic intervention for management of patients with heart failure; however, more work needs to be done to improve the safety and efficacy of this therapy.

Gene Therapy

Genetic therapy has been tested in animal models and represents an emerging therapeutic option for management of heart failure. Genetic modulation in myocytes can be accomplished in 2 ways: (1) transfer of recombinant genes into myocytes to express proteins that are deficient in HF patients (2) transfer of interference RNA (RNAi) into myocytes to inhibit the expression of pathological genes or pathways responsible for pathogenesis and/or progression of HF. The recombinant genes can be transferred into the myocytes with the help of viral vectors like adenoviruses, adenoassociated viruses and lentivirus. These vectors can be delivered to the target cells by intracoronary catheter delivery, intramyocardial injection or pericardial injection. The potential targets for gene therapy are summarized below:

a. *SERCA 2a:* Sarcoplasmic reticulum (SR) is an intracellular organelle which stores and regulates the uptake and release of calcium during contraction and relaxation of cardiac myocytes. When the depolarization wave reaches the T-tubules during systole, it opens the L-type calcium channels causing the entry of small amount of calcium into the myocytes. This leads to activation of ryanodine receptors (calcium release channels) and release of large amount of calcium into the cytosol from the SR causing contraction of cardiomyocytes. At the end of systole, the intracytosolic calcium is taken up into the SR via an ATPase calcium pump named SERCA 2a. This leads to relaxation of the cardiac myocytes during diastole. Hence, appropriate functioning of SERCA 2a is critical in maintaining calcium homeostasis during myocardial contraction and relaxation. It has been observed that the expression and/or function of SERCA 2a is down regulated in cardiomyocytes isolated from HF patients (Periasamy and Huke 2001). Overexpression of SERCA 2a in rat models of heart failure resulted in improved metabolism in cardiomyocytes, normalisation of heart volumes and increased survival (del Monte et al 2001).
b. *Phospholamban*: Reduced functioning of SERCA 2a seen in HF patients is partly mediated by another protein named 'Phospholamban'. The dephosphorylated form of phospholamban inhibits the action of SERCA 2a. Phosphorylation of phospholamban by PKA (Protein Kinase A) and calmodulin kinase II (CK2) in response to β-adrenergic stimulation and calcium release respectively activates the phospholamban and enhances the reuptake of calcium by SERCA 2a. Mutation of phospholamban in transgenic mice which prevents its activation by PKA results in dilated cardiomyopathy and HF (Schmitt et al 2003). Use of antisense phospholamban adenovector to suppress the expression of its

dephosphorylated form or the use of adeno-asssociated virus to increased the expression of pseudophosphorylated phospholamban mutant has shown to improve contractility, prevent remodeling and prevent the onset of dilated cardiomyopathy (del Monte et al 2002, Hoshijima et al 2002).

c. *β-adrenergic receptors*: As it has been discussed above, cardiomyocytes from failing myocardium show a 50% reduction in the density and responsiveness of beta adrenergic receptors (BAR). In a study by Shah et al, intracoronary delivery of an adenovirus containing β-2 adrenergic receptor genes in rabbit models resulted in a 10-fold increase in the expression of β-2 adrenergic receptors. This led to improvement in global LV contractility at baseline and in response to isoproterenol infusion (Shah et al 2000). However, it is critical to control the amount of expression of BAR in cardiomyocytes. Overexpression of BAR by more than 100 times in experimental animals resulted in myocyte necrosis, apoptosis, fibrotic cardiomyopathy and HF (Liggett et al 2000).
d. *β-adrenergic receptor kinase*: This enzyme causes phosphorylation of BAR and leads to their desensitization. In experimental studies, animals receiving transgenes which encoded for a peptide inhibitor of β-adrenergic receptor kinase showed an improvement in baseline LV function (Shah et al 2001).
e. *Adenylyl cyclase*: As mentioned above, activation of β-adrenergic receptors leads to activation of adenylyl cyclase VI (AC6) and an increase in the level of intracellular cAMP. cAMP leads to activation of PKA (protein kinase A) which regulates calcium homeostasis in the myocytes. Over expression of AC6 in murine models results in an increase in the cAMP levels. This results in increased responsiveness of cardiomyocytes to catecholamines, improved global LV function, reduced LV hypertrophy and improved survival (Roth et al 2002).
f. *V2 vasopressin receptor*: Activation of V2 vasopressin receptor causes stimulation of adenylyl cyclase and hence increased in the level of cAMP in the cells. Transcoronary or direct intracardiac injection of recombinant adenovirus for V2 vasopressin receptors resulted in increased expression of these receptors on the cardiac myocytes (Weig et al 2000). The activation of these receptors by arginine vasopressin (AVP) which is found in increased levels in heart failure causes increased myocardial contractility.

Neurohormones

Use of naturally occurring vasodilators like adrenomedullin and relaxin is being tried for management of heart failure patients. Adrenomedullin is a peptide which causes vascular dilatation and enhances myocardial contractility. Infusion of adrenomedullin in HF patients resulted in an increase in cardiac index and decrease in pulmonary capillary wedge pressure (Nagaya et al 2000). Similarly, infusion of relaxin in patients with systolic failure with normal or elevated blood pressure resulted in substantial improvement in dyspnea. At 60 days, there was also a trend towards reduced cardiovascular death and readmission (Teerlink et al 2009).

BIBLIOGRAPHY

1. Abraham WT, Fisher WG, Smith AL, Delurgio DB, Leon AR, Loh E, et al. Cardiac resynchronization in chronic heart failure. N Engl J Med. 2002;346:1845-53.
2. A comparison of antiarrhythmic-drug therapy with implantable defibrillators in patients resuscitated from near-fatal ventricular arrhythmias. The Antiarrhythmics versus Implantable Defibrillators (AVID) Investigators. N Engl J Med. 1997;337:1576-83.
3. Athanasuleas CL, Buckberg GD, Stanley AW, Siler W, Dor V, DiDonato M, et al. Surgical ventricular restoration: The RESTORE Group experience. Heart Fail Rev. 2004;9:287-97.
4. Aziz T, Burgess M, Rahman AN, Campbell CS, Yonan N. Cardiac transplantation for cardiomyopathy and ischemic heart disease: differences in outcome up to 10 years. J Heart Lung Transplant. 2001;20:525-33.
5. Baldasseroni S, Opasich C, Gorini M, Lucci D, Marchionni N, Marini M, et al. Left bundle-branch block is associated with increased 1-year sudden and total mortality rate in 5517 outpatients with congestive heart failure: A report from the Italian network on congestive heart failure. Am Heart J. 2002;143:398-405.
6. Baran DA, Zucker MJ, Arroyo LH, Alwarshetty MM, Ramirez MR, Prendergast TW, et al. Randomized trial of tacrolimus monotherapy: Tacrolimus in combination, tacrolimus alone compared (the TICTAC trial). J Heart Lung Transplant. 2007;26:992-7.
7. Bardy GH, Lee KL, Mark DB, Poole JE, Packer DL, Boineau R, et al. Amiodarone or an implantable cardioverter-defibrillator for congestive heart failure. N Engl J Med. 2005;352:225-37.
8. Bigger JT Jr. Prophylactic use of implanted cardiac defibrillators in patients at high risk for ventricular arrhythmias after coronary-artery bypass graft surgery. Coronary Artery Bypass Graft (CABG) Patch Trial Investigators. N Engl J Med. 1997;337:1569-75.
9. Bounous EP, Mark DB, Pollock BG, Hlatky MA, Harrell FE Jr, Lee KL, et al. Surgical survival benefits for coronary disease patients with left ventricular dysfunction. Circulation. 1988;78:I151-7.
10. Bourge RC, Abraham WT, Adamson PB, Aaron MF, Aranda JM Jr, Magalski A, et al. Randomized controlled trial of an implantable continuous hemodynamic monitor in patients with advanced heart failure: The COMPASS-HF study. J Am Coll Cardiol. 2008;51:1073-9.
11. Bristow MR, Saxon LA, Boehmer J, Krueger S, Kass DA, De Marco T, et al. Cardiac-resynchronization therapy with or without an implantable defibrillator in advanced chronic heart failure. N Engl J Med. 2004;350:2140-50.
12. Buxton AE, Lee KL, Fisher JD, Josephson ME, Prystowsky EN, Hafley G. A randomized study of the prevention of sudden death in patients with coronary artery disease. Multicenter Unsustained Tachycardia Trial Investigators. N Engl J Med. 1999;341:1882-90.
13. Can I, Tholakanahalli VN. Current status of implantable cardioverter-defibrillator therapy in heart failure. Curr Heart Fail Rep. 2009;6:199-209.
14. Chachques JC, Jegaden O, Mesana T, Glock Y, Grandjean PA, Carpentier AF. Cardiac bioassist: Results of the French multicenter cardiomyoplasty study. Asian Cardiovasc Thorac Ann. 2009;17:573-80.
15. Cleland JG, Daubert JC, Erdmann E, Freemantle N, Gras D, Kappenberger L, et al. The effect of cardiac resynchronization on morbidity and mortality in heart failure. N Engl J Med. 2005;352:1539-49.
16 Copeland JG, Smith RG, Arabia FA, Nolan PE, Sethi GK, Tsau PH, et al. Cardiac replacement with a total artificial heart as a bridge to transplantation. N Engl J Med. 2004;351:859-67.
17. Curtis LH, Whellan DJ, Hammill BG, Hernandez AF, Anstrom KJ, Shea AM, et al. Incidence and prevalence of heart failure in elderly persons, 1994-2003. Arch Intern Med. 2008;168:418-24.

18. Del Monte F, Harding SE, Dec GW, Gwathmey JK, Hajjar RJ. Targeting phospholamban by gene transfer in human heart failure. Circulation. 2002;105:904-7.
19. Del Monte F, Williams E, Lebeche D, Schmidt U, Rosenzweig A, Gwathmey JK, et al. Improvement in survival and cardiac metabolism after gene transfer of sarcoplasmic reticulum Ca(2+)-ATPase in a rat model of heart failure. Circulation. 2001;104:1424-9.
20. Deng MC, Eisen HJ, Mehra MR, Billingham M, Marboe CC, Berry G, et al. Noninvasive discrimination of rejection in cardiac allograft recipients using gene expression profiling. Am J Transplant. 2006;6:150-60.
21. Desideri A, Cortigiani L, Christen AI, Coscarelli S, Gregori D, Zanco P, et al. The extent of perfusion-F18-fluorodeoxyglucose positron emission tomography mismatch determines mortality in medically treated patients with chronic ischemic left ventricular dysfunction. J Am Coll Cardiol. 2005;46:1264-9.
22. Endo J, Sano M, Fujita J, Hayashida K, Yuasa S, Aoyama N, et al. Bone marrow derived cells are involved in the pathogenesis of cardiac hypertrophy in response to pressure overload. Circulation. 2007;116:1176-84.
23. Epstein AE, Dimarco JP, Ellenbogen KA, Estes NA 3rd, Freedman RA, Gettes LS, et al. ACC/AHA/HRS 2008 guidelines for Device-Based Therapy of Cardiac Rhythm Abnormalities: Executive summary. Heart Rhythm. 2008;5:934-55.
24. Esmore D, Kaye D, Spratt P, Larbalestier R, Ruygrok P, Tsui S, et al. A prospective, multicenter trial of the VentrAssist left ventricular assist device for bridge to transplant: Safety and efficacy. J Heart Lung Transplant. 2008;27:579-88.
25. Feldman T, Kar S, Rinaldi M, Fail P, Hermiller J, Smalling R, et al. Percutaneous mitral repair with the MitraClip system: Safety and midterm durability in the initial EVEREST (Endovascular Valve Edge-to-Edge REpair Study) cohort. J Am Coll Cardiol. 2009;54:686-94.
26. Ferguson JJ 3rd, Cohen M, Freedman RJ Jr, Stone GW, Miller MF, Joseph DL, et al. The current practice of intra-aortic balloon counterpulsation: results from the Benchmark Registry. J Am Coll Cardiol. 2001;38:1456-62.
27. Fraser JK, Schreiber R, Strem B, Zhu M, Alfonso Z, Wulur I, et al. Plasticity of human adipose stem cells toward endothelial cells and cardiomyocytes. Nat Clin Pract Cardiovasc Med 2006;3 Suppl 1:S33-7.
28. Fukamachi K, McCarthy PM. Initial safety and feasibility clinical trial of the myosplint device. J Card Surg. 2005;20:S43-7.
29. Gangemi JJ, Tribble CG, Ross SD, McPherson JA, Kern JA, Kron IL. Does the additive risk of mitral valve repair in patients with ischemic cardiomyopathy prohibit surgical intervention? Ann Surg. 2000;231:710-14.
30. Granfeldt H, Hellgren L, Dellgren G, Myrdal G, Wassberg E, Kjellman U, et al. Experience with the Impella recovery axial-flow system for acute heart failure at three cardiothoracic centers in Sweden. Scand Cardiovasc J. 2009;43:233-9.
31. Hausmann H, Topp H, Siniawski H, Holz S, Hetzer R. Decision-making in end-stage coronary artery disease: Revascularization or heart transplantation? Ann Thorac Surg. 1997;64:1296-1301; discussion 1302.
32. Hochman JS, Buller CE, Sleeper LA, Boland J, Dzavik V, Sanborn TA, et al. Cardiogenic shock complicating acute myocardial infarction—etiologies, management and outcome: A report from the SHOCK Trial Registry. Should we emergently revascularize Occluded Coronaries for cardiogenic shocK? J Am Coll Cardiol. 2000;36:1063-70.
33. Hohnloser SH, Kuck KH, Dorian P, Roberts RS, Hampton JR, Hatala R, et al. Prophylactic use of an implantable cardioverter-defibrillator after acute myocardial infarction. N Engl J Med. 2004;351:2481-8.
34. Hoshijima M, Ikeda Y, Iwanaga Y, Minamisawa S, Date MO, Gu Y, et al. Chronic suppression of heart-failure progression by a pseudophosphorylated mutant of phospholamban via *in vivo* cardiac rAAV gene delivery. Nat Med. 2002;8:864-71.
35. Jessup M, Brozena S. Heart failure. N Engl J Med. 2003;348:2007-18.

36. John R, Kamdar F, Liao K, Colvin-Adams M, Boyle A, Joyce L. Improved survival and decreasing incidence of adverse events with the HeartMate II left ventricular assist device as bridge-to-transplant therapy. Ann Thorac Surg. 2008;86:1227-34; discussion 1234-1225.
37. Jones RH, Velazquez EJ, Michler RE, Sopko G, Oh JK, O'Connor CM, et al. Coronary bypass surgery with or without surgical ventricular reconstruction. N Engl J Med. 2009;360:1705-17.
38. Kadish A, Dyer A, Daubert JP, Quigg R, Estes NA, Anderson KP, et al. Prophylactic defibrillator implantation in patients with nonischemic dilated cardiomyopathy. N Engl J Med. 2004;350:2151-8.
39. Kang HJ, Kim HS, Zhang SY, Park KW, Cho HJ, Koo BK, et al. Effects of intracoronary infusion of peripheral blood stem-cells mobilised with granulocyte-colony stimulating factor on left ventricular systolic function and restenosis after coronary stenting in myocardial infarction: The MAGIC cell randomised clinical trial. Lancet. 2004;363:751-6.
40. Kauffman HM, Cherikh WS, Cheng Y, Hanto DW, Kahan BD. Maintenance immunosuppression with target-of-rapamycin inhibitors is associated with a reduced incidence of de novo malignancies. Transplantation. 2005;80:883-9.
41. Kehat I, Kenyagin-Karsenti D, Snir M, Segev H, Amit M, Gepstein A, et al. Human embryonic stem cells can differentiate into myocytes with structural and functional properties of cardiomyocytes. J Clin Invest. 2001;108:407-14.
42. Kobashigawa JA, Tobis JM, Starling RC, Tuzcu EM, Smith AL, Valantine HA, et al. Multicenter intravascular ultrasound validation study among heart transplant recipients: outcomes after five years. J Am Coll Cardiol. 2005;45:1532-7.
43. Kosiborod M, Lichtman JH, Heidenreich PA, Normand SL, Wang Y, Brass LM, et al. National trends in outcomes among elderly patients with heart failure. Am J Med. 2006;119:616 e611-7.
44. Liggett SB, Tepe NM, Lorenz JN, Canning AM, Jantz TD, Mitarai S, et al. Early and delayed consequences of beta(2)-adrenergic receptor overexpression in mouse hearts: Critical role for expression level. Circulation. 2000;101:1707-14.
45. Makati KJ, Fish AE, England HH, Tighiouart H, Estes NA 3rd, Link MS. Equivalent arrhythmic risk in patients recently diagnosed with dilated cardiomyopathy compared with patients diagnosed for 9 months or more. Heart Rhythm. 2006;3:397-403.
46. Mann DL, Acker MA, Jessup M, Sabbah HN, Starling RC, Kubo SH. Clinical evaluation of the CorCap Cardiac Support Device in patients with dilated cardiomyopathy. Ann Thorac Surg. 2007;84:1226-35.
47. Miller LW, Pagani FD, Russell SD, John R, Boyle AJ, Aaronson KD, et al. Use of a continuous-flow device in patients awaiting heart transplantation. N Engl J Med. 2007;357:885-96.
48. Morgan JA, John R, Rao V, Weinberg AD, Lee BJ, Mazzeo PA, et al. Bridging to transplant with the HeartMate left ventricular assist device: The Columbia Presbyterian 12-year experience. J Thorac Cardiovasc Surg. 2004;127:1309-16.
49. Moss AJ, Hall WJ, Cannom DS, Daubert JP, Higgins SL, Klein H, et al. Improved survival with an implanted defibrillator in patients with coronary disease at high risk for ventricular arrhythmia. Multicenter Automatic Defibrillator Implantation Trial Investigators. N Engl J Med. 1996;335:1933-40.
50. Moss AJ, Hall WJ, Cannom DS, Klein H, Brown MW, Daubert JP, et al. Cardiac-resynchronization therapy for the prevention of heart-failure events. N Engl J Med. 2009;361:1329-38.
51. Moss AJ, Zareba W, Hall WJ, Klein H, Wilber DJ, Cannom DS, et al. Prophylactic implantation of a defibrillator in patients with myocardial infarction and reduced ejection fraction. N Engl J Med. 2002;346:877-83.
52. Mouquet F, Pfister O, Jain M, Oikonomopoulos A, Ngoy S, Summer R, et al. Restoration of cardiac progenitor cells after myocardial infarction by self-proliferation and selective homing of bone marrow-derived stem cells. Circ Res. 2005;97:1090-2.

53. Murry CE, Field LJ, Menasche P. Cell-based cardiac repair: reflections at the 10-year point. Circulation. 2005;112:3174-83.
54. Nagaya N, Satoh T, Nishikimi T, Uematsu M, Furuichi S, Sakamaki F, et al. Hemodynamic, renal, and hormonal effects of adrenomedullin infusion in patients with congestive heart failure. Circulation. 2000;101:498-503.
55. Periasamy M, Huke S. SERCA pump level is a critical determinant of Ca(2+)homeostasis and cardiac contractility. J Mol Cell Cardiol. 2001;33:1053-63.
56. Perin EC, Dohmann HF, Borojevic R, Silva SA, Sousa AL, Mesquita CT, et al. Transendocardial, autologous bone marrow cell transplantation for severe, chronic ischemic heart failure. Circulation. 2003;107:2294-302.
57. Robson R, Cecka JM, Opelz G, Budde M, Sacks S. Prospective registry-based observational cohort study of the long-term risk of malignancies in renal transplant patients treated with mycophenolate mofetil. Am J Transplant. 2005;5:2954-60.
58. Rose EA, Gelijns AC, Moskowitz AJ, Heitjan DF, Stevenson LW, Dembitsky W, et al. Long-term mechanical left ventricular assistance for end-stage heart failure. N Engl J Med. 2001;345:1435-43.
59. Roth DM, Bayat H, Drumm JD, Gao MH, Swaney JS, Ander A, et al. Adenylyl cyclase increases survival in cardiomyopathy. Circulation. 2002;105:1989-94.
60. Scheidt S, Wilner G, Mueller H, Summers D, Lesch M, Wolff G, et al. Intra-aortic balloon counterpulsation in cardiogenic shock. Report of a cooperative clinical trial. N Engl J Med. 1973;288:979-84.
61. Schmitt JP, Kamisago M, Asahi M, Li GH, Ahmad F, Mende U, et al. Dilated cardiomyopathy and heart failure caused by a mutation in phospholamban. Science. 2003;299:1410-13.
62. Shah AS, Lilly RE, Kypson AP, Tai O, Hata JA, Pippen A, et al. Intracoronary adenovirus-mediated delivery and overexpression of the beta(2)-adrenergic receptor in the heart: Prospects for molecular ventricular assistance. Circulation. 2000;101:408-14.
63. Shah AS, White DC, Emani S, Kypson AP, Lilly RE, Wilson K, et al. *In vivo* ventricular gene delivery of a beta-adrenergic receptor kinase inhibitor to the failing heart reverses cardiac dysfunction. Circulation. 2001;103:1311-16.
64. Siegenthaler MP, Frazier OH, Beyersdorf F, Martin J, Laks H, Elefteriades J, et al. Mechanical reliability of the Jarvik 2000 Heart. Ann Thorac Surg. 2006;81:1752-8; discussion 1758-1759.
65. Sjauw KD, Engstrom AE, Vis MM, van der Schaaf RJ, Baan J Jr, Koch KT, et al. A systematic review and meta-analysis of intraaortic balloon pump therapy in ST-elevation myocardial infarction: Should we change the guidelines? Eur Heart J. 2009;30:459-68.
66. Starling RC, Jessup M, Oh JK, Sabbah HN, Acker MA, Mann DL, et al. Sustained benefits of the CorCap Cardiac Support Device on left ventricular remodeling: Three year follow-up results from the Acorn clinical trial. Ann Thorac Surg. 2007;84:1236-42.
67. Stevenson LW, Miller LW, Desvigne-Nickens P, Ascheim DD, Parides MK, Renlund DG, et al. Left ventricular assist device as destination for patients undergoing intravenous inotropic therapy: a subset analysis from REMATCH (Randomized Evaluation of Mechanical Assistance in Treatment of Chronic Heart Failure). Circulation. 2004;110:975-81.
68. Stewart S, Winters GL, Fishbein MC, Tazelaar HD, Kobashigawa J, Abrams J, et al. Revision of the 1990 working formulation for the standardization of nomenclature in the diagnosis of heart rejection. J Heart Lung Transplant. 2005;24:1710-20.
69. Taylor DO, Edwards LB, Boucek MM, Trulock EP, Aurora P, Christie J, et al. Registry of the International Society for Heart and Lung Transplantation: Twenty-fourth official adult heart transplant report—2007. J Heart Lung Transplant. 2007;26:769-81.
70. Teerlink JR, Metra M, Felker GM, Ponikowski P, Voors AA, Weatherley BD, et al. Relaxin for the treatment of patients with acute heart failure (Pre-RELAX-AHF): A multicentre, randomised, placebo-controlled, parallel-group, dose-finding phase IIb study. Lancet. 2009;373:1429-39.

71. Thiele H, Sick P, Boudriot E, Diederich KW, Hambrecht R, Niebauer J, et al. Randomized comparison of intra-aortic balloon support with a percutaneous left ventricular assist device in patients with revascularized acute myocardial infarction complicated by cardiogenic shock. Eur Heart J. 2005;26:1276-83.
72. Upadhyay GA, Choudhry NK, Auricchio A, Ruskin J, Singh JP. Cardiac resynchronization in patients with atrial fibrillation: A meta-analysis of prospective cohort studies. J Am Coll Cardiol. 2008;52:1239-46.
73. Urbich C, Dimmeler S. Endothelial progenitor cells functional characterization. Trends Cardiovasc Med. 2004;14:318-22.
74. Uretsky BF, Sheahan RG. Primary prevention of sudden cardiac death in heart failure: will the solution be shocking? J Am Coll Cardiol. 1997;30:1589-97.
75. Weig HJ, Laugwitz KL, Moretti A, Kronsbein K, Stadele C, Bruning S, et al. Enhanced cardiac contractility after gene transfer of V2 vasopressin receptors *in vivo* by ultrasound-guided injection or transcoronary delivery. Circulation. 2000;101:1578-85.

Chapter

12

Artificial Cardiac Pacemaker–Its Structure, Implantation and Working

Fraz Ahmed, Mahira Parveen

Abstract. Many abnormal heart rhythms can be treated with a pacemaker. A pacemaker generates electric pulses that regulate heartbeats. Thanks to advances in technology, pacemakers are very light and can adapt to your body needs from moment to moment, beating faster during exercise and slowing down at rest. The procedure to insert a pacemaker is fairly simple and safe. Complications are rare, but knowing about them may help you to detect them early if they happen. After the procedure, you can go back to your regular activities after a short period of healing time.

Keywords. Pacemaker, cardiac pacemaker implantation, artificial pacemaker, permanent pacemaker, internal pacemaker, cardiac resynchronization therapy, crt, biventricular pacemaker.

INTRODUCTION

The heart is the most important muscle in the body. It is composed of atrial and ventricle muscle that make up the myocardium and specialized fibers that can be subdivided into excitation and conduction fibers. Heart has a right and a left side. Each side has two chambers: An atrium and a ventricle. Blood comes from the body to the right atrium. From there, it is pumped to the right ventricle. The right ventricle pumps the blood to the lungs. In the lungs, the blood is loaded with oxygen. From the lungs, the blood goes to the left atrium and then to the left ventricle. From there, it is pumped to the rest of the body and the cycle repeats. The combined contraction of the atria and ventricles is a heartbeat. The heart has its own internal electrical system that controls the rate and rhythm of heartbeat.

With each heartbeat, an electrical signal spreads from the top of the heart i.e. the sinus node or sinoatrial (SA) node in the right atrium and travels through fibers that are similar to electric cables to the bottom i.e. the atrioventricular node, or AV node. From the AV node, the electric current spreads to the ventricles and causes them to contract and pump blood. As the signal spreads from the top of the heart to the bottom, it coordinates the timing of heart cell activity. The cardiac electrical system regulates the frequency of the heart beat (i.e. it sets the heart rate), and it coordinates the contraction of the heart muscle, so that the heart beats efficiently. A normal heart rate varies between 60 and 100 beats per minute while a person is at rest (Guyton and Hall 1996).

WHAT IS A PACEMAKER?

A pacemaker is a small, sophisticated battery-operated electronic device that is surgically implanted in the body to regulate the heartbeats. It monitors and analyzes the heart's rhythm and, when necessary, it delivers a controlled, rhythmic electric stimulus to the heart muscle in order to maintain an effective cardiac rhythm for long periods of time, ensuring effective hemodynamic performance (Sanders and Lee 1996).

THE HISTORY AND DEVELOPMENT OF CARDIAC PACING

In early 1928, Dr Mark C Lidwal made a portable apparatus which work like pacemaker (Geddes 1990). In 1932, Hyman designed the first experimental heart pacemaker (Hyman 1932). Hyman's pacemaker was powered by a hand-wound, spring-driven generator that provided 6 min of pacemaking without rewinding. Dr Hopps worked with Dr WG Bigelow and Dr JC Callaghan at the Banting Institute in the University of Toronto, developing the world's first external artificial pacemaker in 1951. While experimenting with radio frequency heating to restore body temperature, Hopps made an unexpected discovery: If a heart stopped beating due to cooling, it could be started again by artificial stimulation using mechanical or electric means. In this experiment, he placed an electrode on an open chest of a dog through the heart. Along with this he placed another electrode on the dog's body surface. This device was too large to be implanted inside of the human body and transvenous catheter electrodes were used (Woollons 1995). The origin of modern cardiac pacing started when the first pacemaker, developed by Dr Rune Elmqvist, was used in a patient in 1958 by Dr Ake Senning (Elmqvist and Senning 1959). Later in 1959, an electrical engineer Wilson Greatbatch and the cardiologists, Dr WM Chardack and Dr Andrew Gage at the Veterans Administration Hospital in Buffalo, NY, developed the first fully viable implantable pacemaker (Greatbatch 1962), using primary cells as a power source. It was known as the Chardack-Greatbatch implantable pacemaker. Basically, this pacemaker includes a blocking oscillator, which is a special type of wave generator used to produce a narrow pulse. The blocking oscillator is closely related to the more common two-transistor astable circuit, except that it uses only one amplifying device—a transistor (Greatbatch and Holmes 1971). Later in 1964, Berkovits introduced the demand concept, which is the basis of all modern pacemakers. Dual-chamber pacemakers were introduced in the 1960s (Castellanos et al 1968a,b). More sophisticated dual-chamber pacemakers that sense intrinsic activity and pace in both chambers were developed in late 1977.

New Features in Modern Pacemakers

The advances in IC designs have resulted in increasingly sophisticated pacing circuitry, providing, for instance, diagnostic analysis, adaptive rate response, and programmability.

Detection and Sensing Circuitry

A modern pacemaker consists of a telemetry system, an analog sense amplifier, analog output circuitry, and a microprocessor acting as a controller. Nevertheless, the sense amplifier plays a fundamental role in providing information about the current state of the heart. State-of-the-art implantable pulse generators or cardiac pacemakers include real-time sensing capabilities that are designed to detect and monitor intracardiac signal events (e.g. Rwaves in the ventricle). A sense amplifier and its subsequent detection circuitry, together called the front-end, derive only a single event (characterized by a binary pulse) and feed this to a microcontroller that decides on the appropriate pacing therapy to be delivered by the stimulator. Over the years, huge effort has been put into the improvement of sense amplifier and detection circuitry (Schaldach and Furman 1975).

WHY PACEMAKERS ARE USED?

Normally, the signal for a heartbeat begins in the heart's sinus node, the body's natural pacemaker, located in the upper portion of your heart's right atrium. From the sinus node, the signal normally travels to the atrioventricular node (AV node) between the two atria, and then downward to the ventricles. Once the signal arrives at the ventricles, it triggers a contraction of the heart muscle and produces a heartbeat. The indication for implanting a permanent pacemaker and selection of the appropriate mode of operation are mainly based on the type of cardiac disease involved such as failure of impulse formation. as the followings (Sutton and Bourgeois 1991):

- *Sick sinus syndrome*: In this condition, your sinus node either beats too slowly or does not increase its rate in response to exercise and causes a slow heartbeat (bradycardia).
- *Heart block (AV- block):* In this condition, signals from the sinus node either are blocked completely, or are delayed significantly, as they pass through the AV node to the ventricles.
- Less often, a pacemaker is used to treat the following conditions (Sutton and Bourgeois 1991).
- Certain abnormally rapid heart rhythms, called tachyarrhythmias.

- Fainting caused by abnormal nerve impulses that slow the heart, a condition called neurocardiogenic syncope.
- Certain forms of cardiomyopathy (diseases of the heart muscle).
- Certain abnormal heart rhythms (arrhythmias) after a heart transplant.
- Heart block can happen as a result of aging, damage to the heart from a heart attack, or other conditions that interfere with the heart's electrical activity.
- Certain nerve and muscle disorders also can cause heart block, including muscular dystrophy.
- Aging or heart disease damages the sinus node's ability to set the correct pace for your heartbeat. Such damage can cause slower than normal heartbeats or long pauses between heartbeats.
- Certain heart medicines, such as beta blockers may slow the heartbeat too much.

Heart muscle problems that cause electrical signals to travel too slowly through your heart muscle.

Some pacemakers can be used to stop a heart rate that is too fast (tachycardia) or that is irregular. Other types of pacemakers can be used in severe heart failure. These are called biventricular pacemakers. They match up the beating of both sides of the heart. The disorder occurs when an electrical signal is slowed or disrupted as it moves through the heart.

DIAGNOSTIC TESTS

There are a number of diagnostic tests available to detect arrhythmias, following which pacemakers are implanted. Some diagnostic tests are as follows (Bronzino 2000).

EKG (Electrocardiogram)

An EKG is a simple, painless test that detects and records the heart's electrical activity. The test shows how fast the heart is beating and its rhythm (steady or irregular). An EKG also records the strength and timing of electrical signals as they pass through each part of the heart. The test can help diagnose bradycardia and heart block. A standard EKG only records the heartbeat for a few seconds. But it cannot detect arrhythmias that may not happen during the test. To diagnose heart rhythm problems that come and go, portable EKG monitors are used. The two most common types of portable EKGs are Holter and Event monitors.

Holter Monitor: It records the heart's electrical activity for a full 24- or 48-hour period. Normal daily activities are done wearing the Holter monitor. This allows the monitor to record your heart for a longer time than a standard EKG.

Event Monitor: It is similar to a Holter monitor. It is wore as an event monitor while doing normal activities. However, an event monitor only records the heart's electrical activity at certain times while wearing it. For many event monitors, there is a manual start button to initiate the monitor when symptoms are felt, while other event monitors start automatically when they sense abnormal heart rhythms. An event monitor should be worn for 1 to 2 months, or as long as it takes to get a recording of the heart during symptoms.

Echocardiography

Echocardiography (echo) uses sound waves to create a moving picture of your heart. The test provides information about the size and shape of your heart and how well your heart chambers and valves are working. Echo also can identify areas of poor blood flow to the heart, areas of heart muscle that aren't contracting normally, and injury to the heart muscle caused by poor blood flow.

Electrophysiology Study

For electrophysiology study, a thin, flexible wire is passed through a vein in the groin (upper thigh) or arm to the heart. The wire records the heart's electrical signals. The wire is used to electrically stimulate the heart. This allows to study how the heart's electrical system responds. The electrical stimulation helps pinpoint where the heart's electrical system is damaged.

Stress Test

Some heart problems are easier to diagnose when the heart is working hard and beating fast. During stress testing, doing exercise (or medicine are used if unable to do exercise) in order to make the heart work hard and beat fast while heart tests, such as an EKG or echo, are done.

FUNCTIONS OF PACEMAKER

The functions of pacemaker are as follows:

- Speed up a slow heart rhythm.
- Help control an abnormal or fast heart rhythm.
- Make sure the ventricles contract normally if the atria are quivering instead of beating with a normal rhythm (a condition called atrial fibrillation).
- Coordinate the electrical signaling between the upper and lower chambers of the heart.
- Coordinate the electrical signaling between the ventricles. Pacemakers that do this are called cardiac resynchronization therapy (CRT) devices. CRT devices are used to treat heart failure.
- Prevent dangerous arrhythmias caused by a disorder called long QT syndrome.
- Pacemakers also can monitor and record your heart's electrical activity and heart rhythm.

Newer pacemakers can monitor your blood temperature, breathing rate, and other factors and adjust your heart rate to changes in your activity (Harthorne 2001).

There are two different types of output pulses (e.g. monophasic and biphasic) which stimulate the heart. The output stimulus provided by the pulse generator is the amount of electrical charge transferred during the stimulus (current). For effective pacing, the output pulse should have an appropriate width and sufficient energy to depolarize the myocardial cells close to the electrode. Generally, a pacemaker can provide a stimulus in both chambers of the heart. During AV block, ventricular pacing is required because the seat of disease is in the AV node or His-Purkinje system. However, in case of a sick sinus syndrome, the choice of pacemaker will be one that will stimulate the right atrium.

TYPES OF PACEMAKERS

Generally pacemakers are of two types—temporary and permanent.

- *Temporary pacemakers* are used to treat temporary heartbeat problems, such as a slow heartbeat that is caused by a heart attack, heart surgery, or an overdose of medicine. They are also used during emergencies. They are used until a permanent pacemaker can be implanted or until the temporary condition goes away. The persons having a temporary pacemaker have to stay in the hospital as long as the device is in place. Temporary pacemakers are of two types—transcutaneous pacemakers and transvenous pacemakers. They are used only in medical emergencies and are not permanent pacemakers.
- *Permanent pacemakers* are used to control long-term heart rhythm problems.

Further, pacemaker can be divided into two types depending upon the mechanism of action:

- A demand pacemaker monitors the heart rhythm. It only sends electrical pulses to the heart if the heart is beating too slow or if it misses a beat. In 1964, Berkovits introduced the demand concept, which is the basis of all modern pacemakers.
- Rate-responsive pacemakers can use several technologies to determine the optimal heart rate, but two in particular have proven quite useful. The sensor system consists of an activity device sensor that detects some relevant parameter from the body (e.g. sinus node rate, body motion, respiration rate, pH, and blood pressure) and an algorithm in the pacemaker, which is able to adjust the pacemaker response in accordance with the measured quantity. The more the patient's body is moving, faster the heart rate should be. The other is the breathing sensor, which measures the patient's rate of breathing. The faster the breathing, the faster the heart rate should be. Either of these technologies allows rate-responsive pacemakers to mimic the moment-to-moment changes in heart rate seen in patients with normal cardiac electrical systems. Modern rate-responsive (also called frequency-response) pacemakers are capable of adapting to a wide range of sensor information relating to the physiological needs and/or the physical activity of the patient (Schaldach and Furman 1975).

COMPONENTS AND STRUCTURE OF PACEMAKER

Functionally, a pacemaker is a thin titanium box comprising of following various parts (Schaldach and Furman 1975).

Generator

The pulse generator is a tiny computerized electronic chip hermetically sealed in a titanium container that contains information to control the heartbeat along with a battery. The electronic chip in a pulse generator senses the heart's beat and then sends out electric signals accordingly, in order to regulate heartbeats and maintain a normal rate.

Battery

There has been a huge development in the primary power source for pacemakers from the earlier short-lasting to the present long-lasting and durables batteries. Usually when the battery is weak in any electronic device then it is replaced, but in the case of pacemaker, it is welded and sealed in a can and cannot be replaced as individual component. Thus, when the battery becomes weak or when any part of the pacemaker does not function properly, the complete pacemaker has to be replaced.

Earlier mercury batteries were used which could not be sealed resulted in fluid leakage into the pacemaker and caused electrical shorting and device failure early in use. Previously, nuclear pacemakers and nickel-cadmium batteries were also used. Presently, lithium iodide batteries are used as they have a high energy density and provide stable voltage. They can store a large amount of power in a relatively smaller space and have a long shelf life due to their low self-discharge rate.

A pacemaker utilizes the energy stored in batteries to stimulate the heart. Pacing is the most significant drain on the pulse generator power source. The battery capacity is commonly measured in units of charge (ampere-hours). Many factors will affect the longevity of the battery, including primary device settings like pulse amplitude and duration and pacing rate. Pacemaker batteries last between 5 and 15 years (average 6 to 7 years), depending on how active the pacemaker is.

Circuit

Earlier pacemakers used a combination of individual resistors, transistors and capacitors connected together with wire or were placed on printed circuit boards. Nowadays, highly complex and integrated microprocessors based systems are used. They are essentially small computers having RAM and ROM, etc. Hence, they smaller in both size and weight and also consumes comparatively lesser power. They are far better than the earlier ones in features, reliability, flexibility and longevity. They have large data storage capabilities to track the function of the device as well as many different patient parameters like total number of cardiac events, the rate of these events, whether these were pased or intrinsic, and highrate episodes, etc. They can also store intracardiac electrograms and function as event monitors with the ability to playback the paced or sensed events.

Connector Block

The pacemaker wire is connected to the pacemaker circuit by the connector blocks or header. Although there are many different sizes and styles of connector blocks, all the types have in common a method for securing the wire to the pacemaker and a method for making a secure electrical connection. Nonfunctioning of the pacing system may result if the wires are not fitted properly or the wrong type of connector block is used because the electric connection cannot be made. Most pacemakers use setscrews or spring connectors or both to connect the lead to the pacemaker and make electrical connections.

Types of Connector Blocks

- Two set screws design: For each lead (total of 4 in the bipolar dual chamber device), one for the anode and cathode. Each screw must be tightened to hold the lead and provide a secure electrical connection.
- One set screw design: For each lead to hold the distal pin (cathode). The anode is connected electrically by a spring loaded band. A unipolar pacemaker would have only a single screw for each lead without the need for an anodal screw or spring anode connection
- Nonscrew design: Uses spring loaded bands to contact both the cathode and the anode. A plastic component is pressed in by hand that then grips the lead connector to prevent it from coming out of the connector block.

Leads

The pacemaker leads are more than simple "wires". They are too complex and highly engineered devices that consist of many components and each part of the lead is highly specialized. Many different types of leads have evolved in an effort to reduce the size and increase the reliability of this critical pacing component . It is a flexible insulated electrical wire. One end is attached to the generator and the other end is passed through a vein into the heart. Most pacemakers today use two leads—one placed in the right atrium and the other in the right ventricle (Mond 1999).

The Five Basic Types of Leads

- *Unipolar design:* A single coil covered by an insulator.
- *Coaxial bipolar design:* Two concentric coils separated by a layer of insulation.
- *Parallel bipolar design:* Similar to an electrical cord with the two conductors side by side.
- *Coated coil bipolar design:* Insulates each individual filament so they may be wound together giving the look and feel of a unipolar lead.
- *Cable design:* Has no lumen for stylet. It must be positioned through a special sheath delivery system, however it can be made much thinner than other leads.

Electrode

Generally all the pacemaker leads have one or more electrically active surfaces referred to as the electrode(s). The purpose of the electrode is to deliver an electrical stimulus, detect intrinsic cardiac electrical activity, or both. The composition, shape and size of an electrode may vary quite widely from one model lead to another. Many modern electrodes used for pacing are designed to elute an antiinflammatory drug such as the steroid dexamethasone sodium phosphate. Eluting such a drug at the electrode surface has been shown to reduce the amount of acute inflammation and thus the amount of fibrosis at the electrode myocardial interface. Less fibrosis allows the electrode to remain in closer contact with the excitable myocardial cells.

This provides a greater charge density and has the effect of reducing the amount of electrical current required to stimulate the muscle. The result is lower battery drain and increased longevity of the pacemaker by allowing the pacemaker output to be reduced. The anode (also known as the "ring electrode") is larger that the cathode at the end of the lead and is positioned about 1 cm or more back from the cathode. Changes in the spacing between these two electrodes can affect the sensing function, with closer spacing minimizing oversensing of electrical signals from other sources.

Materials Used to Make Electrode

- Elgiloy
- Polished platinum
- Microporous platinum (platinized or "black" platinum)
- Macroporous platinum (mesh)
- Vitreous carbon
- Iridium-oxide
- Platinum-iridium
- Titanium nitride.

Insulation

One of the most important components of any lead system is the insulation. The insulation prevents electrical shorting between the conductor coils within the lead, prevents stimulation of tissues other than the heart, and allows smooth passage of the lead into the vein. Failure of the insulation may result in a number of different problems, the most important of which is failure to pace. Previously, 80A Pellathane™ polyurethane was used as insulator between the two coils in the coaxial bipolar leads. The newest methodology to insulate leads is known as "coated coil" insulation. This technology bonds an insulating coat to each individual filament of the wire, that are then wound together in a design known as coradial construction. The whole wire is then covered with a standard insulator. Even if this outer coating is breached, the individual filaments remain electrically isolated.

Types of Insulation Commonly Used

- Silicone/silastic
- 80A polyurethane
- 55D polyurethane
- Other polyurethanes
- Teflon "coated coil" technology.

Conductor Coil

The metal portion of the wire that carries the electrical impulse from the pacemaker to the heart and the signal from the heart back to the pacemaker is the conductor coil. Most coils are made of multi-filar (several strands) components. This provides strength and flexibility as compared with a solid wire. As the conductor coils are constantly flexed in and around the heart as well as under the clavicle or rib margin, fractures may occur. This may lead to a complete or intermittent loss of pacing. Multiple conductor coils may be present in a lead. The more coils that are present, the more complex the lead construction and therefore the less reliable the lead. Some newer conductor designs are being used that consist of a cable like wire rather than a coil.

Types of Conductor Coil

- Multi-filar design: It is made up of several thin filiments of wire twisted together providing both strength and flexibility.
- Single-filar design: It is similar to a coat hanger. It can be fractured easily by repeated bending and flexing.

Fixation

Once the lead is placed, there is usually some type of fixation mechanism present to prevent the lead from dislodging. Early lead designs did not have a fixation mechanism and were often referred to as "kerplunk" leads since they were heavy and stiff thus dropping into position. Newer leads have either a passive mechanism that entangles the lead into the trabeculae, or a helix that can be screwed into the myocardium. The helix may be extendible and retractable, or may be fixed to the end of the lead.

Types of Fixation Mechanisms

- Plain leads had no fixation device and were held in place by their weight and stiffness.
- Tines were added to act as a "grappling hook" to reduce dislodgment.
- Fins are a variation of tines. These may be less likely to become entangled in the valve.
- Fixed helix active fixation leads screw into the myocardium by rotating the entire lead. The helix is always out.
- Extendable helix leads have a mechanism to extend and retract the screw.
- Preformed "J" lead for simplified atrial placement.

Connector

The portion of the lead that connects it to the pacemaker is known as the connector.

Types of Connectors

- 6 mm unipolar
- 6 mm inline bipolar
- 5 mm unipolar
- 5 mm inline bipolar
- 5 mm bifurcated bipolar
- 3.2 mm unipolar
- 3.2 mm inline bipolar
- Medtronic/CPI type (no seals, long pin)
- Cordis type (seals, long pin)
- VS-1/IS-1 (seals, short pin)

- LV-1 (proprietary Guidant design)
- IS-4 for connecting quadrapolar leads.

Pacing System

All electrical circuits must have a cathode (negative pole) and an anode (positive pole). In general, there are two types of pacing systems with reference to where the anode is located. One type of system uses the metal can of the pacemaker as the anode (+), and the distal electrode of the wire as the cathode (–). This is referred to as a Unipolar system, as the lead has only one electrical pole. In the other type of system both the anode (+) and the cathode (–) are on the pacing lead. This is referred to as a Bipolar system. In all pacing systems the distal pole that is in contact with the heart muscle is negative.

Types of Pacing System

- *Unipolar pacing system*: The lead tip is the cathode and the pacemaker case is the anode.
- *Bipolar pacing system*: The lead tip is the cathode and the anode is a ring slightly behind the cathode. The pacemaker case is not part of the pacing circuit.

WORKING OF PACEMAKERS

The pacemaker monitors and helps to control the heartbeat. The electrodes detect heart's electrical activity (in the right atrium and right ventricle) and transmit that information through the wires to the computer in the pacemaker generator. The generator, which is a computer analyzes the heart's electrical signals, and uses that information to decide whether, when, and where to pace. If the heart rate becomes too slow, the generator transmits a tiny electrical signal to the heart, thus stimulating the heart muscle to contract. This is called pacing. The wires in a biventricular pacemaker carry pulses between an atrium and both ventricles and the generator. The pulses help coordinate electrical signaling between the two ventricles. This type of pacemaker also is called a cardiac resynchronization therapy (CRT) device (Sanders and Lee 1996).

Thus, pacemakers do not take over the work of the heart – the heart still does its own beating – But instead, pacemakers merely help to regulate the timing of the heart beat. Newer pacemakers also can monitor your blood temperature, breathing, and other factors and adjust your heart rate to changes in your activity. The pacemaker's computer can be programmed with an external device.

- Pacemakers have one to three wires that are each placed in different chambers of the heart.
- The wires in a single-chamber pacemaker usually carry pulses between the right ventricle (the lower right chamber of your heart) and the generator.
- The wires in a dual-chamber pacemaker carry pulses between the right atrium (the upper right chamber of your heart) and the right ventricle and the generator. The pulses help coordinate the timing of these two chambers' contractions.

IMPLANTATION OF PACEMAKER

Placing a pacemaker requires minor surgery. The surgery usually is done in a hospital or special heart treatment laboratory. Before the surgery, an intravenous (IV) line will be inserted into one of the veins through the arm or hand. Fluids and medicines are administered directly into the vein through the IV line. The most common location for a pulse generator to be placed is below the left or right collarbone. First, the skin in this area is shaved, cleaned and numbed with a local anesthetic. Antibiotics are provided to prevent infection.

The leads are placed through a small cut (usually about 3 inches long) made in the skin of the chest below the collarbone or abdomen. Using live X-rays (fluoroscopy) to see the area, the leads are passed through the incision into the vein and then into the heart. Then the pacemaker's small metal box is slipped through the cut, and is place just under the skin, and is connected to the leads connecting the heart. The box contains the pacemaker's battery and generator. Once the pacemaker is in place, it is tested to make sure it works properly and then the cut is closed with stitches. The entire surgery takes a few hours.

Once a pacemaker is implanted, it is important to program it. Pacemakers today are extremely flexible devices, and can vary their function according to the precise needs of the patient. As pacemaker generators are essentially tiny computers and like any computer, before they can be optimally useful their software needs to be "tweaked" to suit the individual user. Pacemakers can be programmed non-invasively, with a hand-held device that communicates with the pacemaker through the skin. The programming can be repeated as often as necessary if the patient's underlying heart rhythm problem changes.

POSTIMPLANTATION OF PACEMAKER

Periodic pacemaker checks are necessary, to measure the function of the device and the amount of energy left in the battery. When the battery begins to get low, the doctor schedules an elective pacemaker replacement. This procedure is similar to the implantation procedure, except that usually the pacemaker leads do not need to be replaced. Under local anesthesia, the incision is opened, the generator is detached from the leads and thrown away, a new generator is attached, and the incision is then closed (This is not merely a "battery change," though doctors sometimes call it that. No batteries are changed; instead, the entire old generator is discarded and a brand new one is placed).

COMPLICATIONS WHICH MAY OCCUR WITH PACEMAKERS SURGERY

The pacemaker surgery is generally safe. The chance of having any problems is very low. However, as with any invasive procedure, complications can occur. These include:

- Swelling, bleeding, bruising, or infection in the area where the pacemaker was placed
- Blood vessel or nerve damage
- A collapsed lung
- A bad reaction to the medicine used during the procedure
- Abnormal heart rhythms
- Infection
- Excessive bleeding
- Perforation of the heart muscle
- Stroke or heart attack
- Punctured lung
- Formation of a blood clot inside the skin pocket.

Over a long period of time, a pacemaker can stop working properly because:

- Wires get dislodged or broken
- Battery gets weak or fails
- Heart disease progresses
- Other devices the disrupt the electrical signaling
- Generator failure (extremely rare)
- Lead failure (less rare)
- Pacemaker electrodes can dislodge
- An electrode tip can fracture
- The insulation on a pacemaker lead can break
- The connection between a pacemaker lead and the pulse generator can loosen
- The pacemaker can fire at the wrong time
- The skin where the pacemaker is implanted can erode (wear away).

Following the suggested maintenance schedule usually means that pacemaker problems will be detected before they become serious. However, it is important for patients to be aware of the symptoms of bradycardia, symptoms that might indicate a pacemaker malfunction. Once again, these symptoms include weakness, easy fatigability, lightheadedness, dizziness, or loss of consciousness. Patients experiencing any of these symptoms should notify their doctor. A simple telephone check of the pacemaker is usually enough to rule out a pacemaker problem (Sanders and Lee 1996).

SOME DEVICES CAN INTERFERE WITH PACEMAKERS

After the implantation of pacemaker, close or prolonged contact with electrical devices or devices that have strong magnetic fields should be avoided. Devices that can interfere with a pacemaker are as follows:

- Magnetic resonance imaging, or MRI (Lauck et al 1995)
- Shock-wave lithotripsy to get rid of kidney stones
- Electrocauterization to stop bleeding during surgery (Lauck et al 1995)
- Radiation therapy for cancers can damage the circuits of a pacemaker
- Cell phones, if held in close proximity to the pacemaker (Dawson et al 2002)

- MP3 players (i.e. iPods)
- Household appliances, such as microwave ovens
- High-tension wires (Dawson et al 2002)
- Metal detectors (Dawson et al 2002)
- Industrial welders
- Electrical generators.

These devices can disrupt the electrical signaling of your pacemaker and stop it from working properly. How likely a device is to disrupt your pacemaker depends on how long you're exposed to it and how close it is to your pacemaker. Household appliances can be used, but close and prolonged exposure should be avoided, as it may interfere with your pacemaker.

PACEMAKER CODES

In order to understand the "language" of pacing, it is necessary to comprehend the coding system that was developed originally by the International Conference on Heart Disease (commonly known as the ICHD), and subsequently modified by the NASPE/BPEG (North American Society of Pacing and Electrophysiology/British Pacing and Electrophysiology group) alliance, most recently in 2002. The latter is often referred to as the NBG. The purpose of this coding system is to allow one to communicate the expected behavior of a pacing device to a health care worker or pacemaker technician quickly and accurately. Failure to understand these codes is common, especially as they relate to the more complex device functions. However, if one cannot communicate with a consultant quickly and accurately in this manner, improper evaluation of the pacemaker performance may result, with subsequent misdiagnosis and possible improper treatment of the patient (Table 12.1).

Table 12.1: Five-letter pacemaker codes

Position	1st	2nd	3rd	4th	5th
Category	**Chamber(s) Paced**	**Chamber(s) Sensed**	**Mode of Response**	**Adaptive Rate**	**Chambers being Multisite Paced**
Letters	**V**–Ventricle **A**–Atrium **D**–Double (V and A) **O**–None	**V**–Ventricle **A**–Atrium **D**–Double (V and A) **O**–None	**T**–Triggered **I**–Inhibited **D**–Double (Inhibited and Triggered) **O**–None	**O**–Not active **R**–Rate modulation sensor is active	**O**–None **V**–Ventricle **A**–Atrium **D**–Double (Ventricle and Atrium)

COMMON UNITS FOR PACEMAKERS

Voltage

Basic unit	:	volt (V)
Other unit used	:	millivolt (mV)
Conversion	:	1V = 1,000 mV or 1 mV $= \frac{1}{1,000} V = 10^{-3} V$

Current

Basic unit	:	ampere (A)
Used stimulus amplitude	:	milliampere (mA)
Conversion	:	1A = 1,000 mA or 1 mA $= \frac{1}{1,000} A = 10^{-3} A$
Battery current drain	:	microampere (μA)
Conversion	:	1A = 1,000 μA or 1 μA $= \frac{1}{1,000,000} A = 10^{-6} A$

Resistance

Basic unit	:	ohm (Ω)
Other unit used	:	kilo-ohm (k Ω)
Conversion	:	1 Ω = 1,000 k Ω or 1 k Ω $= \frac{1}{1,000} \Omega = 10^{-3} \Omega$

BIBLIOGRAPHY

1. Bronzino HD. The Biomedical Engineering Handbook, 2nd ed. Boca Raton, FL: CRC, 2000, vol. 1.
2. Castellanos A, Lemberg L, Rodriguez-Tocker L, Berkovits BV. Atrial synchronized pacemaker arrhythmias: Revisited. Amer Heart J. 1968;76:199-208 .
3. Castellanos A, Lemberg L, Salhanick L, Berkovits BV. Pacemaker Vectorcardiography. Amer Heart J 1968;75:6-18.
4. Dawson TW, Caputa K, Stuchly MA, Kavet R. Pacemaker interference by 60-Hz contact currents. IEEE Trans Biomed Eng. 2002;49(8):878-86.
5. Elmqvist R, Senning A. An Implantable Pacemaker for the Heart, CN Smyth, Ed. London, UK: Tliffe and Sons. 1959;pp.253-4.
6. Geddes LA. Historical highlights in cardiac pacing. IEEE Eng Med Biol Mag. 1990;2(2):12-18.
7. Greatbatch W. Medical cardiac pacemaker. US Patent. 3 057 356.
8. Greatbatch W, Holmes CF. History of implantable devices. IEEE Eng Med Biol Mag. 1991;10(3):38-49.
9. Guyton AC, Hall JE. Textbook of Medical Physiology, 9th ed. Philadelphia, PA: Saunders. 1996.
10. Harthorne JW. Pacemakers and store security devices. Cardiol Rev. 2001;9(1):10-17.
11. Hyman AS. Resuscitation of the stopped heart by intracardial therapy," Arch Intern Med. 1932;50:283-5.

12. Lauck G, von Smekal A, Wolke S, Seelos KC, Jung W, Manz M, et al. Effects of nuclear magnetic resonance imaging on cardiac pacemakers. Pacing Clin Electrophysiol. 1995;18(8):1549-55.
13. Mond HG. Recent advances in pacemaker lead technology. Cardiac Electrophysiol Rev. 1999;3(1):5-9.
14. Sanders RS, Lee MT. Implantable pacemakers. Proc IEEE. 1996;84(3):480-6.
15. Schaldach M, Furman S. Advances in Pacemaker Technology. New York: Springer-Verlag. 1975.
16. Sutton R, I. Bourgeois I. The Foundations of Cardiac Pacing, Part I. Mt. Kisco, NY: Futura. 1991.
17. Woollons DJ. To beat or not to beat: The history and development of heart pacemakers. Eng Sci Educ J. 1995;4(6):259-68.

Index

Page numbers followed by *f* refer to figure and *t* refer to table

K

L

M

N

O

P